Cognitive Dimensions of Major Depressive Disorder

Cognitive Dimensions of Major Depressive Disorder

Edited by

BERNHARD T. BAUNE

Cato Chair & Head of Department of Psychiatry
Melbourne Medical School, Faculty of Medicine, Dentistry and Health Sciences,
Personalised Psychiatry & Director of Mental Health Research, North Western
Mental Health, Royal Melbourne Hospital, The University of Melbourne,
Australia

AND

CATHERINE HARMER

Psychopharmacology and Emotion Research Laboratory (PERL)
Department of Psychiatry, University of Oxford, UK

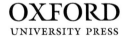

OXFORD
UNIVERSITY PRESS

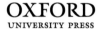

OXFORD

UNIVERSITY PRESS

Great Clarendon Street, Oxford, OX2 6DP,
United Kingdom

Oxford University Press is a department of the University of Oxford.
It furthers the University's objective of excellence in research, scholarship,
and education by publishing worldwide. Oxford is a registered trade mark of
Oxford University Press in the UK and in certain other countries

First Edition published in 2019

Impression: 1

Published in the United States of America by Oxford University Press
198 Madison Avenue, New York, NY 10016, United States of America

British Library Cataloguing in Publication Data

Data available

Library of Congress Control Number: 2019936525

ISBN 978–0–19–881094–0

Printed and bound by
CPI Group (UK) Ltd, Croydon, CR0 4YY

Preface

The causes of depression are largely unknown; however, both environmental and biological processes and their interplay have been long identified to be core underlying contributing factors. More recently, large-scale genomic studies leave us with clear-cut evidence that depression involves numerous neuronal processes. Given the nature of depression as a brain disorder, it is an important challenge for research and clinical application to understand the mechanisms and processes that drive a brain in a depressed state. This way of thinking about depression, which goes substantially beyond a unitary and categorical diagnostic approach to defining the disorder, implies a dimensional and multifaceted understanding of the condition. Indeed, processes of cognitive function, emotion processing, and social cognitive function are essential dimensions of depression that have been closely linked to the pathophysiology of depression. Have these dimensions of depression had the opportunity to form the basis of novel treatments?

This book is written to inform the reader about recent advances in the diagnostic and therapeutic opportunities revealed by a dimensional approach that focuses on cognition. The symptom dimensions of depression include: a) cognitive function; (b) emotion processing; and (c) social cognitive processing, and these are regarded as comprehensively describing large parts of the clinical symptoms as well as the pathophysiology of the brain-based disorder of depression. The focus on cognitive and emotional dimensions of depression offers promising extended and novel diagnostic and treatment approaches, ranging from pharmacological to psychological interventions targeting those dimensions of depression.

This new approach emphasizes depression as a multidimensional cognitive processing disorder from which a variety of interventions may be derived. Not only is the clinical and biological understanding of depression seen in a new light, but also treatments and, most importantly, the targets and outcomes are redefined with this approach. Functional outcomes in terms of workplace productivity and psychosocial function are closely related targets of such treatments.

The reader is invited to rethink the nature as well as the treatment of depression by shifting the usual focus to a mechanistic and functional approach to the brain disorder 'depression'. It is intended that the inspiration that led the editors and authors to create this book shines through the structure, content, and messaging of the book to leave the reader with an extended and modified understanding and treatment approach to depression.

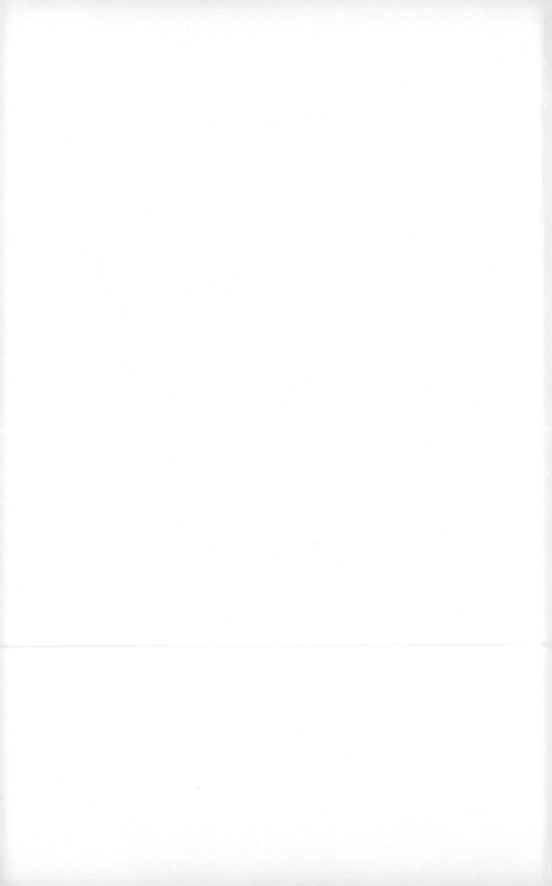

Contents

List of Abbreviations

ACC	Anterior cingulate cortex
AMN	Autobiographic memory network
AN	Affective network
ASM	Attentional scope model
ATD	Acute tryptophan depletion
ATL	Anterior temporal lobe
2BT	Two-Back Test
BD	Bipolar disorder
BDI	Beck Depression Inventory
BLT	Bright light therapy
BOLD	Blood oxygen level-dependent
CBT	Cognitive behavioural therapy
CCN	Cognitive control network
CEN	Control executive network
CNMATA	Cognitive neuropsychological model of antidepressant treatment action
CNS	Central nervous system
COMT	Catechol-O-methyl transferase
CRT	Choice Reaction Time
CT	Cognitive training
dACC	Dorsal anterior cingulate cortex
DECODE	Depression-associated Cognitive Deficits
DLPFC	Dorsolateral prefrontal cortex
DMN	Default mode network
DMPFC	Dorsomedial prefrontal cortex
DSCD	Digit Symbol Coding Test
DSM-5	*Diagnostic and Statistical Manual of Mental Disorders, 5th edition*
DSST	Digit Symbol Substitution Test
ECT	Electroconvulsive therapy
EEG	Electroencephalogram
EMA	Ecological momentary assessment
EPO	Erythropoietin
ESM	Experience sampling method
FC	Functional connectivity
FDA	Food and Drug Administration

fMRI	Functional magnetic resonance imaging
FRN	Feedback-related negativity
GR	Glucocorticoid receptor
HADS	Hospital Anxiety and Depression Scale
HC	Healthy control
HDAC	Histone deacetylase
HPA	Hypothalamic–pituitary–adrenal
HPQ-Global	Health and Work Performance Questionnaire–Global Improvement
$HRSD_{17}$	17-item Hamilton Rating Scale for Depression
$5\text{-}HT_{1A}$	Serotonin 1A receptor
IAPS	International Affective Picture System
ICD	*International Classification of Diseases*
IDS	Inventory for Depressive Symptomatology
IL	Interleukin
LDX	Lisdexamfetamine dimesylate
LEAPS	Lam Employment Absence and Productivity Scale
LIFE-RIFT	Longitudinal Interval Follow-Up Evaluation Range of Impaired Functioning Tool
LTP	Long-term potentiation
MADRS	Montgomery and Asberg Depression Rating Scale
MBD	Methyl-CpG binding domain
MDD	Major depressive disorder
MDE	Major depressive episode
mGluR	Metabotropic glutamate receptor
MPFC	Medial prefrontal cortex
MR	Mineralocorticoid receptor
MSIF	Multidimensional Scale of Independent Functioning
n-3 PUFA	Omega-3 polyunsaturated fatty acid
NAcc	Nucleus accumbens
NCI	Neurocognitive Index
NIT	Negative ion treatment
NMDA	N-methyl-D-aspartate
NRI	Noradrenergic receptor inhibitor
OFC	Orbitofrontal cortex
P&P	Paper-and-pencil
PD	Prisoner's Dilemma
PDQ	Perceived Deficit Questionnaire
PFC	Prefrontal cortex
PFI	Psychosocial Functioning Inventory
PHQ-9	Patient Health Questionnaire-9

QIDS	Quick Inventory of Depressive Symptomatology
QIDS-SR	Quick Inventory of Depressive Symptomatology—Self Report
Q-LES-Q-SF	Quality of Life, Enjoyment and Satisfaction Questionnaire—Short Form
QOL	Quality of life
RAVLT	Rey Auditory Verbal Learning Test
RBANS	Repeatable Battery for the Assessment of Neuropsychological Status
RCI	Reliable Change Index
RCT	Randomized controlled trial
RewP	Reward positivity
rMDD	Remitted major depressive disorder
RMET	Reading the Mind in the Eyes Test
ROI	Region of interest
RST	Response style theory
rTMS	Repetitive transcranial magnetic stimulation
SAD	Seasonal affective disorder
SAMe	S-adenosyl methionine
SASS	Social Adaptation Self-Evaluation Scale
SAS-SR	Social Adjustment Scale Self-report
SCSR	Subgenual cingulate cortex/septal region
SD	Standard deviation
SDS	Sheehan Disability Scale
SF-12/36	Short Form Health Survey, 12 or 36 items
sgACC	Subgenual anterior cingulate cortex
SN	Salience network
SNP	Single nucleotide polymorphism
SNRI	Serotonin and noradrenaline reuptake inhibitor
SOFAS	Social and Occupational Functioning Assessment Scale
SSRI	Selective serotonin reuptake inhibitor
STS	Superior temporal sulcus
tDCS	Transcranial direct current stimulation
TMT	Trail Making Test
TNF-α	Tumour necrosis factor-alpha
ToM	Theory of mind
TSA	Threat to social acceptance
UG	Ultimatum Game
UPSA	UCSD Performance-Based Skills Assessment
VMPFC	Ventromedial prefrontal cortex
VS	Ventral striatum
VTA	Ventral tegmental area

WHO	World Health Organization
WHODAS 2.0	World Health Organization Disability Assessment Schedule 2.0
WHOQOL	World Health Organization Quality of Life
WSAS	Work and Social Adjustment Scale

List of Contributors

Tatjana Aue
Biological and Social Emotion
Psychology Unit, Department of
Psychology, University of Bern,
Switzerland

Bernhard T. Baune
Melbourne Medical School, Faculty
of Medicine, Dentistry and Health
Sciences; Mental Health Research,
NorthWestern Mental Health, Royal
Melbourne Hospital, The University of
Melbourne, Australia

Thomas Beblo
Department of Research, Clinic
of Psychiatry and Psychotherapy,
Evangelisches Klinikum Bethel,
Remterweg, Bielefeld, Germany

Beatrice Bortolato
Local Health Unit 10, Portogruaro,
Psychiatry Department, Italy

Andre F. Carvalho
Department of Psychiatry, University
of Toronto, Toronto, Ontario, Canada

Lorenz B. Dehn
Department of Research, Clinic
of Psychiatry and Psychotherapy,
Evangelisches Klinikum Bethel,
Remterweg, Bielefeld, Germany

Koen Demyttenaere
University Psychiatric Center KU
Leuven, University of Leuven,
Faculty of Medicine, Department of
Neurosciences, Psychiatry Research
Group, Belgium

Rebecca Elliott
Neuroscience and Psychiatry Unit,
Faculty of Biology, Medicine and
Health, University of Manchester, UK

Anna Fall
Sorbonne Universités, UPMC Univ
Paris 06, Inserm, CNRS, APHP,
Institut du cerveau et de la moelle
(ICM)- Hôpital Pitié Salpêtrière,
Boulevard de l'hôpital, Paris, France

Katharina Foerster
Department of Psychiatry, University
of Muenster, Germany

Philippe Fossati
Sorbonne Universités, UPMC Univ
Paris 06, Inserm, CNRS, APHP,
Institut du cerveau et de la moelle
(ICM)- Hôpital Pitié Salpêtrière,
Boulevard de l'hôpital,F-75013,
Paris, France

Cynthia H. Y. Fu
Centre for Affective Disorders,
Institute of Psychiatry, Psychology and
Neuroscience, King's College London,
London, UK

Franziska K. Goer
Neuroscience and Psychiatry Unit,
Faculty of Biology, Medicine
and Health, University of
Manchester, UK

Tracy L. Greer
Department of Psychiatry, UT
Southwestern Medical Center, Center
for Depression Research and Clinical
Care, Dallas, Texas, USA

Catherine Harmer
Psychopharmacology and Emotion
Research Laboratory (PERL),
Department of Psychiatry, University
of Oxford, UK

John E. Harrison
Alzheimer's Center, VUmc,
Amsterdam, The Netherlands;
Institute of Psychiatry, Psychology
and Neuroscience, King's College
London, UK

Nathan Herrmann
Neuropsychopharmacology Research
Group, Hurvitz Brain Sciences
Program, Sunnybrook Research
Institute, Toronto, ON, Canada

Sophie Hinfray
Hôpitaux Universitaires Paris Ouest,
Service de Psychiatrie de l'adulte et du
sujet âgé, Paris, France

Silke Joergens
Department of Psychiatry, University
of Muenster, Germany

Jeethu K. Joseph
Clinical Data Specialist, Department
of Psychiatry, UT Southwestern
Medical Center, Center for Depression
Research and Clinical Care, Dallas,
Texas, USA

Alexander Kaltenboeck
Psychopharmacology and Emotion
Research Laboratory (PERL),
Department of Psychiatry, University
of Oxford, UK

Muzaffer Kaser
Clinical Lectureship, National Institute
for Health Research, London, UK,
University of Cambridge, School of
Clinical Medicine, Department of
Psychiatry, Cambridge, UK

Raymond W. Lam
Department of Psychiatry, University
of British Columbia, Canada

Cédric Lemogne
Hôpitaux Universitaires Paris Ouest,
Service de Psychiatrie de l'adulte et du
sujet âgé, Paris, France

Roger S. McIntyre
Mood Disorders Psychopharmacology
Unit (MDPU), Toronto Western
Hospital, University Health Network,
Toronto, ON, Canada

John D. Medaglia
Department of Psychology, Drexel
University, Philadelphia, USA

Natalie T. Mills
Discipline of Psychiatry, School of
Medicine, University of Adelaide,
Adelaide, Australia

Loren Mowszowski
School of Psychology, Faculty of
Science, The University of Sydney,
Sydney, Australia

Sharon Naismith
School of Psychology, Faculty of
Science, The University of Sydney,
Sydney, Australia

Georgia O'Callaghan
Mood Brain & Behavior Unit, Emotion
& Development Branch, National
Institute of Mental Health, National
Institutes of Health, Bethesda,
MD, USA

Hadas Okon-Singer
Department of Psychology, University
of Haifa, Haifa, Israel,
The Integrated Brain and Behavior
Research Center (IBBR), University of
Haifa, Haifa, Israel

Zihang Pan
Mood Disorders Psychopharmacology
Unit (MDPU), Toronto Western
Hospital, University Health Network,
Toronto, ON, Canada

Genevieve Rayner
Florey Institute of Neuroscience and
Mental Health, Melbourne, Australia

Thalia Richter
Department of Psychology, University
of Haifa, Haifa, Israel,
The Integrated Brain and Behavior
Research Center (IBBR), University of
Haifa, Haifa, Israel

Oliver J. Robinson
Institute of Cognitive Neuroscience,
University College London, UK

Jean-Yves Rotge
Sorbonne Universités, UPMC Univ
Paris 06, Inserm, CNRS, APHP,
Institut du cerveau et de la moelle
(ICM)- Hôpital Pitié Salpêtrière,
Boulevard de l'hôpital, Paris, France

Barbara J. Sahakian
University of Cambridge, School
of Clinical Medicine, Department
of Psychiatry and the Behavioural
and Clinical Neuroscience Institute,
Cambridge, UK

Anjali Sankar
Department of Psychiatry,
Yale School of Medicine,
New Haven, CT, USA

Maria Serra-Blasco
Department of Psychiatry, Parc
Taulí Foundation, Barcelona,
Catalonia, Spain

Alexander J. Shackman
Department of Psychology and
Neuroscience and Cognitive Science
Program, University of Maryland,
College Park, MD, USA

Marco Solmi
University of Padua, Neurosciences
Department, Psychiatry Unit,
Padua, Italy

Argyris Stringaris
Mood Brain & Behavior Unit, Emotion
& Development Branch, National
Institute of Mental Health, National
Institutes of Health, Bethesda,
MD, USA

Brendon Stubbs
Department of Psychological
Medicine, Institute of Psychiatry,
Psychology and Neuroscience, King's
College London, London, United
Kingdom

Michael Weightman
Discipline of Psychiatry, School of
Medicine, University of Adelaide,
Adelaide, Australia

Claudia Woolf
Older People's Mental Health Service,
St Vincent's Hospital Sydney, Australia
and School of Psychology, Faculty of
Science, The University of Sydney,
Sydney, Australia

1

Functional and Psychosocial Consequences of Major Depressive Disorder

Tracy L. Greer and Jeethu K. Joseph

Introduction

Depression is recognized across the globe as a chronic illness that significantly impacts functioning, and it has consistently remained among the leading diseases associated with disability (1). While recent data on the global burden of disease suggests that overall health is improving globally—a positive finding—there is an increased number of years of life with functional health loss, underscoring the need to pay close attention to functional outcomes associated with all chronic health conditions (1), including depression.

Importantly, patients increasingly voice the desire to include function as a measurable component of defining wellness, both in the context of evaluating the efficacy of treatment(s), as well as serving as a potential indicator of impending relapse. Furthermore, patients often endorse functional improvement as being as important as, or even more important than, the reduction of depressive symptoms (2). In fact, a recent study showed that approximately 25% of depressed individuals who achieved scores of 8–12 on the 17-item Hamilton Rating Scale for Depression (HRSD$_{17}$), indicating a mild level of depressive symptom severity, considered themselves to be in remission, despite not achieving the typical criterion of symptomatic remission (HRSD$_{17}$ score of 7 or less) (3). Self-endorsed remitted individuals were significantly more likely to have better psychosocial function, quality of life, coping skills, and features of positive mental health (e.g. optimism and self-confidence) compared to those with similar symptom levels who did not consider themselves to be in remission. Indeed, it is increasingly recognized that there can be discordance between depressive symptom severity and functional status, with functional impairments frequently observed despite achievement of symptomatic remission. For example, Sheehan and colleagues (4) showed that, among patients with major depressive disorder (MDD) who received duloxetine antidepressant treatment, 38% achieved symptomatic remission (HRSD$_{17}$ score of 7 or less), 32% achieved functional remission (Sheehan Disability Scale [SDS] score of 6 or less) and fewer—23%—achieved both. Given the emphasis placed on functioning by patients, the extensive burden of disease, and the known discordance between symptomatology and functioning, it is critical that we better understand and target functioning as a treatment endpoint to improve the daily lives of individuals with depression.

How Functional Outcomes in Depression are Defined and Assessed

Before describing how depression impacts function, it is important to provide some context as to how it is currently defined and measured. One of the major issues impacting our understanding of functioning in depression is the wide variety of terms used to define it, and the similarly vast number of assessments employed to measure it. Several terms, such as 'quality of life', 'health-related quality of life', 'functioning', 'psychosocial functioning', and 'life satisfaction', are used interchangeably, which is not surprising given some of the overlaps in constructs. However, it is helpful to differentiate these constructs when possible so that the impact of both disease and treatment can be consistently evaluated. The WHOQOL (World Health Organization Quality of Life) Group (5) defines quality of life as 'an individual's perception of their position in life in the context of the culture and value systems in which they live and in relation to their goals, expectations, standards, and concerns' (p. 1405). This can be differentiated from a psychosocial function, which has been defined as a 'person's ability to perform daily tasks and to interact with others and with society in a mutually satisfying manner' (p. S10) (6). While this differentiation can allow for some distinction in the characteristics associated with the evaluation of each, such as opportunities for more objective and role-specific (e.g. marital, occupational, physical, etc.) evaluation of psychosocial functioning (6), many existing scales still blend these issues and there is, as yet, no consistently adopted nomenclature in the field.

Existing scales vary with respect to: 1) time-period assessed (with the majority evaluating the past week); 2) rater (e.g. patient/participant, clinician, and, more rarely, collateral sources such as a family member or other caregiver); 3) specificity of information (e.g. global versus a specific domain, such as work; oftentimes, scales will provide both global and domain-specific scores); and 4) assessment of perceived quality versus performance in various functional areas. In addition, some scales have been developed specifically for patients with depression, whereas others are more generally focused to evaluate non-specific chronic disease burden. Measures of disability/functional disability often assess how a disease state impacts role functioning and activity within several life domains. Table 1.1 provides an overview of the breadth of available measures.

The vast majority of assessments are self-report questionnaires that measure patient-reported outcomes, although there are some clinician-rated measures

Table 1.1 Commonly utilized functional assessments

Measure	Purpose and characteristics	Intended audience
Quality of life		
Quality of Life (QOLS) (40)	15-item self-report. Measures five conceptual domains of quality of life: 1) Material and physical wellbeing 2) Relationships with other people 3) Social, community, and civic activities, personal development and fulfilment, and recreation	Adults
Quality of Life, Enjoyment and Satisfaction Questionnaire—Short Form (Q-LES-Q-SF) (41)	16-item self-report. Broad measure of quality of life. Helps obtain degree of enjoyment and satisfaction experienced in various areas of daily functioning	Adults
Short Form Health Survey (SF-12 or SF-36) (42)	12- or 36-item self-report. Measures quality of life across eight areas: 1) Physical functioning 2) Bodily pain 3) Role limitations owing to health problems or to personal or emotional problems 4) Emotional wellbeing 5) Social functioning 6) Energy/fatigue 7) General health perceptions Includes single item of perceived change in health	Adults

(*continued*)

Table 1.1 Continued

Measure	Purpose and characteristics	Intended audience
World Health Organization Quality of Life—BREF (WHOQOL-BREF) (43)	26-item self-report. Measures across five scales, assessing for various components of quality-of-life cross-culturally. Domains include: 1) Physical health 2) Psychological 3) Social relationships 4) Environment	Primarily adults
Performance/functioning		
Lam Employment Absence and Productivity Scale (LEAPS) (44)	Ten-item self-report. Designed to collect information on how participants are functioning at work. Can be scored by the participants themselves. Not a diagnostic tool, but it can be used with Patient Health Questionnaire (PHQ-9) or Quick Inventory of Depressive Symptomatology—Self Report (QIDS-SR). Can also monitor changes in functioning over time	
Longitudinal Interval Follow-Up Evaluation Range of Impaired Functioning Tool (LIFE-RIFT) (45)	Four-item semistructured clinician interview. Measures functional impairment in four domains: 1) Work 2) Interpersonal relations 3) Recreation 4) Global satisfaction	Ages 17 and older
Multidimensional Scale of Independent Functioning (MSIF) (46)	Twenty-five-item clinician-structured interview and self-report measure. Rates functional disability in three areas: 1) Role responsibility 2) Presence and level of support 3) Performance quality	Adults
Psychosocial Functioning Inventory (PFI) (47)	Eighty-one-item clinician-administered multiscale measure. Ten primary and two composite scales that cover: 1) Affective well-being 2) Role functioning 3) Environmental 4) System dependency dimensions	Adolescent to geriatric

Sheehan Disability Scale (SDS) (48)	Adults	Three-item self-report. Developed to assess functional impairment in three domains: 1) Work/school 2) Social life 3) Family life
Social Adaptation Self-Evaluation Scale (SASS) (49)	Adults	Twenty-one-item self-report. Developed to evaluate patient social motivation and behaviour in depression. Covers the different aspects of: 1) Social interactions 2) Global social attitude 3) Self-perception
Social Adjustment Scale Self-report (SAS-SR) (50)	17 and older	The 54-item self-report scale of social adjustment. (Two shorter versions are available: 24-item and 14-item screener) Measures instrumental and expressive performance over the past 2 weeks in six role areas: 1) Work (paid, unpaid homemaker, or student) 2) Social and leisure activities 3) Relationships with extended family 4) Role as a marital partner, parental role, and role within family Includes perceptions of economic functioning. Overall performance at expected tasks, friction with others, interpersonal relationships, and feelings/satisfaction is covered.
Social and Occupational Functioning Assessment Scale (SOFAS) (51)	Adults	Single-item clinician-rated scale to determine the participant's overall level of functioning. Focuses on social and occupational functioning independently from the overall severity of symptoms. Also includes impairments caused by physical and mental disorders. Can be used to rate functioning for current or other time periods

(continued)

Table 1.1 Continued

Measure	Purpose and characteristics	Intended audience
UCSD Performance-Based Skills Assessment (UPSA) (7)	Multiple-item clinician interview. Various role-play-based tasks that take approximately 45 minutes to administer. There is also a brief version that takes approximately 15 minutes to administer. Tasks evaluate functional capacity and skills involved in five domains of functioning: 1) Household chores 2) Communication 3) Finance 4) Transportation 5) Planning recreation activities	Adults
Work and Social Adjustment Scale (WSAS) (52)	Six-item self-report. Measures functional impairment attributable to an identified problem. Measures: 1) Employment status 2) Hours missed from work owing to health reasons 3) Hours missed from work owing to other reasons such as vacation 4) Number of hours worked in the last week 5) Impairment from health conditions while working 6) Impairment in regular daily activities other than work	Adults
World Health Organization Disability Assessment Schedule 2.0 (WHODAS 2.0) (39)	Thirty-six-item self-report or clinician interview. Used to determine standard disability levels across cultures. Can be used across all disorders. Six domains of functioning: 1) Cognition 2) Mobility 3) Self-care 4) Getting along 5) Life activities 6) Participation	Adults

available as well. Less frequently, objective, performance-based measures such as the UCSD Performance-Based Skills Assessment (UPSA) have been utilized. Originally examined predominantly in schizophrenia, the UPSA utilizes a role-play format to examine performance in five domains of functioning: 1) household chores; 2) communication; 3) finance; 4) transportation; and 5) planning recreational activities (7). It has been more recently utilized in depression, with a recent study identifying an increase of between 6 and 7 points as being a clinically important difference in individuals with MDD (8). Health approaches that can include passive monitoring of functional outcomes such as social behaviours are emerging techniques that are promising novel approaches to evaluation in this area (9). The emergence of performance-based and passive monitoring methodologies may have important implications for improving our understanding of functioning in depression by increasing the opportunity to evaluate more 'real-world' information that may more accurately represent one's interaction with the environment and that may be less prone to the potential bias associated with self-reported assessment of functioning (10).

The Importance of Assessing Function in Depression

Depression has been associated with a broad range of functional impairments, including reduced satisfaction with life, higher utilization of health services, greater disability, high rates of unemployment, and significant 'presenteeism', or reduced productivity while at work (11, 12). While functional impairment does tend to increase with higher depressive symptom severity, even subthreshold depressive symptoms can negatively impact function. Both diagnosed depression and subthreshold depressive symptoms have been shown to disrupt physical, social, and health-related functioning in ways that are comparable to, or even exceed, disruptions associated with many other chronic diseases, such as hypertension, diabetes, coronary artery disease, angina, arthritis, back problems, pulmonary disorders, or gastrointestinal disorders (13). Functional impairments are further enhanced when depression is comorbid with other chronic diseases (14, 15).

Functional impairments are observed in several different life environments, including home, work, school, and community, and all of the various social interactions that occur within those environments, such as with family, friends, coworkers, and classmates (10, 16, 17). Thus, these impairments are broadly and pervasively experienced, and they also appear to be frequently sustained, even in the presence of symptomatic improvement or even resolution. Kennedy et al. (18) note that there is a particularly sparse literature on functional outcomes associated with the longer-term course (5 years or more) of depression, and that there is quite a bit of variability in the number of depressed persons exhibiting long-term functional impairments across studies, with ranges of one-third to two-thirds of depressed persons exhibiting poor social adjustment, low levels of satisfaction and enjoyment, and impaired relationships with friends and partners at the most severe levels. Potential differences in rates were attributed to factors such as variability in assessments used and follow-up time periods, as well as other factors such as exposure to psychotherapy, which may have particular benefit on social outcomes.

The functional impairments experienced by depressed patients can range from minimally disruptive to life-altering. Table 1.2 illustrates some of the subjective experiences associated with functional impairments in depression, and some of the resulting consequences that may be realized if functional impairments are not resolved. In all life areas, impairments can result in undesirable consequences that may occur sporadically and that are perhaps minimally disruptive (e.g. increased arguments with a spouse, missed payments), but, without intervention, they can progress to more significant consequences that are even more impactful, such as divorce or bankruptcy.

Recently, the impact of depression on workplace functioning has received significant attention. Significant personal costs of depression in the workplace can be characterized by situations such as relationship strain between coworkers/employers and decreased self-esteem owing to reduced performance and feelings of inadequacy, and sometimes disciplinary actions, including termination of employment and the

Table 1.2 Examples of commonly endorsed functional impairments in MDD across life domains

Life domain	Subjective experiences	Objective consequences
Social	• Feeling withdrawn and uninterested in social activities • Feeling that you have let friends down • Feelings of isolation	• Declining social invitations • Reduced social interactions • Loss of relationships
Household/ daily life	• Unable to keep up with finances or household chores	• Missed payments • Financial distress/bankruptcy • Sanitary issues
Work/ academic	• Difficulty meeting deadlines • Interpersonal conflict/feeling you have let coworkers down • Decreased fulfilment	• Disciplinary actions • Job loss • Drop out of school
Family	• Feeling that you have let the family down • Feeling of burden to other family members	• Divorce • Custody issues
Health-related	• Increased pain • Decreased self-care	• Medical comorbidities • Difficulty with seeking care • Difficulty with treatment adherence

associated consequences (e.g. loss of income, loss of health insurance) that can result in additional personal stressors. High rates of disability and unemployment are observed in MDD and increasing depressive symptom severity tends to increase these rates as well (19). Employers incur costs associated with employees' presenteeism and missed days of work (12, 20), with about 48–50% of costs of depression estimated as being workplace costs (21). Societal costs are in turn realized, with estimates of MDD yielding an economic burden of approximately $210.5 billion dollars in the USA as of 2010 (21), and similarly high costs worldwide (6).

Relevant Contributors to Functional Impairments in Depression

Depression is known to be associated with increased psychiatric and medical comorbidities that can additively impact functioning. Furthermore, specific symptoms of depression, sometimes evaluated beyond the context of core depressive symptoms, such as pain, sleep, cognitive function, and anxiety, have been independently associated with impaired functioning (22). Cognitive dysfunction, for example, has been proposed as a mediator of functioning in depression that warrants specific evaluation and treatment approaches (23, 24). Indeed, specific symptoms that are not resolved with antidepressant treatment may result in lingering functional impairment. For example, inadequately treated pain can result in reduced social and occupational functioning, even in the presence of remission of depressive symptoms (25). Additional emphasis, both clinical and investigative, regarding potential contributors to functional disruption above and beyond depressive symptomatology will help advance our understanding of functional outcomes and appropriate treatment. Consideration should be given to the potential need for specific measurement and treatment of these symptoms.

Treatment Effects on Functional Outcomes

A variety of antidepressant treatments have been shown to improve psychosocial functioning and quality of life (26), including several classes of antidepressants (17), cognitive therapy (27), and exercise (28). Some evidence suggests that functioning improves to a lesser extent and more slowly than depressive symptoms (27), although recent data show that some individuals can achieve functional improvements early in the course of treatment, and such improvements can positively impact longer-term clinical course (29–32). However, functional impairments frequently persist throughout the long-term course of depression (33, 34), although maintenance treatment (as observed with venlafaxine ER in secondary analyses from the PREVENT study) can maintain functional gains achieved during acute phase therapy (35). Despite some promising observations with treatment, even when improvements are realized, functioning often remains below that of non-depressed individuals (16). This suggests the need for targeted treatments that specifically improve functional outcomes, as well as the need for assessment of functioning during treatment of depression and ongoing monitoring. Additionally, targeted selection of antidepressant treatments with known effects on specific symptoms, such as cognitive impairment or pain, may be needed to achieve functional improvements (22).

Future Directions

Although recommended approaches toward the goal of consistent definition and utilization of functional assessment have been suggested throughout the past several years (e.g. the use of single-item measures to capture functioning and quality of life [36] or larger, multidimensional scales that combine evaluation of function and symptom severity, such as the Remission from Depression Scale [37]), none has yet been routinely adopted. Development of a consensus approach to defining and evaluating function would significantly enhance clinical care and research in this area. Some additional suggested approaches toward this goal are currently under way. For example, an international Working Group, led by the International Consortium for Health Outcomes Measurement, has been convened to recommend a standard approach to the evaluation of outcomes in depression and anxiety disorders. They recommend the use of the World Health Organization Disability Schedule 2.0 (WHODAS 2.0) (38) to measure physical, social, and occupational functioning on an annual basis, and a single item from the Patient Health Questionnaire-9 that evaluates the extent to which patients attribute difficulties with daily life functioning to their depressive symptoms to be used to measure functioning during ongoing treatment (39). It will be important to determine how widely adopted such an approach may be. Additionally, continued emphasis on specific symptoms known to be highly related to functional outcomes (e.g. cognition) and targeted treatment approaches that specifically aim to improve functional outcomes will hopefully meaningfully improve this extremely important aspect of depression.

References

1. GBD 2015 DALYs and HALE Collaborators. Global, regional, and national disability-adjusted life-years (DALYs) for 315 diseases and injuries and healthy life expectancy (HALE), 1990-2015: a systematic analysis for the Global Burden of Disease Study 2015. Lancet 2015;388(10053):1603–58.

2. Zimmerman M, McGlinchey J, Posternak M, Friedman M, Attiullah N, Boerescu D. How should remission from depression be defined? The depressed patient's perspective. Am J Psychiatry 2006a;163(1):148–50.

3. Zimmerman M, Martinez J, Attiullah N, Friedman M, Toba C, Boerescu DA. Why do some depressed outpatients who are not in remission according to the hamilton depression rating scale nonetheless consider themselves to be in remission? Depression Anxiety 2012;29(10):891–5.

4. Sheehan DV, Harnett-Sheehan K, Spann ME, Thompson HF, Prakash A. Assessing remission in major depressive disorder and generalized anxiety disorder clinical trials with the discan metric of the Sheehan disability scale. Int Clin Psychopharmacol 2011;26(2):75–83.

5. The WHOQOL Group. The World Health Organization Quality of Life assessment (WHOQOL): position paper from the World Health Organization. Social Sci Med 1995;41(10):1403–9.

6. Lam RW, Filteau MJ, Milev R. Clinical effectiveness: the importance of psychosocial functioning outcomes. J Affective Dis 2011;132(1):S9–S13.

7. Patterson TL, Goldman S, Mckibbin CL, Hughs T, Jeste DV. UCSD Performance-based skills assessment: development of a new measure of everyday functioning for severely mentally ill adults. Schizophrenia Bull 2001;27(2):235–45.

8. Harvey PD, Jacobson W, Zhong W, et al. Determination of a clinically important difference and definition of a responder threshold for the UCSD performance-based skills assessment (UPSA) in patients with major depressive disorder. J Affective Dis 2017;213:105–11.

9. Clifford GD, Clifton D. Wireless technology in disease management and medicine. Annu Rev Med 2012;63:479–92.

10. Coryell W, Scheftner W, Keller M, Endicott J, Maser J, Klerman GL. The enduring psychosocial consequences of mania and depression. Am J Psychiatry 1993;150(5):720–7.

11. Hermann H, Patrick DL, Diehr P, et al. Longitudinal investigation of depression outcomes in primary care in six countries: the LIDO study. Functional status, health service use and treatment of people with depressive symptoms. Psychol Med 2002;32:889–902.

12. Stewart WF, Ricci JA, Chee E, Hahn SR, Marganstein D. Cost of lost productive work time among US workers with depression. JAMA 2003;289:3135–3144.

13. Wells KB, Stewart A, Hays RD, et al. The functioning and well-being of depressed patients: results from the Medical Outcomes Study. JAMA 1989;262(7): 914–19.

14. Moussavi S, Chatterji S, Verdes E, Tandon A, Patel V, Ustun B. Depression, chronic diseases, and decrements in health: results from the World Health Surveys. Lancet 2007;370(9590):851–8.

15. Druss BG, Hwang I, Petukhova M, Sampson NA, Wang PS, Kessler RC. Impairment in role functioning in mental and chronic medical disorders in the United States: results from the National Comorbidity Survey Replication. Mol Psychiatry 2009;14(7):728–37.

16. Miller IW, Keitner GI, Schatzberg AF, et al. The treatment of chronic depression, part 3: psychosocial functioning before and after treatment with sertraline or imipramine. J Clin Psychiatr 1998;59(11):608–19.

17. Hirschfeld RM, Montgomery SA, Keller MB, et al. Social functioning in depression: a review. J Clin Psychiatry 2000;61(4):268–75.

18. Kennedy N, Foy K, Sherazi R, McDonough M, McKeon P. Long-term social functioning after depression treated by psychiatrists: a review. Bipolar Disorder 2007;9(1–2):25–37.

19. Birnbaum HG, Kessler RC, Kelley D, Ben-Hamadi R, Joish VN, Greenberg PE. Employer burden of mild, moderate, and severe major depressive disorder: mental health services utilization and costs, and work performance. Depression Anxiety 2010;27(1):78–89.

20. Evans VC, Chan SSL, Iverson GL, Bond DJ, Yatham LN, Lam RW. Systematic review of neurocognition and occupational functioning in major depressive disorder. Neuropsychiatry 2013;3(1):97–105.

21. Greenberg PE, Fournier AA, Sisitsky T, Pike CT, Kessler RC. The economic burden of adults with major depressive disorder in the United States (2005 and 2010). J Clin Psychiatry 2015;76(2):155–62.

22. Greer TL, Kurian BT, Trivedi MH. Defining and measuring functional recovery from depression. CNS Drugs 2010;24(4):267–84.

23. McIntyre RS, Cha DS, Soczynska JK, et al. Cognitive deficits and functional outcomes in major depressive disorder: determinants, substrates, and treatment interventions. Depression Anxiety 2013;30(6):515–27.

24. Lam RW, Kennedy SH, McIntyre RS, Khullar A. Cognitive dysfunction in major depressive disorder: effects on psychosocial functioning and implications for treatment. Can J Psychiatry Revue Canadienne de Psychiatrie 2014;59(12):649–54.

25. Harada E, Satoi Y, Kuga A, et al. Associations among depression severity, painful physical symptoms, and social and occupational functioning impairment in patients with major depressive disorder: a 3-month, prospective, observational study. Neuropsychiatr Dis Treatment 2017;13:2437–45.

26. Sheehan DV, Nakagome K, Asami Y, Pappadopulos EA, Boucher M. Restoring function in major depressive disorder: a systematic review. J Affective Dis 2017;215:299–313.

27. Dunn TW, Vittengl JR, Clark LA, Carmody T, Thase ME, Jarrett RB. Change in psychosocial functioning and depressive symptoms during acute-phase cognitive therapy for depression. Psycholog Med 2012;42(2):317–26.

28. Greer TL, Trombello JM, Rethorst CD, et al. Improvements in psychosocial functioning and health-related quality of life following exercise augmentation in patients with treatment response but nonremitted major depressive disorder: results from the TREAD study. Depression Anxiety 2016;33(9):870–81.

29. Jha MK, Greer TL, Grannemann BD, Carmody T, Rush AJ, Trivedi MH. Early normalization of quality of life predicts later remission in depression: findings from the CO-MED trial. J Affective Dis 2016;206:17–22 .

30. Jha MK, Minhajuddin A, Greer TL, Carmody T, Rush AJ, Trivedi MH. Early improvement in psychosocial function predicts longer-term symptomatic remission in depressed patients. PLoS One 2016b ;11(12):e0167901.

31. Jha MK, Minhajuddin A, Greer TL, Carmody T, Rush AJ, Trivedi MH. Early improvement in work productivity predicts future clinical course in depressed outpatients: findings from the CO-MED trial. Am J Psychiatry 2016;173(12): 1196–204.

32. Jha MK, Teer RB, Minhajuddin A, Greer TL, Rush AJ, Trivedi MH. Daily activity level improvement with antidepressant medications predicts long-term clinical outcomes in outpatients with major depressive disorder. Neuropsychiatr Dis Treatment 2017;13:803–13.

33. Hirschfeld RM, Dunner DL, Keitner G, et al. Does psychosocial functioning improve independent of depressive symptoms? A comparison of nefazodone, psychotherapy, and their combination. Biol Psychiatry 2002;51(2):123–33.

34. Judd LL, Schettler PJ, Solomon DA, et al. Psychosocial disability and work role function compared across the long-term course of bipolar I, bipolar II and unipolar major depressive disorders. J Affect Disord 2008;108(1–2):49–58.

35. Watanabe K, Thase ME, Kikuchi T, et al. Long-term function and psychosocial outcomes with venlafaxine extended release 75–225 mg/day versus placebo in the PREVENT study. Int Clin Psychopharmacol 2017;32(5):271–80.

36. Zimmerman M, Ruggero CJ, Chelminski I, et al. Developing brief scales for use in clinical practice: the reliability and validity of single-item self-report measures of depression symptom severity, psychosocial impairment due to depression, and quality of life. J Clin Psychiatry 2006;67(10):1536–41.

37. Zimmerman M, Martinez JH, Attiullah N, et al. A new type of scale for determining remission from depression: the Remission from Depression Questionnaire. J Psychiatric Res 2013;47(1):78–82.

38. World Health Organization. Measuring Health and Disability: Manual for WHO Disability Assessment Schedule (WHODAS 20). Geneva: World Health Organization, 2010.

39. Obbarius A, van Maasakkers L, Baer L, et al. Standardization of health outcomes assessment for depression and anxiety: recommendations from the ICHOM Depression and Anxiety Working Group. Quality of Life Res 2017;26(12):3211–25.

40. Burckhardt CS, Anderson KL. The Quality of Life Scale (QOLS): reliability, validity, and utilization. Healthy Quality Life Outcomes 2003;1(60).

41. Endicott J, Nee J, Harrison W, Blumenthal R. Quality of Life Enjoyment and Satisfaction Questionnaire. Psychopharmacol Bull 1993;29(2):321–6.

42. Ware JE, Sherbourne CD. The MOS 36-ltem Short-Form Health Survey (SF-36). Med Care 1992;30(6):473–83.

43. World Health Organization Quality of Life BREF. Handbook of Disease Burdens and Quality of Life Measures. Geneva: World Health Organization; 2010: p. 4354.

44. Lam RW, Michalak EE, Yatham LN. A new clinical rating scale for work absence and productivity: validation in patients with major depressive disorder. BMC Psychiatry 2009;9(1):78.

45. Leon AC, Solomon DA, Mueller TI, Turvey CL, Endicott J, Keller MB. The Range of Impaired Functioning Tool (LIFE-RIFT): a brief measure of functional impairment. Psychol Med 1999;29(4):869–78.

46. Jaeger J, Berns SM, Czobor P. The Multidimensional Scale of Independent Functioning: a new instrument for measuring functional disability in psychiatric populations. Schizophrenia Bull 2003;29(1):153–67.

47. Flanagan JC. A research approach to improving our quality of life. Am Psychol 1978;33:138–47.

48. Sheehan DV, Harnett-Sheehan K, Raj BA. The measurement of disability. Int Clin Psychopharmacol 1996;3:89–95.

49. Bosc M, Dubini A, Polin V. Development and validation of a social functioning scale, the Social Adaptation Self-evaluation Scale. Eur Neuropsychopharmacol 1997;7(1):S57–70.

50. Weissman MM. Assessment of social adjustment by patient self-report. Arch Gen Psychiatry 1976;33(9):1111.

51. Rybarczyk B. Social and Occupational Functioning Assessment Scale (SOFAS). Encyclopedia of Clinical Neuropsychology, 2011: p. 2313.

52. Mundt JC, Marks IM, Shear MK, Greist JM. The Work and Social Adjustment Scale: a simple measure of impairment in functioning. Br J Psychiatry 2002;180(5):461–4.

2

Opportunities and Challenges of the Phenotypic Heterogeneity of Major Depressive Disorder

Koen Demyttenaere

Heterogeneity in the Concept Major Depressive Disorder

Major depressive disorder (MDD) is often defined based on the *Diagnostic and Statistical Manual of Mental Disorders* (DSM) criteria where five out of nine symptoms (with depressed mood or diminished interest and pleasure being mandatory) should be present during at least the same 2-week period and representing a change from previous functioning, causing a clinically significant distress or impairment (1). This DSM definition obviously has its usefulness but also poses multiple challenges. It has been shown that, based on the nine DSM criteria, 227 unique profiles are possible. Moreover, the fact that several criteria are compound criteria (interest or pleasure, increased or decreased sleep, increased or decreased appetite, psychomotor retardation or agitation, …) further adds to the heterogeneity: by cutting these criteria further down, 945 unique profiles or symptom constellations are possible (2, 3).

Another problem with the DSM definition is that 'the symptoms cause a clinically significant distress or impairment in social, occupational, or other important areas of functioning': this is, however, not well defined and hence is open to subjectivity. It is, for example, not easy to disentangle 'causality' and 'consequence' in a patient being fired at work, developing depressive symptoms which then impair his or her functioning. It seems reasonable to state that, in a depressive patient, all domains of life (occupational, social, family life) are impaired. Using the Sheehan Disability Scale as a measure of impairment and considering that, for depression, most depressed patients show scores between 5 and 8 (moderate or severe impairment) (4). When defining that there should be at least a moderate impairment in all domains of functioning (score of at least 4 for occupational and social and family functioning), it was shown that 28% of the patients presenting with at least five out of the nine DSM symptoms did not fulfil 'a clinically significant impairment in functioning' (5, 6).

Most patients suffering from depression also present a range of other symptoms and it is difficult to define which symptoms are core, or comorbid (sometimes reaching thresholds for other disorders), or associated. When looking at the history of antidepressant marketing it becomes obvious that this has been the focus of the pharmaceutical industry during the past decades and that this resulted in a better understanding of the relation between the various symptom clusters and hence of the clinical reality of our patients (Figure 2.1). The selective serotonin reuptake inhibitors (SSRIs) focus a lot on the comorbid anxious symptoms and comorbid anxiety disorders, with paroxetine the guide in this field. It is, moreover, remarkable that, once the indication of MDD is obtained, most pharmaceutical companies focus on generalized anxiety disorder as the next indication. The serotonin and noradrenaline reuptake inhibitors (SNRIs) focus especially on somatic symptoms, with duloxetine most specifically focusing on painful physical symptoms (and the SSRIs also focusing on premenstrual dysphoric disorder) and desvenlafaxine also focusing on vasomotor symptoms associated with menopause. Agomelatine focuses on anhedonia and the lack of positive affect and vortioxetine focuses on the cognitive symptoms in depression. There is pharmacological and neurobiological evidence for these claims and some clinical evidence for each of these effects, although in most cases the evidence for the specificity of mode of action and specificity of effect is limited. Figure 2.1 puts anxiety symptoms and somatic symptoms closer to each other and also puts anhedonia and cognitive symptoms closer to each other. Indeed, it is well known that anxious patients show more somatic symptoms and show more intolerance to somatic side-effects of medication. In a large factor analysis on the data from STAR*D and GENDEP, the best fitted model was a six-factor solution: positive

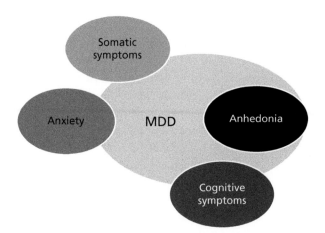

Figure 2.1   Core and associated symptoms in patients with major depressive disorder (MDD).

affect and cognitive functioning were clustered together in one factor, suggesting their closer relationship, and this factor was the most predictive for outcome (7).

Heterogeneity in Assessment Tools

A variety of assessment tools are used, each assessing a variety of symptoms. Some scales (e.g. Patient Health Questionnaire-9 [PHQ-9]) closely reflect DSM criteria while others have a much larger scope. Some scales focus on the clinical reality, e.g. the Hamilton Rating Scale for Depression (HRSD) includes a range of anxiety and neurovegetative symptoms, which reflects the reality of many patients having comorbid symptoms but limits its use in patients with comorbid somatic disorders where some symptoms may overlap and blur changes during treatment (8–10). In an attempt to overcome this problem, other scales mainly focus on the emotional or psychological symptoms of depression (e.g. the Hospital Anxiety and Depression Scale [HADS]) (11). Other scales focus on the sensitivity to change, e.g. the Montgomery Asberg Depression Rating Scale (MADRS) selected those 10 items that improved most during treatment with a variety of antidepressants (with various modes of action) (12).

Randomized controlled trials (RCTs) are still considered the gold standard but it may not be forgotten that, in the real word, the magnitude of the drug effect is less well known: it was shown that, in an outpatient practice, only 8% of patients with MDD could have been enrolled in a RCT (owing to inclusion and exclusion criteria) and, in the more naturalistic FINDER study, only 10% could have been enrolled in a RCT (13, 14).

Whether observer-rating or self-rating scales or the similarities and discrepancies between them should be taken into account is another debate (15, 16). Max Hamilton, who could be considered to have a conflict of interest, once declared: 'Clinical trials should be conducted in such a way that they resemble ordinary clinical practice as much as possible. This is one of the reasons why I have some antipathy to self-rating scales. In ordinary clinical practice, the physician ascertains the changes in a patient's condition by asking him questions and receiving replies thereto. Observer rating scales fit in very well with this procedure; self-rating scales provide an excellent excuse for the investigator to avoid interviewing his patient … ' (10).

In an attempt to have more ecologically valid assessments, experience sampling methods (ESM; having multiple self-rating assessments per day via an app) were recently introduced to have assessments less prone to overgeneralization. Whether this ESM has significant clinical advantages is still to be proven. Another trend toward more naturalistic assessments is moving from more subjective assessment tools (observer- or self-rating questionnaires) to real-life experimental tasks: Pizzagalli developed a 'probabilistic reward task based on a differential reinforcement schedule that allowed to objectively assess participants' propensity to modulate behavior as a function of reward' (17). But whether this economically driven reward task really represents anticipatory and consumatory hedonic tone is still debatable. The THINC® cognition tool is another example where (subjective) patient-reported assessment (PDQ, Perceived Deficit Questionnaire) is combined with objective tests, including the Digit Symbol Coding Test (DSCD), Choice Reaction Time (CRT), the Trail Making Test (TMT), and the Two-Back Test (2BT) (18). However, again, intrinsic motivation of the patient precedes performance on these tests.

There is often confusion on their use: sometimes they are used as screening or as diagnostic tools, sometimes they are used as measures of severity, and sometimes they are used to assess changes during treatment (Table 2.1).

A network analysis restricted to the 15 Inventory of Depressive Symptomatology—Clinician rated (IDS-C) symptoms of major depression representing the DSM criteria (decreased or increased appetite was taken as one item) showed that the centrality (connectedness of each symptom with all others) was highest for loss of energy, loss of interest, change in appetite, concentration problems, and mild insomnia (2, 19, 20). The same network analysis was done for all the 28 IDS-C symptoms (decreased or increased appetite and decreased or increased weight were twice taken as one item) and the analysis could not find a difference in centrality between items representing DSM criteria and items not representing DSM criteria: loss of energy, sadness, sympathetic arousal, loss of interest, and loss of pleasure now showed the highest centrality. These findings suggest that the distinction between DSM depression criteria and *International Classification of Diseases* (ICD) depression symptoms is artificial. Moreover, an investigation of the relative importance of individual depressive symptoms on overall impairment showed that sad mood, concentration problems, fatigue, loss

Table 2.1 Diversity in assessment scales

Observer rating	Self-rating
HRSD (17)	Carroll (21)
MADRS (10)	MADRS-S (9)
DSM (9)	PHQ-9 (9)
IDS (30)	IDS-S (30)
QIDS (16)	QIDS-S (16)
	Zung SDS (20)
	BDI (21)
	HADS 7

For abbreviations see text.

of interest, and being slowed down contributed most to overall impairment, again not showing a differential impact of DSM depression criteria and ICD depression symptoms (26).

Heterogeneity in Treatment Response

The largest meta-analysis of 6–8-week randomized placebo-controlled trials showed a response rate of 53.8% for antidepressants and 37.3% for placebo (27). Response rate in STAR*D level 1, where all patients were treated with citalopram for 12 weeks (but this patient population had a higher number of previous episodes), was 47% (28). However, when taking into account some sociodemographic variables (education more or less than 14 years, employed or unemployed, and gender) and some clinical variables (anxious or not anxious depression, episode duration more or less than 1 year), response rates varied between 31% and 63%, illustrating again the importance of the heterogeneity of the depressed patient population (29). Moreover, in RCTs study design plays a dramatic role: a meta-analysis investigating this aspect found response rates for antidepressants and placebo of 51.7% and 34.3%, respectively, in two-arm trials, of 57.7% and 44.6%, respectively, in three-arm trials (two antidepressant arms and one placebo arm), and of 65.4% in two-arm trials with just two active antidepressants, again underscoring the importance of expectations (chance on placebo 50%, 33%, or 0%) in patients as well as in physicians (30). Patient preference for treatment modality has also been shown to influence outcome dramatically. An example is the study where patient preference was assessed (48% preferred psychotherapy, 18% preferred antidepressants, and 34% had no preference ... and patients were then randomized to pharmacotherapy or psychotherapy): matched patients (preferring psychotherapy and getting psychotherapy or preferring antidepressants and getting antidepressants) or patients without a preference had a good outcome while those who were mismatched had a significantly worse outcome (31). Another example illustrating the power of beliefs and hence heterogeneity was a meta-analysis on the escitalopram database, where all studies, including the Quality of Life, Enjoyment and Satisfaction Questionnaire (Q-LES-Q), were analysed to see whether baseline attitude toward taking medication influences outcome: in patients receiving placebo, response rates were, respectively, 34%, 36%, and 56% for those having a rather negative, a neutral, or a rather positive baseline attitude; for active medication (escitalopram, duloxetine, or venlafaxine) the percentages were 51%, 56%, and 69% (32). Antidepressants always performed better than placebo, but the effect of differences in baseline attitude was as large as the difference between active medication and placebo. A last example illustrating how heterogeneity blurs results with treatment is the failed sertraline, hypericum, and placebo trial, where neither sertraline nor hypericum did better than placebo. An interesting aspect of this study was that, at the end, the question was asked of patients, as well as of physicians, whether they could guess on which treatment arm the patient was. For both patients and physicians, guessing that the patient was on sertraline or on hypericum resulted in a highly statistically significant better outcome than when they were guessing that the patient was taking placebo; interestingly, patients had the numerically highest remission rates when they guessed they were taking hypericum, while patients had the numerically highest remission rates when their physician guessed they were taking sertraline (33, 34).

Conclusion

It is our firm belief that personalized (or precision) medicine should first take into account the heterogeneity in the depressed patient population, the heterogeneity of the psychometric scales uses to assess changes, and, last but not least, patient expectations, attitudes, and beliefs before it can keep its promise of improving outcomes in our depressed patients through possible biological markers.

References

1. American Psychiatric Association. Diagnostic and Statistical Manual of Mental Disorders. 5th ed. (DSM-5) Washington, DC: American Psychiatric Press, 2013.

2. Fried EI, Nesse RM. Depression is not a consistent syndrome: an investigation of unique symptom patterns in the STAR* D study. J Affect Dis 2015;172:96–102.

3. Fried EI. The 52 symptoms of major depression: lack of content overlap among seven common depression scales. J Affect Dis 2017; 208:191–7.

4. Sheehan DV, Harnett-Sheehan K, Raj BA. The measurement of disability. Int Clin Psychopharmacol 1996;11 (Suppl. 3):89–95.

5. Spitzer RL, Wakefield JC. DSM-IV diagnostic criterion for clinical significance: does it help solve the false positives problem? Am J Psychiatry 1999;156:1856–64.

6. Demyttenaere K, Enzlin P, Dewé W, et al. Compliance with antidepressants in a primary care setting, 2: the influence of gender and type of impairment. J Clin Psychiatry 2001;62 (Suppl. 22):34–7.

7. Uher R, Perlis RH, Henigsberg N, et al. Depression symptom dimensions as predictors of antidepressant treatment outcome: replicable evidence for interest-activity symptoms. Psychol Med 2012;42:967–80.

8. Spitzer RL, Kroenke K, Williams JBW. Validation and utility of a self-report version of PRIME-MD—the PHQ primary care study. JAMA 1999;282:1737–44.

9. Kroenke K, Spitzer RL, Williams JBW. The PHQ-9. Validity of a brief depression severity measure. J Gen Interrn Med 2001;16:606–13.

10. Hamilton M. A rating scale for depression. J Neurol Neurosurg Psychiatry 1960;23:56–62.

11. Zigmond AS, Snaith RP. The hospital anxiety and depression scale. Acta Psychiatr Scand 1983;67:361–70.

12. Montgomery SA, Åsberg M. A new depression scale designed to be sensitive to change. Br J Psychiatry 1979;134:382–9.

13. Zimmerman M, Mattia JL, Posternak MA. Are subjects in pharmacological trials of depression representative of patients in routine clinical practice? Am J Psychiatry 2002;159 (3):469–73.

14. Demyttenaere K, Verhaeghen A, Dantchev N, et al. 'Caseness' for depression and anxiety in a depressed outpatient population: symptomatic outcome as a function of baseline diagnostic categories. Prim Care Companion J Clin Psychiatry 2009;11(6):307–15.

15. Snaith P. What do depression rating scales measure? Br J Psychiatry 1993;163:293–8.

16. Möller HJ. Rating depressed patients: observer- vs self-assessment. Eur Psychiatry 2000;15:160–72.

17. Pizzagalli DA, Jahn AL, O'Shea JP. Toward an objective characterization of an anhedonic phenotype: a signal detection approach. Biol Psychiatry 2005;57:319–27.

18. McIntyre RS, Best MW, Bowie CR, et al. The THINC-integrated tool (THINC-it) screening assessment for cognitive dysfunction: validation in patients with major depressive disorder. J Clin Psychiatry 2017;78 (7):873–81.

19. Rush AJ, Giles DE, Schlesser MA, Fulton CL,Weissenburger J, Burns C. The Inventory for Depressive Symptomatology (IDS): preliminary findings. Psychiatry Res 1986;18:65–87.

20. Rush AJ, Trivedi MH, Ibrahim HM, et al. The 16-item Quick Inventory of Depressive Symptomatology rating (QIDS-C), and self-report (QIDS-SR): a psychometric evaluation in patients with major depression. Biol Psychiatry 2003;54(5):573–83.

21. Carroll BJ, Feinberg M, Smouse PE, Rawson SG, Greden JF. The Carroll rating scale for depression. I. Development, reliability and validation. Br J Psychiatry 1981;138:194–200.

22. Svanborg P, Asberg M. A comparison between the Beck Depression Inventory (BDI) and the self-rated version of the Montgomery-Asberg Depression Rating Scale (MADRS) J Affect Dis. 2001;64:203–16.

23. Rush JA, Hiser W, Giles DE. A comparison of self-reported versus clinician-rated symptoms of depression. J Clin Psychiatry 1987;48:246–8.

24. Zung WWK, Durham NC. A self-rating depression scale. Arch Gen Psychiatry 1965;12:61–70.

25. Beck AT, Ward CH, Mendelson M, Mock J, Erbaugh J. An inventory of measuring depression. Arch Gen Psychiatry 1961;4:53–61.

26. Fried EI, Nesse RM. The impact of individual depressive symptoms on impairment of psychosocial functioning. PLOS one 2014;9:e90311.

27. Papakostas GI, Fava M. Does the probability of receiving placebo influence clinical trial outcome? A meta-regression of double-blind, randomized trials in MDD. Eur Neuropsychopharmacol 2009;19:34–40.

28. Trivedi MH, Rush AJ, Wisniewski SR, et al.; the STAR*D study team. Evaluation of outcomes with citalopram for depression using measurement-based care in STAR*D: implications for clinical practice. Am J Psychiatry 2006;163(1):28–40.

29. Jain FA, Hunter AM, Brooks JO 3rd, Leuchter AF. Predictive socioeconomic and clinical profiles of antidepressant response and remission. Depress Anxiety 2013;30(7):624–30.

30. Sinyor M, Levitt AJ, Cheung AH, et al. Does inclusion of a placebo arm influence response to active antidepressant treatment in RCTs? Results from pooled and meta-analyses. J Clin Psychiatry 2010;71(3):270–9.

31. Kwan BM, Dimidjian S, Rizvi SL. Treatment preference, engagement, and clinical improvement in pharmacotherapy versus psychotherapy for depression. Behav Res Ther 2010;48:799–804.

32. Demyttenaere K, Reines EH, Lönn SL, Lader M. Satisfaction with medication is correlated with outcome but not persistence in patients treated with placebo, escitalopram, or serotonin-norepinephrine reuptake inhibitors: a post hoc analysis. The Primary Care Companion to CNS Disorders 2011;13(4):PCC.10m01080.

33. Chen JA, Papakostas GI, Youn SJ, et al. Association between patient beliefs regarding assigned treatment and clinical response: reanalysis of data from the Hypericum Depression Trial Study Group. J Clin Psychiatry 2011;72:1669–76.

34. Chen JA, Vijapura S, Papakostas GI, et al. Association between physician beliefs regarding assigned treatment and clinical response: re-analysis of data from the Hypericum Depression Trial Study Group. Asian J Psychiatry 2015;13:23–9.

3

Major Depressive Disorder as a Disorder of Cognition

Muzaffer Kaser and Barbara J. Sahakian

Impact of Cognitive Dysfunction in Depression

Cognitive dysfunction is a major clinical feature in depressive disorders (1). Patients with depression often report difficulties in concentration or memory (2), and almost half of patients continue to have residual cognitive symptoms between episodes. However, clinicians tend to focus more on mood and sleep problems than cognition (3). Survey results revealed that 50% of depressed patients had never been asked about their cognitive symptoms by a healthcare professional (4). Almost all participants reported that cognitive symptoms had a negative impact on their quality of life and work. Fifteen per cent of patients said that they had lost their job owing to persistent cognitive difficulties. At the workplace, depression is a primary contributor to absenteeism and presenteeism (5). Presenteeism associated with depression refers to the fact that people return to work but cannot achieve previous performance because of the residual symptoms. Self-reported cognitive deficits in fully employed patients were associated with interference in the workplace, with attention and planning domains being most affected (6). Poorer cognitive functioning interferes with employment status in currently depressed and remitted depressed individuals (7). At the population level, better cognitive function is associated with better wellbeing (8).

Assessment of cognitive function at the time of clinical presentation has predictive value for functional outcomes. In a prospective study, Jaeger et al. (9) showed that patients with poorer neurocognitive test performance at baseline had more functional impairments at the 6-month follow-up. Similarly, persistent deficits in attention and mental flexibility were reported in a prospective study spanning 12 months. Seventy-five per cent of patients in the sample continued to have employment and relational functioning deficits (10).

Definition and Extent of Cognitive Dysfunction in Patients with Depression

Extensive studies reported poorer cognitive performance in patients with depression compared to healthy controls (11, 12). Affected domains included attention, working memory, episodic memory, and a range of executive functions (e.g. planning, cognitive flexibility, response inhibition, and decision-making). Some studies reported marked cognitive impairment while others showed unaffected cognition in depression (13). There are inconsistencies regarding the domains affected and the magnitude of deficits. Young people may not exhibit marked impairments during the first episode, or some tests may not be sensitive enough to detect deficits. It should be noted that depression is a common mental health problem affecting a heterogeneous group of people.

In a meta-analysis of 113 studies investigating executive function deficits in depression, healthy controls performed better than the patients in every single parameter, even for the single test outcomes analysed (12). Despite mixed results in individual tests, overall deficits in executive function are one of the most replicated cognitive findings in patients with depression. Substantial variability in assessment methods, sample characteristics, and domains assessed explained the findings in the relatively few studies that failed to find cognitive deficits. Standardized testing tools can provide more reliable information. A meta-analysis (14) that included the studies using a single neuropsychological battery, CANTAB (www.cambridgecognition.com), showed that patients with current depression showed moderate cognitive deficits in executive function, attention, and memory tasks. The magnitude of deficits was comparable between currently depressed and remitted depressed patients and was independent of medication use.

Severity of Cognitive Impairment in Depression

Setting the criteria for cognitive dysfunction in depression is not a straightforward task. For instance, dementia researchers use a rather consistent and well-established cut-off 1.5 standard deviations below the normal population to identify mild cognitive impairment. On the other hand, cognitive dysfunction in patients with schizophrenia usually manifests with two standard deviations below healthy volunteers. At the group level, the magnitude of cognitive deficits in depression is smaller than those in schizophrenia or mild cognitive impairment. However, while the majority of people with schizophrenia or mild cognitive impairment are not in employment, those with depression may still be in work. Therefore, the overall impact of depression on society is possibly more pronounced because of the effects of cognitive impairments on work functioning.

A major problem with the definition of cognitive dysfunction is the fact that even a relatively small impairment in cognition may impact on functionality at work and home. Gualtieri and Morgan (15) reported that 21% of patients with major depressive disorder (MDD) show a cognitive performance of two standard deviations below the average for two or more domains. Of 285 patients examined, 110 (38.6%) had impairment in at least one of the cognitive domains. Another study defined standard cut-off scores and standard deviations for each domain akin to conventional IQ measures. In this sample, 61% of unmedicated patients with MDD had impairments in at least one cognitive domain (16). In a recent study, 44.4% of patients with MDD had cognitive composite scores at least one standard deviation below the scores of average healthy volunteers (17). A task force report by the International Society of Bipolar Disorders made several recommendations for future clinical trials that may have implications for unipolar depression research. One of the recommendations is that patients with 0.5 standard deviations below average should be categorized as a cognitively impaired group in future clinical trials (18).

Rarely are premorbid measures of cognition available since people are generally not given cognitive tests prior to the onset of depression. Therefore, predicted levels of performance may need to be estimated from measures of premorbid IQ or years of education. For example, a high-functioning individual in a cognitively demanding job (e.g. an academic, CEO, or a software developer) would normally score well above average before the depressive episode. When tested after depression, scores may fall in the normal range rather than the above-normal range. Although the individual scores in the average range, the decline is very likely to cause dysfunction for a professional whose job is heavily dependent on cognitive abilities, including decision-making, problem-solving, and planning.

Is the Cognitive Impairment Fully Reversible in Remission from the Depressive Episode?

A growing body of evidence suggests that cognitive impairment in depression is a distinct entity rather than an epiphenomenon of low mood state (19). Persistence of cognitive problems in the remission phase and the impact on functional outcomes highlight the importance of investigating the deficits in remitted depression (20). Meta-analysis of findings revealed that patients with remitted depression had cognitive impairments in multiple domains, with small to medium effect sizes (21). Duration and number of episodes, residual symptoms, age, or gender, had no effect on these impairments. It should be noted that most of the studies were cross-sectional and few studies assessed the same patient group both in a depressive episode and after they are remitted (22, 23).

Cognitive Neuropsychological Model of Depression

Cognitive domains affected in depression are not limited to attention, memory, or executive functions. Dysfunction in emotional processing and hypersensitivity to negative feedback could also contribute to poorer performance in neuropsychological tests. Patients with depression tend to respond to negative stimuli more quickly than positive stimuli (24). Healthy participants, in contrast, tend to have bias toward positive cues. The negative affective biases were demonstrated in the presence of emotionally valenced words (24) and in attentional control tasks involving faces (25). In an experimental setting, depressed participants perform significantly worse when they receive negative feedback on their performance. This so-called catastrophic response to negative feedback seems to interfere with the top-down control mechanism over emotional processes in the brain. In other terms, this could be a manifestation of impaired hot cognition and cold cognition. Hot cognition refers to processes involving emotional and reward-related stimuli. Hot cognition operates when participants are presented emotionally salient stimuli (emotional words, faces, etc.) or when the feedback on their performance is linked to an affective state (e.g. fulfilment or sense of failure). Cold cognition is used to define non-emotional cognitive abilities (26).

The interplay between emotional processing, cognitive control, and other relevant factors is formulated in the Cognitive Neuropsychological Model of Depression (Figure 3.1). According to this model, bottom-up affective biases and top-down attentional biases (owing to dysfunctional cognitive control) help to maintain the depressive state (27, 28). The model accommodates the vulnerability factors such as genetic influences, adverse life events, and the mechanisms that pharmacological or psychological treatments tap into. Conventional cognitive behavioural therapy aims to break negative schemata through techniques that help patients to challenge negative thoughts. In the context of the classical cognitive model this could be identified as patients with depression using their cold cognitive control over their top-down negative biases.

This model proposes that antidepressants or psychological interventions do not have a direct effect on mood, but they exert their effects via modulation of negative biases (27). Cognitive behavioural therapy and antidepressant medication can alter the way that the brain processes affective stimuli and help to mitigate the negative biases, eventually leading to improved cognitive control and remission of the mood symptoms. A series of studies suggested that antidepressants could reverse the negative emotional bias in the first week of treatment (29). Some of the findings in the model can be traced at neuroimaging or pharmacological challenge studies. For instance, negative biases in depressed patients were associated with activation in the anterior cingulate cortex (30). There is also neuroimaging insight into the neural mechanisms underlying the interaction between dysfunctional emotional processing and impaired cognitive control (31), although further studies are required.

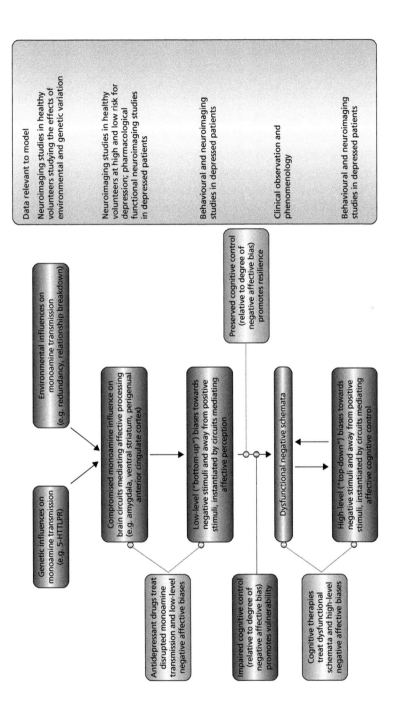

Figure 3.1 The Extended Cognitive Neuropsychological Model of Depression. The boxes represent the factors that contribute to the development and maintenance of the depressive state, including the boxes that represent factors that contribute to the treatment of and recovery from depression (cognitive therapies, antidepressant drugs, and resilience factors). The right column is a guide for the evidence from different levels. 5-HTTLPR, Serotonin transporter-linked polymorphic region.

Reprinted by permission from Springer: *Springer Nature*, 37, 1, Roiser JP, Elliott R, Sahakian BJ, Cognitive mechanisms of treatment in depression, pp. 117–136. Copyright © 2011, Springer.

Cognitive Dysfunction in Depression is an Unmet Treatment Need

Cognitive dysfunction in depression is a clear unmet need (32). According to the results from a survey of depressed patients in the UK, almost all had cognitive symptoms with significant impact on their work and social life. Strikingly, half of the respondents were never asked about their cognitive symptoms by the healthcare professionals (4). Currently, the organization of health systems and clinical guidelines do not specifically consider cognitive dysfunction as a treatment target for depression. A recent study showed that there is limited knowledge of cognitive dysfunction in depression amongst UK clinicians (33). The major challenge is the lack of specific treatments for cognitive dysfunction in depression (32). Patients suffering from enduring cognitive difficulties after remission of mood symptoms seek help to address these. But when they present to their GPs or psychiatrists, the treatment options are very limited. Untreated cognitive symptoms may persist, leading to further deterioration and relapses (34).

Defining cognition as a target for treatment in depression is an important step, but it will require many parties working together. This view has been increasingly acknowledged by the experts in the field as well as policy-makers. The report by the National Academies of Sciences, Engineering, and Medicine on cognitive dysfunction highlighted the challenges and future directions (35). Recommendations from this expert-led initiative can be used as a roadmap. Firstly, we need reliable, practical assessment tools that are sensitive to change. Treatments to address cognitive deficits need to be assessed with objective tests providing consistent measures of cold cognition as well as hot cognition. Subjective measures and functional outcomes are regarded as a priority by regulators as they focus on the real-life impact of any intervention. A major challenge is to evaluate the cognitive efficacy of the treatments reliably. Proposed solutions included using translational cognitive biomarkers and introducing novel trial designs with stratification so that they can address heterogeneity. It is also important to learn from the developments in other psychiatric conditions, such as schizophrenia. However, both neuropsychological and functional assessments need to be tailored accordingly for depression, including both 'hot' and 'cold' cognitive measures. Moving forward, flexibility in the selection of objective measures will allow for maximum progression in the field of treatment development for cognitive and motivational dysfunction in neuropsychiatric disorders, including MDD.

Many clinical trials still do not include cognitive outcomes as primary measures. A recent meta-analysis of studies investigating the cognitive effects of monoaminergic antidepressants documented the paucity of research in the field (36). Only nine placebo-controlled trials were deemed suitable for inclusion in the meta-analysis. The meta-analysis showed a positive effect of antidepressants on psychomotor speed and delayed recall, although the effect size was small. Heterogeneity was high, consistency between study measures was low, and the study samples varied (elderly versus non-elderly). Another study published after the meta-analysis investigated the cognitive effects of three different antidepressants (venlafaxine, escitalopram, and paroxetine) in a large patient sample (n=712) (37). There were no significant changes in cognitive functions compared to baseline, while most patients' mood symptoms improved. Further longitudinal treatment studies are needed that would include cognitive functions as primary outcomes.

Modafinil as an Add-on Treatment for Cognition and Work-Related Motivation

To date, some experimental studies have investigated potential treatments to address cognition in depression. Review of all treatment studies is beyond the scope of this chapter, but we would like to highlight the example of modafinil based on the studies, some of which were conducted in our laboratory. Modafinil is a wakefulness-promoting agent with established procognitive efficacy in healthy volunteers (38) and in patients with schizophrenia (39), first-episode psychosis (40), and adults with attention deficit hyperactivity disorder (41). In a recent study using CANTAB, we showed that modafinil improved working memory and episodic memory in patients with remitted depression (42). The results are promising and suggest investigating the potential of modafinil further.

Modafinil has other beneficial effects on mood, fatigue, and motivation that may help patients with depression. In a meta-analysis of randomized controlled trials in unipolar and bipolar depression, we showed that modafinil augmentation therapy was associated with improvements in mood and fatigue (43). Modafinil increased task-related motivation while participants performed cognitive tests (38). Those effects may have implications for restoring work-related dysfunction associated with depression. Another report from our group showed that modafinil can mitigate the bias toward negative emotional faces (44).

What Does the Future Hold? Large-Scale Studies, Deep and Frequent Phenotyping

As described earlier, studies with small sample sizes may not be grasping the complexities of cognitive functions in depression. Repeated testing in large samples can help to understand the link between cognitive dysfunction and depression. It can also allow researchers to identify appropriate functional outcome measures.

A preliminary study in a UK Biobank sample of more than 140,000 participants showed an association between history of severe depression and poorer cognitive performance (45). Future studies investigating the temporal stability of cognitive functions and their relationship with depression are warranted. The use of online cognitive testing holds potential for large-scale studies. Self-reported depression that is widely used in large-scale studies is subjective and may not correspond to clinically diagnosed depression. Cohorts with clinician-confirmed diagnostic assessments can provide more reliable information on the link between depression and cognitive functions (46). Prospective cohort studies that incorporate neurocognitive testing can also be valuable (47).

While the evidence on cold cognitive functions in depression is well established, more studies are needed to clarify the role of emotional, social, and reward processing in depression and perhaps help determine possible treatment targets. Reliable and sensitive measures are needed. The EMOTICOM battery consists of neurocognitive tests tapping into behavioural features such as affective processing, reward learning, motivation, and social cognition (48). These domains are frequently affected in depression. The performance in EMOTICOM tests was not dependent on the general intellectual functioning as they showed weak correlations with IQ and education levels. The EMOTICOM battery can be used to assess the hot cognitive functions in patients with depression comprehensively.

Cognitive training of cold cognition may prove of benefit in depression. Using game apps on mobile devices, episodic memory was improved in patients with schizophrenia (49) and in patients with amnestic mild cognitive impairment (50). A possible direction may be to use procognitive medication such as modafinil in combination with game-based cognitive training to produce even greater improvements in episodic memory for depressed patients.

Technological advances allow us to use wearables and smartphones to obtain more detailed cognitive, physical, and subjective measures from people with depression. According to a recent expert opinion panel (35), frequent monitoring of mood, cognition, and other relevant parameters can work as screening tools to identify people with higher risk of poorer functioning associated with depression. Then, clinically depressed patients can be invited to more detailed 'deep phenotyping' evaluations. This approach has already been adopted in some dementia studies (51). In line with the increasing volume of data, machine learning methods and computational modelling will prove beneficial for early detection, assessing treatment efficacy, and monitoring relapse.

References

1. Clark L, Chamberlain SR, Sahakian BJ. Neurocognitive mechanisms in depression: implications for treatment. Annu Rev Neurosci 2009; 32:57–74.

2. Conradi HJ, Ormel J, De Jonge P. Presence of individual (residual) symptoms during depressive episodes and periods of remission: a 3-year prospective study. Psycholog Med 2011;41(6):1165–74.

3. Demyttenaere K, Donneau AF, Albert A, Ansseau M, Constant E, van Heeringen K. What is important in being cured from depression? Discordance between physicians and patients. J Affective Dis 2015;174:390–6.

4. Clark Health Communications. Survey of British adults diagnosed with depression on behalf of Clark Health Communications. 2015 http://www.comres.co.uk/wp-content/uploads/2015/09/Clark-Health-Communications_Cognitive-Dysfunction-in-Depression.pdf

5. Druss BG, Schlesinger M, Allen Jr HM. Depressive symptoms, satisfaction with health care, and 2-year work outcomes in an employed population. Am J Psychiatry 2001;158(5):731–4.

6. Lawrence C, Roy A, Harikrishnan V, Yu S, Dabbous O. Association between severity of depression and self-perceived cognitive difficulties among full-time employees. The Primary Care Companion for CNS Disorders 2013;15(3) pii: PCC.12m01469.

7. Baune BT, Miller R, McAfoose J, Johnson M, Quirk F, Mitchell D. The role of cognitive impairment in general functioning in major depression. Psychiatry Res 2010;176(2):183–9.

8. Beddington J, Cooper CL, Field J, et al. The mental wealth of nations. Nature 2008;455(7216):1057–60.

9. Jaeger J, Berns S, Uzelac S, Davis-Conway S. Neurocognitive deficits and disability in major depressive disorder. Psychiatry Res 2006;145(1):39–48.

10. Godard J, Baruch P, Grondin S, Lafleur MF. Psychosocial and neurocognitive functioning in unipolar and bipolar depression: a 12-month prospective study. Psychiatry Res 2012;196(1):145–53.

11. Zakzanis KK, Leach L, Kaplan E. On the nature and pattern of neurocognitive function in major depressive disorder. Neuropsychiatry, Neuropsychol Behav Neurol 1998;11(3):111–19.

12. Snyder HR. Major depressive disorder is associated with broad impairments on neuropsychological measures of executive function: a meta-analysis and review. Psychol Bull 2013;139(1):81–132.

13. Grant MM, Thase ME, Sweeney JA. Cognitive disturbance in outpatient depressed younger adults: evidence of modest impairment. Biolog Psychiatry 2001; 50(1):35–43.

14. Rock PL, Roiser JP, Riedel WJ, Blackwell AD. Cognitive impairment in depression: a systematic review and meta-analysis. Psychol Med 2014;44(10):2029–40.

15. Gualtieri CT, Morgan DW. The frequency of cognitive impairment in patients with anxiety, depression, and bipolar disorder: an unaccounted source of variance in clinical trials. J Clin Psychiatry 2008;69(7):1122–30.

16. Iverson GL, Brooks BL, Langenecker SA, Young AH. Identifying a cognitive impairment subgroup in adults with mood disorders. J Affective Dis 2011;132(3):360–7.

17. McIntyre RS, Best MW, Bowie CR, et al. The THINC-Integrated Tool (THINC-it) Screening Assessment for Cognitive Dysfunction: validation in patients with major depressive disorder. J Clin Psychiatry 2017;78(7):873–81.

18. Miskowiak KW, Burdick KE, Martinez-Aran A, et al. Methodological recommendations for cognition trials in bipolar disorder by the International Society for Bipolar Disorders Targeting Cognition Task Force. Bipolar Dis 2017; 19(8):614–26.

19. Hasselbalch BJ, Knorr U, Kessing LV. Cognitive impairment in the remitted state of unipolar depressive disorder: a systematic review. J Affective Dis 2011;134(1):20–31.

20. McIntyre RS, Xiao HX, Syeda K, et al. The prevalence, measurement, and treatment of the cognitive dimension/domain in major depressive disorder. CNS Drugs 2015;29(7):577–89.

21. Bora E, Harrison BJ, Yücel M, Pantelis C. Cognitive impairment in euthymic major depressive disorder: a meta-analysis. Psychol Med 2013;43(10):2017–26.

22. Beats BC, Sahakian BJ, Levy R. Cognitive performance in tests sensitive to frontal lobe dysfunction in the elderly depressed. Psychol Med 1996;26(3):591–603.

23. Boeker H, Schulze J, Richter A, Nikisch G, Schuepbach D, Grimm S. Sustained cognitive impairments after clinical recovery of severe depression. J Nervous Mental Disease 2012;200(9):773–6.

24. Elliott R, Sahakian BJ, McKay AP, Herrod JJ, Robbins TW, Paykel ES. Neuropsychological impairments in unipolar depression: the influence of perceived failure on subsequent performance. Psychol Med 1996;26(5):975–89.

25. Harmer CJ, Favaron E, Massey-Chase R, et al. Effect of acute antidepressant administration on negative affective bias in depressed patients. Am J Psychiatry 2009;166:1178–84.

26. Roiser JP, Sahakian BJ. Hot and cold cognition in depression. CNS Spectrums 2013;18(3):139–49.

27. Roiser JP, Elliott R, Sahakian BJ. Cognitive mechanisms of treatment in depression. Neuropsychopharmacology 2012;37(1):117–36.

28. Roiser JP, Sahakian BJ. Information processing in mood disorders. In: RJ DeRubeis and DR Strunk (eds). The Oxford Handbook of Mood Disorders, 2017. Oxford: Oxford University Press. (179–189).

29. Harmer CJ, Shelley NC, Cowen PJ, Goodwin GM. Increased positive versus negative affective perception and memory in healthy volunteers following selective serotonin and norepinephrine reuptake inhibition. Am J Psychiatry 2004;161(7):1256–63.

30. Elliott R, Rubinsztein JS, Sahakian BJ, Dolan RJ. The neural basis of mood-congruent processing biases in depression. Arch Gen Psychiatry 2002;59(7):597–604.

31. Tavares JV, Clark L, Furey ML, Williams GB, Sahakian BJ, Drevets WC. Neural basis of abnormal response to negative feedback in unmedicated mood disorders. Neuroimage 2008;42(3):1118–26.

32. Kaser M, Zaman R, Sahakian BJ. Cognition as a treatment target in depression. Psychol Med 2017;47(6):987–9.

33. McAllister-Williams RH, Bones K, Goodwin GM, et al. Analysing UK clinicians' understanding of cognitive symptoms in major depression: a survey of primary care physicians and psychiatrists. J Affective Dis 2017;207:346–52.

34. Mueller TI, Leon AC, Keller MB, et al. Recurrence after recovery from major depressive disorder during 15 years of observational follow-up. Am J Psychiatry 1999;156(7):1000–6.

35. National Academies of Sciences, Engineering, and Medicine. Enabling Discovery, Development, and Translation of Treatments for Cognitive Dysfunction in Depression: Workshop Summary. Washington, DC: National Academies Press; 2015.

36. Rosenblat JD, Kakar R, McIntyre RS. The cognitive effects of antidepressants in major depressive disorder: a systematic review and meta-analysis of randomized clinical trials. Int J Neuropsychopharmacology 2016;19(2):pii: pyv082.

37. Shilyansky C, Williams LM, Gyurak A, Harris A, Usherwood T, Etkin A. Effect of antidepressant treatment on cognitive impairments associated with depression: a randomised longitudinal study. The Lancet Psychiatry2016;3(5):425–35.

38. Müller U, Rowe JB, Rittman T, Lewis C, Robbins TW, Sahakian BJ. Effects of modafinil on non-verbal cognition, task enjoyment and creative thinking in healthy volunteers. Neuropharmacology 2013;64:490–5.

39. Lees J, Michalopoulou PG, Lewis SW, et al. Modafinil and cognitive enhancement in schizophrenia and healthy volunteers: the effects of test battery in a randomised controlled trial. Psychol Med 2017;47(13):2358–68.

40. Scoriels L, Barnett JH, Soma PK, Sahakian BJ, Jones PB. Effects of modafinil on cognitive functions in first episode psychosis. Psychopharmacology 2012;220(2): 249–58.

41. Turner DC, Clark L, Dowson J, Robbins TW, Sahakian BJ. Modafinil improves cognition and response inhibition in adult attention-deficit/hyperactivity disorder. Biol Psychiatry 2004;55(10):1031–40.

42. Kaser M, Deakin JB, Michael A, et al. Modafinil improves episodic memory and working memory cognition in patients with remitted depression: a double-blind, randomized, placebo-controlled study. Biol Psychiatry: Cognitive Neuroscience Neuroimaging 2017;2(2):115–22.

43. Goss AJ, Kaser M, Costafreda SG, Sahakian BJ, Fu CH. Modafinil augmentation therapy in unipolar and bipolar depression: a systematic review and meta-analysis of randomized controlled trials. J Clin Psychiatry 2013;74(11):1101–7.

44. Kaser M, Bland A, Deakin JB, et al. 1006-Effects of modafinil on emotional processing in patients with remitted depression. Biol Psychiatry 2017;81(10):S407.

45. Cullen B, Nicholl BI, Mackay DF, et al. Cognitive function and lifetime features of depression and bipolar disorder in a large population sample: cross-sectional study of 143,828 UK Biobank participants. Eur Psychiatry 2015;30(8):950–8.

46. Sund R. Quality of the Finnish Hospital Discharge Register: a systematic review. Scand J Public Health 2012;40(6):505–15.

47. Lewis G, Kounali DZ, Button KS, et al. Variation in the recall of socially rewarding information and depressive symptom severity: a prospective cohort study. Acta Psychiatrica Scand 2017;135(5):489–98.

48. Bland AR, Roiser JP, Mehta MA, et al. EMOTICOM: a neuropsychological test battery to evaluate emotion, motivation, impulsivity, and social cognition. Frontiers Behav Neurosci 2016;10:25.

49. Sahakian BJ, Bruhl AB, Cook J, et al. The impact of neuroscience on society: cognitive enhancement in neuropsychiatric disorders and in healthy people. Phil Trans R Soc B 2015;370(1677):20140214.

50. Savulich G, Piercy T, Fox C, et al. Cognitive training using a novel memory game on an iPad in patients with amnestic mild cognitive impairment (aMCI). Int J Neuropsychopharmacol 2017;20(8):624–33.

51. Lawson J, Murray M, Zamboni G, et al. Deep and frequent phenotyping: a feasibility study for experimental medicine in dementia. Alzheimers Dement 2017;13(7):1268–9.

4

Cognitive Dysfunction as a Symptom Dimension Across Major Psychiatric Disorders

Zihang Pan and Roger S. McIntyre

Introduction

Affective mood disorders such as major depressive disorder (MDD) and bipolar disorder (BD) are highly prevalent and disabling illnesses associated with significant morbidity and mortality in affected populations (1). MDD and BD are significant contributors to global functional disability and occupational impairment, affecting approximately 350 million individuals globally, with a lifetime prevalence of up to 15% in the general North American population (2). Affective mood disorders present as syndromes consisting of disturbances in mood, dysregulation of thought patterns, changes in energy and metabolism, and impaired cognition. World Health Organization (WHO) projections identify that affective mood disorders will become the leading cause of disease burden globally by 2030 (3). Estimated economic costs of MDD and BD owing to decreased productivity resulted in losses of at least $32.3 billion in Canada and $201.5 billion in the USA in 2016 alone (4). Cognitive dysfunction has been well established over the past two decades as a core characteristic criterion of MDD and BD. Cognitive deficits have also been proven to be effective predictors of functional impairment in occupational and social domains (5, 6).

Despite advances in pharmacotherapy, a significant proportion of patients with MDD and BD remain symptomatic even after optimal treatment with approved first-line agents. Functional impairment, chronicity, and elevated rates of recurrence contribute to the persistence of affective symptoms and cognitive dysfunction in MDD and BD. Cognitive dysfunction, in particular, seems to be a major symptomatic obstacle to overcome in affective mood disorder treatment and recovery.

Major depressive episodes (MDEs) are characteristic of MDD and depressed BD symptomatology. Cognitive functions (i.e. in the domains of learning and memory, executive function, processing speed, attention, and concentration) may become impaired in patients presenting with a MDE. Both MDD and BD have been conceptualized as neuroprogressive illnesses (7, 8). Cognitive dysfunctions, combined with other progressive clinical observations such as anhedonia and depressed mood, are thought to be key factors subserving disability associated with mood disorders (9). Neuroinflammatory pathways are postulated to play key roles in the pathoaetiology of MDD and BD, contributing to mood- and cognition-related neuroprogressive challenges. There is compelling evidence that proinflammatory cytokines are implicated in cognitive disturbances, and this may offer opportunities to identify targets and biomarkers connecting observed cognitive symptoms in MDD and BD with common neurobiological pathways.

Therefore, it is increasingly relevant to refine our knowledge of cognitive disturbances across major psychiatric illnesses and develop translational tools to effectively prevent, manage, and treat affective mood disorders. This chapter provides an overview of cognitive symptoms across MDD and BD and discusses potential neurobiological substrates contributing to cognitive dysfunction.

Cognitive Deficits in Major Depressive Disorder

A domain-based approach is necessary to determine the roles of complex phenomenological features such as cognition. Disturbances in concentration, executive function, decision-making, and learning and memory are part of the *Diagnostic and Statistical Manual of Mental Disorders*, 5th edition (DSM-5) criterion items that determine cognitive deficits in MDD (10). Disparate neurobiological systems, including, but not limited to, impulsivity, reward, arousal, suicidality, anhedonia, motivation, psychomotor functions, and energy and fatigue, can all contribute towards observed changes in cognition in MDD (11, 12).

Cognitive constructs have been classified and operationalized based on various proposed typologies. These typologies seek to define cognition in a way that is meaningful to clinicians and sensitive to assessments. The conventional typology places cognitive functions into the four subdomains of executive function, learning and memory, attention and concentration, and processing speed (13). These subdomains are interconnected and dissociable phenomena with overlapping, as well as distinct, neurobiological substrates.

Psychopathology of cognitive dysfunction in MDD is subserved by abnormalities in the structure, function, and chemical composition of frontotemporal and frontosubcortical circuitry (14, 15). Nodal structures such as the hippocampus, amygdala, and the anterior cingulate cortex are susceptible to volumetric and functional changes as a consequence of MDD illness severity, frequency, and duration (16). Neurochemical changes in individuals with MDD can also be conceptualized from neurosubstrate abnormalities, implicating monoaminergic and catecholaminergic disturbances as they relate to attention and executive function deficits (17).

Circuits of the orbitofrontal cortex, dorsolateral prefrontal cortex, and anterior cingulate cortex (ACC) are particularly relevant to the pathophysiology of MDD. The dorsal ACC, working in concert with the hippocampus and the dorsolateral prefrontal cortex, contributes to the formation of dorsal 'cognitive' networks, which have been postulated to be of particular importance to the study of executive function deficits (18). Ventral affective networks such as the perigenual ACC, the amygdala, and the orbitofrontal cortex, in conjunction with the hippocampus, may work together to establish cognitively-relevant stimuli and output cognitively-appropriate responses, crucial for planning, working memory, and executive functioning (18).

One of the most recognized abnormalities in individuals with MDD is bilateral reduction of hippocampal volume. Such a reduction can be a consequence of decreased neuronal and dendritic density, and/or reduced size in neuronal soma (19). Indeed, hypofrontality of the prefrontal cortex and associated increases in ACC activity are hypothesized to be the link between cortical and subcortical structures that, when aberrant, lead to decreased functional outcomes (15, 20). These alterations mediate deficits in executive function, attention, learning, memory, and the rate and frequency of information processing.

The distinction of 'cold' and 'hot' cognition is an important one to make in evaluating cognitive dysfunctions in MDD (21). 'Cold' cognition refers to cognition that is uncoupled from emotional valence (e.g. aspects of working memory and executive function). Conversely, 'hot' cognition refers to emotionally-valenced or emotionally-linked cognitive processes. An example of 'hot' cognition is rumination, whereby thoughts and memories informed by emotion play significant roles in the decision-making process (22). Disturbances in either 'hot' or 'cold' cognition, depending on the type of neurochemical or neurocircuitry dysregulation, may lead to divergent presentations of cognitive symptoms in individuals with MDD (i.e. motivational anhedonia, psychomotor retardation, learning, and memory impairments).

Additionally, cognitive impairments in individuals with MDD, whether informed by emotional valence or not, may be due to an increase in neural effort. The n-Back test is a validated measure of working memory, whereby the subject is asked to determine whether previous stimuli have been observed. In one study, performance on the n-Back test did not significantly differ between MDD subjects versus healthy controls; instead, differences were observed in the activation and deactivation of nodal substrates between the MDD and non-MDD groups (23). Specifically, the MDD subjects exhibited greater activation of working memory networks as demonstrated by greater n-Back complexity relative to healthy controls (23). These findings imply that MDD individuals require greater neural effort to achieve the same level of cognitive performance as healthy individuals.

There is also evidence that points to abnormal activity in the medial prefrontal cortex as the neurosubstrate basis of increased neural effort in individuals with MDD (23). Brain functions and their corresponding neurobiological substrates are both integrated and segregated and may rely upon a system of reciprocity between integrated and segregated structures. The selective activation of certain regions and deactivation of others, also known as anticorrelation, is critical for proper cognitive functioning (22). Dysregulation of normal reciprocity between nodal structures within the default mode networks, therefore, may act as a crucial link between substrate disturbances and suboptimal functional outcomes manifested as cognitive impairments and reduced cognitive efficiency (24).

The mediators of aberrant neural circuitry, structure, and function are hypothesized to involve imbalance in hormone regulation (i.e. insulin resistance, glucocorticoid abnormalities), neurotrophin dysregulation (i.e. brain-derived neurotrophic factor), immunoinflammatory activation, and oxidative stress (25–28). The reciprocal relationship between mood and metabolic disorders has been well documented (29). Evidence linking diabetes mellitus type 2 and insulin resistance with cognitive deficits has been previously established (30). An imbalance between insulin and counterregulatory neurohormonal systems (i.e. glucocorticoids) may alter proapoptotic intracellular signalling cascades, which could result in neuronal and glial loss and accelerated neurocognitive decline. In addition, metabolic syndrome and obesity have been consistently established to impact cognitive functions negatively (31).

In summary, the pathoaetiology of cognitive dysfunction in MDD relates both structural and functional disturbances in neural circuits as well as connected cognitive networks. Substrates that subserve cognitive performance in MDD are overlapping as well as discrete, and may involve affective, metabolic, and immunoinflammatory processes. Interventional strategies, therefore, must be informed of these underlying pathophysiological changes subserving cognitive deficits in MDD.

Cognitive Deficits in Bipolar Disorder

Cognitive deficits have been well established as a core characteristic symptom domain of BD and have been increasingly recognized as important predictors of occupational and functional outcomes (5). Like cognition in MDD, cognitive dysfunctions in BD can be mood-dependent and -independent. Indeed, cognitive dysfunction persists during the euthymic state in bipolar individuals (32).

Cognitive dysfunctions in the subdomains of verbal memory, attention and concentration, and executive function have been reported in individuals with BD (32). However, there is still a paucity of studies addressing granular details of cognitive deficits in BD (33). In addition, methodological differences between comparative groups, heterogeneity of bipolar sample populations, and variable disease mood states (e.g. mania, hypomania, euthymia, depression) provide challenges in making overarching conclusions regarding cognition in BD.

Extant literature has suggested an association between cognitive impairments and clinical factors such as the degree of affective symptoms, subtype of BD episodes, and onset characteristics (34). One study found that BD I patients obtained significantly lower scores in psychomotor speed, working memory, verbal learning, delayed memory, and executive functioning compared with healthy controls (35). The same study found that BD II patients also showed significantly decreased functioning in psychomotor speed, working memory, and executive control, but not on verbal learning and delayed memory (35). Other studies supported the idea that bipolar individuals have decreased cognitive performance during euthymic states and that BD II patients have a level of cognitive performance intermediate between BD I and healthy control groups in the domain of verbal memory and executive functions (34, 36).

Immune dysfunction has been proposed as a potential mechanism of cognitive impairment in BD (37). Inflammation has been repeatedly characterized as an agent of change in the pathophysiology of mood disorders (38, 39). Indeed, several inflammatory diseases, such as inflammatory bowel disease, psoriasis, rheumatoid arthritis, autoimmune thyroiditis, obesity, and diabetes mellitus type 2, have all been linked with increased rates of BD (40–42).

Several studies have found an elevation in serum proinflammatory cytokines in individuals with BD during periods of depression, mania, and euthymia (43, 44). Elevated proinflammatory cytokines are indicative of systemic low-grade, chronic, and persistent inflammation. Serum immune mediators, including, but not limited to, tumour necrosis factor-alpha (TNF-α), C-reactive protein, interleukin (IL)-1, IL-6, and various chemokines have been found to be elevated in individuals with BD compared to healthy controls (45). Elevated levels of proinflammatory cytokines in individuals with BD are also associated with poorer cognitive function (46–48). Thus, inflammation provides novel opportunities for the treatment of cognitive dysfunctions presented in BD.

Neurobiological Substrates of Cognition in Major Depressive Disorder and Bipolar Disorder

Specific neurobiological substrate pathways subserving the observed impairment of cognitive function in MDD and BD have not been fully elucidated. The well-established abnormalities in monoamine systems in MDD and BD likely contribute, to some extent, to impaired cellular signalling and neurocircuit deficits

(49). Peripheral inflammation and systemic activation of proinflammatory cytokines provide an alternative explanation for the pathogenesis of cognitive symptoms.

Cytokines from the periphery can enter the central nervous system (CNS) following systemic inflammation via leaky regions in the blood–brain barrier. Regions such as the choroid plexus and circumventricular organs are particularly susceptible to inflammatory cytokine entry (50). Upon entry, endothelial cells and perivascular macrophages in the cerebral vasculature can be activated to produce additional local inflammatory mediators such as prostaglandins, nitric oxides, and chemokines (51). These inflammatory signals lead to a positive feedback of the recruitment and activation of immune cells and further induce local cytokine production (51). Activation of peripheral nerve afferents (i.e. trigeminal and vagus nerves) relays cytokine signals to higher brain regions via the nucleus of the solitary tract and the hypothalamus, thus allowing communication between inflammatory signals and neurocircuitry (52).

TNF-α, a pleiotropic cytokine, is of particular interest because of its role as a mediator of CNS function. Elevated levels of TNF-α, along with IL-1 and IL-6, are among the most consistently identified proinflammatory cytokine abnormalities in MDD and BD (53). The soluble form of TNF-α binds to its corresponding receptors TNF-α receptor 1 (TNFR1) and TNF-α receptor 2 (TNFR2). Ligand-receptor binding leads to the activation of transcription factors such as nuclear factor kappa B (NF-κB) and the initiation of downstream apoptotic cascades via activated caspase-3 and caspase-8 complexes (54). In addition, binding of TNF receptors can result in the production of cytokines and other proinflammatory molecules. Under proinflammatory conditions, peripheral production of TNF-α by monocytes results in activated microglia (55). These activated microglia, in turn, become the primary source of TNF-α in the CNS, leading to a positive feedback that exacerbates the inflammatory process. Furthermore, cross-talk between activated microglia and astrocytes and oligodendrocytes leads to increased reuptake and metabolic conversion of glutamate. High levels of glutamate can increase intracellular calcium levels. Excess calcium can damage neuronal cell structures and promote oxidative stress. The degree and severity of cognitive dysfunction is therefore mediated by the spatial and temporal nature of neurotoxicity and apoptosis (56).

Both peripheral and central inflammation can have profound effects on cell–cell signalling, apoptosis, and brain circuitry (7, 57). Depression, cognitive disturbances, motivational anhedonia, and fatigue have all been well-characterized in populations with inflammatory and metabolic disorders (58). The amplification of inflammatory signals, therefore, provides a convincing hypothesis for the pathogenesis of cognitive symptoms in patients with MDD and BD.

Conclusion

The prevailing disease models identify cognition as a core psychopathological disturbance across multiple psychiatric disorders, including, but not limited to, MDD and BD. Cognition is a principal mediator of psychosocial and workplace function, thus cognitive recovery in individuals with MDD and BD is necessary to achieve optimal remission outcomes. The current clinical paradigm is insufficient in addressing cognitive symptom domains. An inflammatory approach to cognition seems promising. Further steps are necessary to elucidate the involvement of neurosubstrates and inflammatory metabolites in the pathogenesis of cognitive impairments in MDD and BD. The growing interest in the development of domain-based approaches to the assessment and treatment of psychiatric conditions provides a pragmatic impetus for therapeutic discovery. Discourse regarding the identification of cognitive symptoms and strategies to understand its underlying neurobiological mechanisms are important steps in the path toward optimally treating and preventing cognitive symptoms across multiple major psychiatric conditions.

References

1. Fagiolini A, Forgione R, Maccari M, et al. Prevalence, chronicity, burden and borders of bipolar disorder. J Affect Disord 2013;148:161–9.

2. Marcus M, Yasamy MT, Ommeren MV, Chisholm D, Saxena S. Depression: a global public health concern. Retrieved July 22, 2012. https://www.who.int/mental_health/management/depression/who_paper_depression_wfmh_2012.pdf

3. Collins PY, Patel V, Joestl SS, et al. Grand challenges in global mental health. Nature 2011;475:27–30.

4. Cha DS, Carmona NE, Subramaniapillai M, et al. Cognitive impairment as measured by the THINC-integrated tool THINC-it.: association with psychosocial function in major depressive disorder. J Affect Disord 2017;222:14–20.

5. Tse S, Chan S, Ng KL, Yatham LN. *Meta-Analysis of Predictors of Favorable Employment Outcomes Among Individuals With Bipolar Disorder*. Wiley Online Library, 2014. https://www.ncbi.nlm.nih.gov/pubmed/24219657

6. Woo YS, Rosenblat JD, Kakar R, Bahk W-M, McIntyre RS. Cognitive deficits as a mediator of poor occupational function in remitted major depressive disorder patients. Clin Psychopharmacol Neurosci 2016;14:1–16.

7. Rosenblat JD, Brietzke E, Mansur RB, Maruschak NA, Lee Y, McIntyre RS. Inflammation as a neurobiological substrate of cognitive impairment in bipolar disorder: evidence, pathophysiology and treatment implications. J Affect Disord 2015;188:149–59.

8. Pan Z, Grovu RC, Cha DS, et al. Pharmacological treatment of cognitive symptoms in major depressive disorder. CNS Neurol Disord Drug Targets 2017;16:891–9.

9. Carvalho AF, Berk M, Hyphantis TN, McIntyre RS. The integrative management of treatment-resistant depression: a comprehensive review and perspectives. Psychother Psychosom 2014;83:70–88.

10. McIntyre RS, Cha DS, Soczynska JK, et al. Cognitive deficits and functional outcomes in major depressive disorder: determinants, substrates, and treatment interventions. Depress Anxiety 2013;30:515–27.

11. McIntyre RS, Woldeyohannes HO, Soczynska JK, et al. Anhedonia and cognitive function in adults with MDD: results from the International Mood Disorders Collaborative Project. CNS Spectr 2016;21:362–6.

12. McIntyre RS, Xiao HX, Syeda K, et al. The prevalence, measurement, and treatment of the cognitive dimension/domain in major depressive disorder. CNS Drugs 2015;29:577–89.

13. Harrison JE, Lam RW, Baune BT, McIntyre RS. Selection of cognitive tests for trials of therapeutic agents. Lancet Psychiatry 2016;3:499.

14. Jiao Q, Ding J, Lu G, et al. Increased activity imbalance in fronto-subcortical circuits in adolescents with major depression. PLoS One 2011;6:e25159.

15. Pizzagalli DA. Frontocingulate dysfunction in depression: toward biomarkers of treatment response. Neuropsychopharmacology 2011;36:183–206.

16. MacQueen GM, Campbell S, McEwen BS, et al. Course of illness, hippocampal function, and hippocampal volume in major depression. FOC 2005;3:146–55.

17. Stahl SM, Zhang L, Damatarca C, Grady M. Brain circuits determine destiny in depression: a novel approach to the psychopharmacology of wakefulness, fatigue, and executive dysfunction in major depressive disorder. J Clin Psychiatry 2003;64(Suppl 14):6–17.

18. Kheirbek MA, Hen R. Dorsal vs ventral hippocampal neurogenesis: implications for cognition and mood. Neuropsychopharmacology 2011;36:373–4.

19. Malykhin NV, Carter R, Seres P, Coupland NJ. Structural changes in the hippocampus in major depressive disorder: contributions of disease and treatment. J Psychiatry Neurosci 2010;35:337–43.

20. Zeng L-L, Shen H, Liu L, et al. Identifying major depression using whole-brain functional connectivity: a multivariate pattern analysis. Brain 2012;135:1498–507.

21. Roiser JP, Sahakian BJ. Hot and cold cognition in depression. CNS Spectr 2013;18:139–49.

22. Hamilton JP, Furman DJ, Chang C, Thomason ME, Dennis E, Gotlib IH. Default-mode and task-positive network activity in major depressive disorder: implications for adaptive and maladaptive rumination. Biol Psychiatry 2011;70:327–33.

23. Harvey P-O, Fossati P, Pochon J-B, et al. Cognitive control and brain resources in major depression: an fMRI study using the n-back task. Neuroimage 2005;26:860–9.

24. Cha DS, De Michele F, Soczynska JK, et al. The putative impact of metabolic health on default mode network activity and functional connectivity in neuropsychiatric disorders. CNS Neurol Disord Drug Targets 2014;13:1750–8.

25. Li M, Soczynska JK, Kennedy SH. Inflammatory biomarkers in depression: an opportunity for novel therapeutic interventions. Curr Psychiatry Rep 2011;13: 316–20.

26. Ryan JP, Sheu LK, Critchley HD, Gianaros PJ. A neural circuitry linking insulin resistance to depressed mood. Psychosom Med 2012;74:476–82.

27. Andreazza AC. Combining redox-proteomics and epigenomics to explain the involvement of oxidative stress in psychiatric disorders. Mol Biosyst 2012;8:2503–12.

28. McAfoose J, Baune BT. Evidence for a cytokine model of cognitive function. Neurosci Biobehav Rev 2009;33:355–66.

29. McIntyre RS, Rasgon NL, Kemp DE, et al. Metabolic syndrome and major depressive disorder: co-occurrence and pathophysiologic overlap. Curr Diab Rep 2009;9:51–9.

30. Baker LD, Cross DJ, Minoshima S, et al. Insulin resistance and Alzheimer-like reductions in regional cerebral glucose metabolism for cognitively normal adults with prediabetes or early type 2 diabetes. Arch Neurol 2011;68:51–7.

31. Hidese S, Ota M, Matsuo J, et al. Association of obesity with cognitive function and brain structure in patients with major depressive disorder. J Affect Disord 2018;225:188–94.

32. Bourne C, Aydemir Ö, Balanzá-Martínez V, et al. Neuropsychological testing of cognitive impairment in euthymic bipolar disorder: an individual patient data meta-analysis. Acta Psychiatr Scand 2013;128:149–62.

33. Sole B, Martínez-Arán A, Torrent C, Bonnin CM. Are bipolar II patients cognitively impaired? A systematic review. Psycholog Med 2011;41:1791–803.

34. Martínez-Arán A, Vieta E, Reinares M, et al. Cognitive function across manic or hypomanic, depressed, and euthymic states in bipolar disorder. Am J Psychiatry 2004;161:262–70.

35. Dittmann S, Hennig-Fast K, Gerber S, et al. Cognitive functioning in euthymic bipolar I and bipolar II patients. Bipolar Disord 2008;10:877–87.

36. Torrent C, Martínez-Arán A, Daban C, et al. Cognitive impairment in bipolar II disorder. Br J Psychiatry 2006;189:254–9.

37. Barbosa IG, Rocha NP, Huguet RB, et al. Executive dysfunction in euthymic bipolar disorder patients and its association with plasma biomarkers. J Affect Disord 2012;137:151–5.

38. Rosenblat JD, McIntyre RS. Are medical comorbid conditions of bipolar disorder due to immune dysfunction? Acta Psychiatr Scand 2015;132:180–91.

39. Rosenblat JD, Cha DS, Mansur RB, McIntyre RS. Inflamed moods: a review of the interactions between inflammation and mood disorders. Prog Neuropsychopharmacol Biol Psychiatry 2014;53:23–34.

40. Perugi G, Quaranta G, Belletti S, et al. General medical conditions in 347 bipolar disorder patients: clinical correlates of metabolic and autoimmune-allergic diseases. J Affect Disord 2015;170:95–103.

41. Hsu C-C, Chen S-C, Liu C-J, et al. Rheumatoid arthritis and the risk of bipolar disorder: a nationwide population-based study. PLoS One 2014;9:e107512.

42. McIntyre RS, Konarski JZ, Misener VL, Kennedy SH. Bipolar disorder and diabetes mellitus: epidemiology, etiology, and treatment implications. Ann Clin Psychiatry 2005;17:83–93.

43. Brietzke E, Stertz L, Fernandes BS, et al. Comparison of cytokine levels in depressed, manic and euthymic patients with bipolar disorder. J Affect Disord 2009;116:214–17.

44. Barbosa IG, Machado-Vieira R, Soares JC, Teixeira AL. The immunology of bipolar disorder. Neuroimmunomodulation 2014;21:117–22.

45. Barbosa IG, Bauer ME, Machado-Vieira R, Teixeira AL. Cytokines in bipolar disorder: paving the way for neuroprogression. Neural Plast 2014;2014:360481.

46. Dickerson F, Stallings C, Origoni A, et al. C-reactive protein is elevated in schizophrenia. Schizophr Res 2013;143:198–202.

47. Doganavsargil-Baysal O, Cinemre B, Aksoy UM, et al. Levels of TNF-α, soluble TNF receptors sTNFR1, sTNFR2, and cognition in bipolar disorder. Hum Psychopharmacol 2013;28:160–7.

48. Hope S, Hoseth E, Dieset I, et al. Inflammatory markers are associated with general cognitive abilities in schizophrenia and bipolar disorder patients and healthy controls. Schizophr Res 2015;165:188–94.

49. Stahl SM. Enhancing outcomes from major depression: using antidepressant combination therapies with multifunctional pharmacologic mechanisms from the initiation of treatment. CNS Spectr 2010;15:79–94.

50. Pan W, Kastin AJ. Interactions of cytokines with the blood–brain barrier: implications for feeding. Curr Pharm Des 2003;9:827–31.

51. Rosenblat JD, McIntyre RS. Bipolar disorder and immune dysfunction: epidemiological findings, proposed pathophysiology and clinical implications. Brain Sci 2017;7:pii: E144.

52. Ericsson A, Kovács KJ, Sawchenko PE. A functional anatomical analysis of central pathways subserving the effects of interleukin-1 on stress-related neuroendocrine neurons. J Neurosci 1994;14:897–913.

53. Clark IA, Alleva LM, Vissel B. The roles of TNF in brain dysfunction and disease. Pharmacol Ther 2010;128:519–48.

54. Tracey D, Klareskog L, Sasso EH, Salfeld JG, Tak PP. Tumor necrosis factor antagonist mechanisms of action: a comprehensive review. Pharmacol Ther 2008;117:244–79.

55. Qin L, Wu X, Block ML, et al. Systemic LPS causes chronic neuroinflammation and progressive neurodegeneration. Glia 2007;55:453–62.

56. Bortolato B, Carvalho AF, Soczynska JK, Perini GI, McIntyre RS. The involvement of TNF-α in cognitive dysfunction associated with major depressive disorder: an opportunity for domain specific treatments. Curr Neuropharmacol 2015;13:558–76.

57. Pan Z, Rosenblat JD, Swardfager W, McIntyre RS. Role of proinflammatory cytokines in dopaminergic system disturbances, implications for anhedonic features of MDD. Curr Pharm Des 2017;23:2065–72.

58. Lam RW, Kennedy SH, McIntyre RS, Khullar A. Cognitive dysfunction in major depressive disorder: effects on psychosocial functioning and implications for treatment. Can J Psychiatry 2014;59:649–54.

5

Clinical and Functional Characteristics of Cognitive Dysfunction in Major Depressive Disorder

Maria Serra-Blasco and Raymond W. Lam

Introduction

Major depressive disorder (MDD) has a global prevalence rate of 4.7% (1), affecting more than 300 million people around the world. According to the World Health Organization, MDD is the leading contributor to disease burden worldwide, representing 7.5% of all years lived with a disability (2). As with other chronic illnesses, MDD is associated with high personal, economic, and societal costs (3). MDD is often a chronic condition. After a first depressive episode, an individual with MDD has a 50% probability of experiencing a relapse of symptoms in the future, and this risk of relapse increases with every subsequent depressive episode. In addition, a high percentage of patients do not respond to available treatments for MDD, and even those who do improve might have residual, subclinical symptoms that hamper full recovery.

Cognitive dysfunction is well recognized as a cardinal symptom in MDD that critically affects everyday functioning (4). Cognitive dysfunction may include specific problems in thinking, concentrating, speaking, retaining information, or organizing tasks and activities. Such impairments impede complete recovery from MDD and a return to pre-illness daily functioning. On a conceptual level, cognitive dysfunction can be characterized both subjectively, according to ratings and self-reports by patients with MDD, and objectively, as measured by psychometric testing. In patients with MDD, subjective cognitive complaints are generally poorly correlated with objective measurements of cognitive functioning (5). As a result, individual reports of subjective cognitive dysfunction might be because of factors other than genuine neuropsychological deficits, although those possible factors are beyond the scope of this chapter.

More generally, people with MDD who experience cognitive difficulties tend to have poorer functional outcomes overall (6). Cognitive impairments can also persist despite improvement of mood after treatment (7). Patients with MDD who have persistent cognitive deficits after treatment are less likely to remit and more likely to relapse into depression (8). In this chapter, we will discuss the bidirectional relationships between cognitive dysfunction and clinical characteristics and functional outcomes in MDD, and update recent findings regarding cognitive impairment, functioning, and implications for treatment.

Clinical Characteristics and Cognitive Dysfunction

As with depressive symptomatology, people with MDD do not experience or display neuropsychological deficits as homogeneous phenomena. The presence and extent of cognitive impairments may differ significantly owing to the clinical manifestation of MDD and a person's individual characteristics. For example, the age of first onset of MDD can have significant clinical and cognitive implications: earlier onset of MDD is associated with a more severe course of illness (9), perhaps because of longer exposure to the known neurotoxic effects of MDD (10). In addition, patients with earlier-onset MDD typically experience worse psychosocial adjustment earlier in life (9, 11) and are more likely to have comorbid psychiatric conditions (12). In contrast, patients with late-onset MDD are more likely to have medical comorbidities and to experience psychotic symptoms that can be less responsive to antidepressant medication (13). Although the vast majority of literature points toward greater cognitive deficits (and especially executive dysfunction) in late-onset depression (14), a recent meta-analysis found no direct effect of age at onset of depression on cognitive function (15). However, such disparate findings may be partly due to differing criteria for defining 'early' versus 'late' onset, and to lack of differentiation between late-onset and late-life depression (16), owing in part to lack of clinical consensus in defining these subgroups.

Cognitive dysfunction appears to be more pronounced in elderly patients with MDD, who demonstrate problems with visuoperception, verbal learning, memory, and motor speed (17). These deficits are not due to ageing alone and may persist for up to 4 years despite effective antidepressant treatment. Many studies have suggested that cognitive impairment observed in late-life is more of a 'trait' than a 'state' and might reflect temporal lobe dysfunction caused by chronic disease rather than progressive dementia (16, 18). Nonetheless, older patients with MDD are also more likely to develop dementia, and in such cases depression-associated cognitive dysfunction is potentially a prodrome (19).

The impact of gender on cognitive impairment remains unclear. Although gender is associated with strong effects on brain structure, neurocognitive function, and neurochemistry (20), such differences appear to be weakly related to cognitive dysfunction or restricted to impairments in certain domains only. As an example, men show stronger performance in tasks involving spatial reasoning (21) whereas women score higher in verbal tasks (22). However, some gender effects on cognition have been attributed to interactions with personality traits; for example, greater visuospatial working memory spans in men (23) have been theorized as a possible result of gender differences in spatial-orientation skills combined with protective factors such as low neuroticism and high internal locus of control. Overall, however, there is no strong evidence for gender differences in cognitive domains, whether first-level (e.g. memory and attention) or second-level (e.g. executive functioning), or involving interactions with depressive symptomatology.

Cognition is significantly affected by the illness burden of MDD, as characterized by the number of previous depressive episodes, the total duration of illness (as measured by the time between the onset of the first episode and the assessment date), and the severity of the symptoms. In one of the first studies of the relationship between illness burden and cognitive performance, Basso et al. (24) found that memory impairments were not present in patients experiencing their first episode of MDD, compared to patients with recurrent depression, but other cognitive domains were similarly affected. A decade later, Gorwood et al. (25) found that, in a larger sample of depressed outpatients, memory performance was most strongly related to symptom severity during the intake assessment, but more strongly related to previous history of MDD when patients returned for a second assessment. By the time patients experienced a third depressive episode, coinciding with the timeframe when the risk of relapse substantially increases, significant memory deficits were observed (26). In studies by Preiss et al. (27), the number of previous depressive episodes was notably high in euthymic patients who reported memory deficits, suggesting that subsequent depressive episodes might have negative, cumulative effects on certain cognitive domains. It is important to note, however, that cognitive dysfunction is found even in samples of patients with first-episode MDD (28).

The subtype of MDD also affects cognitive functioning. Patients with melancholic depression display extensive cognitive impairments compared to patients with MDD without melancholic features (29, 30). Such deficits appear to be independent of age, gender, and severity of depressive symptoms. An underlying deficit in mesolimbic-cortical circuitry has been hypothesized as a possible reason for the differential performance of depressed patients with melancholic features, given that such patients have shown a relative lack of motivationally directed behaviour, compared to non-melancholic depressed patients (31).

Some studies have suggested that neuropsychological profiles in psychotic depression may be similar to those in schizophrenia. Consequently, cognitive deficits in patients with MDD with psychotic features are more severe than in those without psychosis (13, 32). Psychotic depression is associated with cognitive deficits in a broad range of domains (33), including sustained attention and response inhibition, verbal declarative memory, verbal working memory, attention shifting, and inhibition. However, patients with psychotic depression have demonstrated intact performance on forward digit-span and verbal fluency tests (34). Therefore, while there is strong evidence that MDD with psychotic depression is associated with profound cognitive deficits (30), further research is needed to determine which specific tasks or domains are consistently impaired.

The severity of depressive symptoms is also positively correlated with cognitive dysfunction. Patients with more severe symptoms of MDD experience stronger negative cognitive biases (35) and more serious impairments in memory, attention, executive functioning, and processing speed (36, 37). More generally, memory and other cognitive capacities involving information-retention appear to be only modestly correlated with symptom severity, and the directional relationship (if any) is not known.

Functional Outcomes and Cognitive Dysfunction

Impairments in daily functioning are among the most common consequences of MDD; they may occur globally or in specific areas, such as one's ability to work, maintain a household, manage one's finances, sustain relationships, or participate in a community. *The Diagnostic and Statistical Manual of Mental Disorders*, 5th edition (DSM-5) requires that symptoms cause significant distress or severely disrupt social or occupational functioning for a diagnosis of MDD (38). However, functional outcomes are not studied comprehensively and treatment trials for MDD rarely include them as primary or even secondary outcomes (39). Rather, treatment efficacy is typically determined by changes in symptom rating scales (most of which include, at most, a single item assessing cognition), with response and remission defined by threshold change and threshold severity of symptoms. However, functional improvement and recovery often does not parallel symptom recovery. The importance of full functional recovery was noted in a STAR*D report in which patients who achieved symptom remission but still had functional impairment after 12 weeks of citalopram treatment had significantly greater odds of relapse at both 6-month and 1-year follow-up than patients with both symptom and functional remission (40).

Cognition is vitally important for everyday functioning. Cognitive dysfunction can disrupt routine and even mundane activities, such as listening or speaking during conversations, performing multistep tasks, or coping with new situations. Deficits in attention and executive functioning can make everyday life even more challenging for depressed patients who are already struggling with apathy, low motivation, or fatigue. Difficulties in planning one's day, organizing one's time, prioritizing/sequencing actions, multitasking, and inhibiting unwanted habits can all significantly interfere with recovery from MDD. Memory deficits could have severe practical consequences for people with MDD if one forgets to take prescribed medications or attend clinical appointments, or if recall of important events and conversations is impaired.

Despite the importance of cognition for functioning, few studies have examined the relationship between cognitive dysfunction and functional outcomes in people with MDD. Only one systematic review has examined studies of cognitive performance and daily functioning in adults with MDD (41). This review highlighted the limited evidence, as only 10 studies were identified that focused on effects of neurocognitive deficits on psychosocial functioning. The results showed that individuals with MDD reported neurocognitive deficits in at least one cognitive domain and that functional impairments in MDD were broadly associated with deficits in executive functioning, attention, psychomotor speed, and certain aspects of memory. However, many of the studies reviewed had significant methodological limitations, including lack of follow-up evaluations, confounding effects of depression severity, and conclusions based only on correlational analyses.

Occupational performance is a particularly important aspect of psychosocial functioning. Many studies show that MDD is associated with pernicious and costly burdens to society owing to increased absenteeism from work and increased presenteeism (that is, attending work but being less productive because of illness-related factors), the latter being more difficult to detect and quantify (42).

Cognitive dysfunction significantly impairs occupational functioning in people still working while depressed. For example, a survey of employed patients with MDD found that 78% of the sample were bothered by poor concentration more than half the time; these patients had high rates of self-reported work impairment, including getting less work done, doing poor-quality work, making more mistakes, and having trouble with work relationships (Figure 5.1).

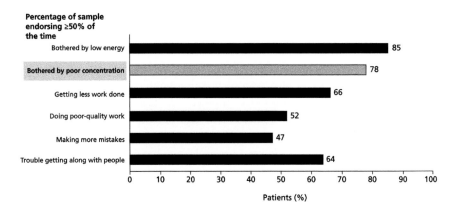

Figure 5.1 Self-reported symptoms and work impairment (based on LEAPS, Lam Employment Absence and Productivity Scale) in a clinic sample of employed patients with MDD (n=297).

Typically, depression-associated cognitive dysfunction disrupts occupational functioning independent of other symptoms. In a sample of employed people with MDD, variability in workplace impairment was attributable to cognitive difficulties experienced subjectively by workers, independent of the severity of depressive symptoms (43). Similarly, in a Korean study of workers with MDD, those with more severe subjective cognitive complaints had higher rates of presenteeism and greater overall work productivity loss, regardless of depression severity (44).

Residual cognitive deficits after treatment for depression (see section on 'Impact of Cognitive Dysfunction for Depression Outcomes and Treatment', below) may continue to impair work functioning and impede return to work. In a survey of workers returning to work after a depression-related absence, 66% of the workers self-reported problems with concentration, memory, or making decisions; however, supervisors reported that 76–86% of workers had these cognitive difficulties (45).

Impact of Cognitive Dysfunction for Depression Outcomes and Treatment

Specific cognitive impairments might also be associated with poor treatment response and with future relapse or recurrence of depressive symptoms. Kalayam and Alexopoulos (46) found that, in a sample of elderly patients with MDD, executive deficits predicted a poor clinical response to antidepressant treatment. Their findings were replicated in a larger sample (47) and demonstrated that markers of executive dysfunction, such as perseveration or disinhibition, increased the risk of poor response to treatment with citalopram. In addition, Dunkin and colleagues (48) found that non-response to fluoxetine could be predicted by performance on tests of executive function, specifically, the number of correct categorical responses on the Wisconsin Card Sorting Test and the number of errors in the interference condition of the Stroop Test.

Executive dysfunction is also associated with a poorer prognosis, not only in young adults (49) but also in geriatric populations. Studies using the Dementia Rating Scale showed that low initiation and high perseveration may predict relapse or recurrence of depressive episodes 2 years later (50). In addition, poor performance on divided-attention tasks may also predict the long-term course of MDD (51) as well as a delayed return to work for people who have sustained severe head trauma (52).

De Raedt and Koster (53) proposed a model to understand attentional biases as critical features that increase the risk of relapse after a depressive episode. Their model postulates that reduced cortical activity in MDD interacts with depressogenic schemes (54) and leads to impairment in exertion of attentional inhibitory control; this, in turn, would interfere with one's ability to disconnect from negative repetitive thoughts, such as ruminations or other unwanted information or ideas.

Cognitive deficits in many cognitive domains can also persist even when other depressive symptoms remit, as shown in several meta-analyses (55, 56). For example, attention and executive functioning remain moderately affected even with symptom remission and are considered more stable traits of a depression phenotype; in contrast, memory is not always significantly impaired in patients with remitted MDD (57). Moreover, there is some evidence that memory improves with amelioration of depressive symptoms, possibly because of other non-specific mechanisms of action derived through various therapeutic strategies.

More recent studies have examined the specific cognitive effects of therapeutic strategies for MDD, including interventions that target cognition directly (such as cognitive remediation) or indirectly (such as pharmacotherapy, aerobic exercise, and others) (58). Cognition-focused techniques such as cognitive remediation have been associated with significant improvements in neuropsychological test performance in patients with MDD. Porter et al. (59), in a sample of patients with treatment-resistant depression, found that amelioration of cognitive difficulties with cognitive remediation predicted improvements in other functional domains in which performance was previously impaired. Harvey et al. (60) augmented cognitive therapy with memory-enhancement training, with results showing improvements in not only memory but also in global functioning, especially in patients without a college education. Oertel-Knöchel et al. (61) conducted a similar study but augmented cognitive therapy with aerobic exercise, which has been shown to enhance neurocognition (62); the combined intervention had beneficial effects on cognition (visual learning, working memory, and processing speed) and subjectively rated quality of life in patients with MDD and schizophrenia.

Pharmacotherapy for MDD can also effectively target cognitive dysfunction in addition to mood symptoms, with some antidepressants showing more evidence for cognition effects than others (63). For example, the multimodal antidepressant vortioxetine is associated with both objective and subjective improvement in cognition relative to placebo (64). These effects were mediated through a direct effect on cognition rather than an indirect effect through improvement in mood. Improving cognition can also translate into improved functioning; vortioxetine significantly improved both general cognitive measures as well as functional performance tests (Figure 5.2) compared to placebo, but duloxetine did not (65). In another study of employed patients with MDD treated with desvenlafaxine, those patients who had clinically significant improvement in cognition also had significantly better clinical and work functioning outcomes, compared to patients who did not experience cognitive improvement (66) (Figure 5.3).

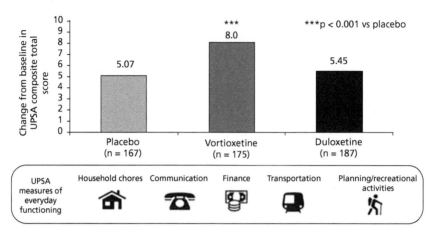

Figure 5.2 Effects of vortioxetine, duloxetine, and placebo on the University of California San Diego Performance-based Skills Assessment (UPSA).

Adapted from *Neuropsychopharmacology,* 40, 8, Mahableshwarkar AR, Zajecka J, Jacobson W, Chen Y, Keefe RS, A randomized, placebo-controlled, active-reference, double-blind, flexible-dose study of the efficacy of vortioxetine on cognitive function in major depressive disorder, pp. 2025–37, 2015. Reproduced under the terms of the Creative Commons Attribution 4.0 International (CC BY 4.0) license. (https://creativecommons.org/licenses/by/4.0/)

Clinical Implications and Conclusions

MDD is a heterogeneous condition, but most affected patients experience cognitive dysfunction regardless of clinical symptoms or characteristics. Problems with attention, memory, and executive function are among the most common cognitive difficulties. Cognitive dysfunction may contribute to or worsen the disease burden and pose potentially severe obstacles to both clinical and functional recovery. Factors that predict cognitive dysfunction and extent of impairment can include older age, early or late onset of MDD, number of previous depressive episodes (especially three or more), melancholic or psychotic features in MDD, and severity of depressive symptoms. Cognitive deficits may persist as residual symptoms, even when other depressive symptoms are remitted, and can impair full occupational and functional recovery.

Given the importance of cognition for optimal psychosocial functioning, clinicians and researchers are advised to expand the focus of treatment for MDD by prioritizing cognitive dysfunction and its effects on other functional outcomes. Specific steps could include screening for and assessing cognitive dysfunction using both subjective (self-rated) and objective (neuropsychological tests) measures (67); assessing global and specific functional impairments using standardized rating scales (39); identifying and implementing treatment strategies that target cognitive deficits, either in themselves or in association with other depressive symptoms (68); and continuous monitoring of cognition, mood symptoms, and functional outcomes throughout the course of treatment (4).

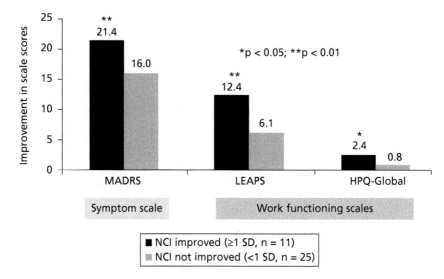

Figure 5.3 Symptom and work functioning outcomes after 8 weeks of treatment with desvenlafaxine in employed patients with MDD with and without significant cognitive improvement (defined as ≥1 standard deviation improvement on a composite score from the CNS-Vital Signs cognitive test battery). MADRS, Montgomery and Asberg Depression Rating Scale; NCI, Neurocognitive Index (composite score from CNS Vital Signs neuropsychological test battery); SD, standard deviation; LEAPS, Lam Employment Absence and Productivity Scale; HPQ-Global, Health and Work Performance Questionnaire-Global Improvement.

Adapted from *Journal of Affective Disorders*, 203, Lam RW, Iverson GL, Evans VC et al. The effects of desvenlafaxine on neurocognitive and work functioning in employed outpatients with major depressive disorder, pp. 55–61. © 2016 Elsevier B.V. All rights reserved.

Investigators planning cognition studies in MDD should also consider common methodological issues, such as heterogeneity in the clinical sample, how cognitive impairment is defined within entry criteria for clinical trials of MDD targeting cognition, and tracking both clinical response and functional outcomes (69). In addition, comparable data from a matched, healthy comparison sample would allow for more rigorous statistical analyses, including controlling for 'cognitive reserve', which includes important variables such as years of education and baseline intellectual ability (70).

References

1. Ferrari AJ, Somerville AJ, Baxter AJ, et al. Global variation in the prevalence and incidence of major depressive disorder: a systematic review of the epidemiological literature. Psychol Med 2013;43(3):471–81.

2. World Health Organization. Depression [Fact sheet; Updated February 2017]. http://www.who.int/mediacentre/factsheets/fs369/en/. Last accessed 14 February 2018.

3. Fineberg NA, Haddad PM, Carpenter L, et al. The size, burden and cost of disorders of the brain in the UK. J Psychopharmacol 2013;27(9):761–70.

4. Lam RW, Kennedy SH, McIntyre RS, Khullar A. Cognitive dysfunction in major depressive disorder: effects on psychosocial functioning and implications for treatment. Can J Psychiatry 2014;59:649–54.

5. Mohn C, Rund BR. Neurocognitive profile in major depressive disorders: relationship to symptom level and subjective memory complaints. BMC Psychiatry 2016;16:108.

6. McCall WV, Dunn AG. Cognitive deficits are associated with functional impairment in severely depressed patients. Psychiatry Res 2003;121(2):179–84.

7. Roca M, Monzón S, Vives M, et al. Cognitive function after clinical remission in patients with melancholic and non-melancholic depression: a 6-month follow-up study. J Affect Disord 2015;171:85–92.

8. Papakostas GI. Cognitive symptoms in patients with major depressive disorder and their implications for clinical practice. J Clin Psychiatry 2014;75(1):8–14.

9. Riddle M, Potter GG, McQuoid DR, Steffens DC, Beyer JL, Taylor WD. Longitudinal cognitive outcomes of clinical phenotypes of late-life depression. Am J Geriatr Psychiatry 2017;25(10):1123–34.

10. Moylan S, Maes M, Wray NR, Berk M. The neuroprogressive nature of major depressive disorder: pathways to disease evolution and resistance, and therapeutic implications. Mol Psychiatry 2013;18(5):595–606.

11. Zisook S, Lesser I, Stewart JW, et al. Effect of age at onset on the course of major depressive disorder. Am J Psychiatry 2007;164(10):1539–46.

12. Baune BT, McAfoose J, Leach G, Quirk F, Mitchell D. Impact of psychiatric and medical comorbidity on cognitive function in depression. Psychiatry Clin Neurosci 2009;63(3):392–400.

13. Schatzberg AF, Posener JA, DeBattista C, Kalehzan BM, Rothschild AJ, Shear PK. Neuropsychological deficits in psychotic versus nonpsychotic major depression and no mental illness. Am J Psychiatry 2000;157(7):1095–100.

14. Pimontel MA, Rindskopf D, Rutherford BR, Brown PJ, Roose SP, Sneed JR. A meta-analysis of executive dysfunction and antidepressant treatment response in late-life depression. Am J Geriatr Psychiatry 2016;24(1):31–41.

15. Disabato BM, Morris C, Hranilovich J, et al. Comparison of brain structural variables, neuropsychological factors, and treatment outcome in early-onset versus late-onset late-life depression. Am J Geriatr Psychiatry 2014;22(10):1039–46.

16. Köhler S, Thomas AJ, Barnett NA, O'Brien JT. The pattern and course of cognitive impairment in late-life depression. Psychol Med 2010;40(4):591–602.

17. Thomas AJ, Gallagher P, Robinson LJ, et al. A comparison of neurocognitive impairment in younger and older adults with major depression. Psychol Med 2009;39(5):725–33.

18. Portella MJ, Marcos T, Rami L, Navarro V, Gastó C, Salamero M. Residual cognitive impairment in late-life depression after a 12-month period follow-up. Int J Geriatr Psychiatry 2003;18(7):571–6.

19. Modrego PJ, Ferrández J. Depression in patients with mild cognitive impairment increases the risk of developing dementia of Alzheimer type: a prospective cohort study. Arch Neurol 2004;61(8):1290–3.

20. Cosgrove KP, Mazure CM, Staley JK. Evolving knowledge of sex differences in brain structure, function, and chemistry. Biol Psychiatry 2007;62(8):847–55.

21. Geary DC, Saults SJ, Liu F, Hoard MK. Sex differences in spatial cognition, computational fluency, and arithmetical reasoning. J Exp Child Psychol 2000;77(4): 337–53.

22. Speck O, Ernst T, Braun J, Koch C, Miller E, Chang L. Gender differences in the functional organization of the brain for working memory. Neuroreport 2000;11(11):2581–5.

23. Coluccia E, Louse G. Gender differences in spatial orientation: a review. J Environ Psychol 2004;24(3):329–40.

24. Basso MR, Bornstein RA. Relative memory deficits in recurrent versus first-episode major depression on a word-list learning task. Neuropsychology 1999;13(4):557–63.

25. Gorwood P, Corruble E, Falissard B, Goodwin GM. Toxic effects of depression on brain function: impairment of delayed recall and the cumulative length of depressive disorder in a large sample of depressed outpatients. Am J Psychiatry 2008;165(6):731–9.

26. Keller MB, Boland RJ. Implications of failing to achieve successful long-term maintenance treatment of recurrent unipolar major depression. Biol Psychiatry 1998;44(5):348–60.

27. Preiss M, Kucerova H, Lukavsky J, Stepankova H, Sos P, Kawaciukova R. Cognitive deficits in the euthymic phase of unipolar depression. Psychiatry Res 2009;169(3):235–9.

28. Ahern E, Semkovska M. Cognitive functioning in the first episode of major depressive disorder: a systematic review and meta-analysis. Neuropsychology 2017; 31:52–72.

29. Bosaipo NB, Foss MP, Young AH, Juruena MF. Neuropsychological changes in melancholic and atypical depression: a systematic review. Neurosci Biobehav Rev 2017;73:309–25.

30. Zaninotto L, Solmi M, Veronese N, et al. A meta-analysis of cognitive performance in melancholic versus non-melancholic unipolar depression. J Affect Disord 2016;201:15–24.

31. Day CV, Gatt JM, Etkin A, DeBattista C, Schatzberg AF, Williams LM. Cognitive and emotional biomarkers of melancholic depression: an iSPOT-D report. J Affect Disord 2015;176:141–50.

32. Gomez RG, Fleming SH, Keller J, et al. The neuropsychological profile of psychotic major depression and its relation to cortisol. Biol Psychiatry 2006;60(5):472–8.

33. Hill SK, Keshavan MS, Thase ME, Sweeney JA. Neuropsychological dysfunction in antipsychotic-naive first-episode unipolar psychotic depression. Am J Psychiatry 2004;161(6):996–1003.

34. Basso MR, Bornstein RA. Neuropsychological deficits in psychotic versus nonpsychotic unipolar depression. Neuropsychology 1999;13(1):69–75.

35. Dohr KB, Rush AJ, Bernstein IH. Cognitive biases and depression. J Abnorm Psychol 1989;98(3):263–7.

36. Snyder HR. Major depressive disorder is associated with broad impairments on neuropsychological measures of executive function: a meta-analysis and review. Psychol Bull 2013;139(1):81–132.

37. McDermott LM, Ebmeier KP. A meta-analysis of depression severity and cognitive function. J Affect Disord 2009;119(1–3):1–8.

38. American Psychiatric Association. Diagnostic and Statistical Manual of Mental Disorders. Fifth edition. Arlington, VA: American Psychiatric Publishing, 2013.

39. Lam RW, Parikh SV, Michalak EE, Dewa CS, Kennedy SH. Canadian Network for Mood and Anxiety Treatments (CANMAT) consensus recommendations for functional outcomes in major depressive disorder. Ann Clin Psychiatry 2015;27:142–9.

40. IsHak WW, Greenberg JM, Cohen RM. Predicting relapse in major depressive disorder using patient-reported outcomes of depressive symptom severity, functioning, and quality of life in the individual burden of illness index for depression (IBI-D). J Affect Disord 2013;151:59–65.

41. Evans VC, Iverson GL, Yatham LN, Lam RW. The relationship between neurocognitive and psychosocial functioning in major depressive disorder: a systematic review. J Clin Psychiatry 2014;75(12):1359–70.

42. Stewart WF, Ricci JA, Chee E, Hahn SR, Morganstein D. Cost of lost productive work time among US workers with depression. JAMA 2003;289(23):3135–44.

43. McIntyre RS, Soczynska JZ, Woldeyohannes HO, et al. The impact of cognitive impairment on perceived workforce performance: results from the International Mood Disorders Collaborative Project. Compr Psychiatry 2015;56:279–82.

44. Kim JM, Chalem Y, di Nicola S, Hong JP, Won SH, Milea D. A cross-sectional study of functional disabilities and perceived cognitive dysfunction in patients with major depressive disorder in South Korea: the PERFORM-K study. Psychiatry Res 2016;239:353–61.

45. Chenier L. Depression in the Workplace. Ottawa: Conference Board of Canada, 2013.

46. Kalayam B, Alexopoulos GS. Prefrontal dysfunction and treatment response in geriatric depression. Arch Gen Psychiatry 1999;56(8):713–18.

47. Alexopoulos GS, Kiosses DN, Heo M, Murphy CF, Shanmugham B, Gunning-Dixon F. Executive dysfunction and the course of geriatric depression. Biol Psychiatry 2005;58(3):204–10.

48. Dunkin JJ, Leuchter AF, Cook IA, Kasl-Godley JE, Abrams M, Rosenberg-Thompson S. Executive dysfunction predicts nonresponse to fluoxetine in major depression. J Affect Disord 2000;60(1):13–23.

49. Withall A, Harris LM, Cumming SR. The relationship between cognitive function and clinical and functional outcomes in major depressive disorder. Psychol Med 2009;39(3):393–402.

50. Alexopoulos GS, Meyers BS, Young RC, et al. Executive dysfunction and long-term outcomes of geriatric depression. Arch Gen Psychiatry 2000;57(3):285–90.

51. Majer M, Ising M, Künzel H, et al. Impaired divided attention predicts delayed response and risk to relapse in subjects with depressive disorders. Psychol Med 2004;34(8):1453–63.

52. van Zomeren AH, van den Burg W. Residual complaints of patients two years after severe head injury. J Neurol Neurosurg Psychiatry 1985;48(1):21–8.

53. De Raedt R, Koster EH. Understanding vulnerability for depression from a cognitive neuroscience perspective: a reappraisal of attentional factors and a new conceptual framework. Cogn Affect Behav Neurosci 2010;10(1):50–70.

54. Beck AT. The evolution of the cognitive model of depression and its neurobiological correlates. Am J Psychiatry 2008;165(8):969–77.

55. Rock PL, Roiser JP, Riedel WJ, Blackwell AD. Cognitive impairment in depression: a systematic review and meta-analysis. Psychol Med 2014;44(10):2029–40.

56. Hasselbalch BJ, Knorr U, Kessing LV. Cognitive impairment in the remitted state of unipolar depressive disorder: a systematic review. J Affect Disord 2011;134(1–3):20–31.

57. Nilsson J, Thomas AJ, Stevens LH, McAllister-Williams RH, Ferrier IN, Gallagher P. The interrelationship between attentional and executive deficits in major depressive disorder. Acta Psychiatr Scand 2016;134(1):73–82.

58. Martínez-Arán A, Torrent C, Solé B, et al. Functional remediation for bipolar disorder. Clin Pract Epidemiol Ment Health 2011;7:112–16.

59. Porter RJ, Bowie CR, Jordan J, Malhi GS. Cognitive remediation as a treatment for major depression: a rationale, review of evidence and recommendations for future research. Aust N Z J Psychiatry 2013;47(12):1165–75.

60. Harvey AG, Lee J, Smith RL, et al. Improving outcome for mental disorders by enhancing memory for treatment. Behav Res Ther 2016;81:35–46.

61. Oertel-Knöchel V, Mehler P, Thiel C, et al. Effects of aerobic exercise on cognitive performance and individual psychopathology in depressive and schizophrenia patients. Eur Arch Psychiatry Clin Neurosci 2014;264(7):589–604.

62. Smith PJ, Blumenthal JA, Hoffman BM, et al. Aerobic exercise and neurocognitive performance: a meta-analytic review of randomized controlled trials. Psychosom Med 2010;72(3):239–52.

63. Rosenblat JD, Kakar R, McIntyre RS. The cognitive effects of antidepressants in major depressive disorder: a systematic review and meta-analysis of randomized clinical trials. Int J Neuropsychopharmacol 2015;19:pii:pyv082.

64. McIntyre RS, Harrison J, Loft H, Jacobson W, Olsen CK. The effects of vortioxetine on cognitive function in patients with major depressive disorder: a meta-analysis of three randomized controlled trials. Int J Neuropsychopharmacol 2016;pii:pyw055.

65. Mahableshwarkar AR, Zajecka J, Jacobson W, Chen Y, Keefe RS. A random-ized, placebo-controlled, active-reference, double-blind, flexible-dose study of the efficacy of vortioxetine on cognitive function in major depressive disorder. Neuropsychopharmacology 2015;40(8):2025–37.

66. Lam RW, Iverson GL, Evans VC, et al. The effects of desvenlafaxine on neurocognitive and work functioning in employed outpatients with major depressive disorder. J Affect Disord 2016;203:55–61.

67. McIntyre RS, Best MW, Bowie CR, et al. The THINC-integrated tool (THINC-it) screening assessment for cognitive dysfunction: validation in patients with major depressive disorder. J Clin Psychiatry 2017;78(7):873–81.

68. Solé B, Jiménez E, Martinez-Aran A, Vieta E. Cognition as a target in major depression: new developments. Eur Neuropsychopharmacol 2015;25(2):231–47.

69. Miskowiak KW, Burdick KE, Martinez-Aran A, et al. Methodological recommendations for cognition trials in bipolar disorder by the International Society for Bipolar Disorders Targeting Cognition Task Force. Bipolar Disord 2017;19(8):614–26.

70. Stern Y. What is cognitive reserve? Theory and research application of the reserve concept. J Int Neuropsychol Soc 2002;8(3):448–60.

6

The Assessment of Cognitive Dysfunction in Major Depressive Disorder

John E. Harrison

Assessing Cognition in Patients with Major Depressive Disorders

A wide variety of measures have been employed to assess cognition in patients with major depressive disorders (MDD). We will review the use of both computerized and traditional 'paper-and-pencil' (P&P) measures. This chapter is not designed to be a comprehensive review and we will restrict ourselves to an account and characterization of the measures that have been included in recent meta-analyses. The studies to which we will refer are listed in Table 6.1.

Table 6.2 summarizes and describes the P&P measures reported in the listed meta-analyses. The computerized tests employed are described in Table 6.3. Each test is listed alphabetically with a column of notes and, where available, details of pharmacological intervention sensitivity, expressed as a treatment effect size.

The P&P tests typically employed are usually drawn from the corpus of clinical psychology and are therefore designed to identify cognitive impairment, but not necessarily the measurement of cognitive change. Critical to the interpretation of an individual's performance in the former context is the availability of normative data against which an individual test score can be compared with, usually, an age-, years of education-, and sex-matched population. Performance in this context is typically described as a z-score or, more typically, as a percentile, with –1.96 standard deviations (SDs) representing the cut-off for conspicuous impairment. Often P&P tests are available in a single format, which can compromise their use as measures of cognitive change, i.e. situations in which repeated assessment is required. However, some P&P measures, such as the Repeatable Battery for the Assessment of Neuropsychological Status (RBANS), have been deliberately designed for repeated use, facilitated by the provision of multiple parallel versions of each test to reduce learning from first exposure impacting later performance (1).

Many of the available computerized testing systems have been designed as measures of cognitive change and, with the accretion of normative data, have also been employed to detect impairment. While there is a good deal of similarity

Table 6.1 Meta-analytic studies

Lead author	Year	Comments
Ahern (29)	2017	A review of cognitive deficits in first-episode patients
Lee (30)	2012	A further review of first-episode deficits
Rock (31)	2014	A review of cognitive deficits revealed by studies employing the CANTAB system
Snyder (32)	2013	A meta-analysis of executive function difficulties observed in patients with MDD

in the content of these systems, there is some distinction between them. The CANTAB system, for example, was designed to contain human analogues of popularly employed preclinical tests (2). Others, such as the system from CNS Vital Signs, features paradigms from both traditional neuropsychology and cognitive psychology (3). The Cognitive Drug Research (4) and CogState systems (5) tend to feature tests drawn exclusively from cognitive psychology.

Table 6.2 P&P cognitive measures employed in studies of depression

Test	Sensitivity [a]
Buschke Selective Reminding	—
California Verbal Learning	—
Category Fluency Test	—
Controlled Oral Word Association Test	—
Digit Span Forward	—
Digit Span Backward	—
Digit Symbol Coding	—
Digit Symbol Substitution Test	0.51
Hopkins Verbal Learning Test	—
Modified Card Sorting Test	—
Rey Auditory Verbal Learning	0.32
Rey Complex Figure	—
Stroop	0.33
Symbol Digit Modalities	—
Trail Making Test Part A	0.29
Trail Making Test Part B	0.31
Visual Reproduction I	—
Visual Reproduction II	—
Wechsler Logical Memory	—
Wisconsin Card Sorting Test	—

[a] Sensivity estimates taken from the FOCUS study.

Table 6.3 Computerized cognitive measures employed in studies of depression

Test	Sensitivity
Detection [1]	0.42[a]
Identification [1]	0.36[a]
One Back [1]	0.08[b]
Groton Maze Learning [1]	0.11[b]
Stockings of Cambridge [2]	—
Spatial Working Memory [2]	—
Intra/Extra Set Shifting [2]	—
Spatial Span [2]	—
Delayed Matching to Sample [2]	—
Paired Associates Learning [2]	—
Pattern Recognition Memory [2]	—
Spatial Recognition Memory [2]	—
Rapid Visual Information Processing [2]	—
Reaction Time [2]	—

[1] CogState assessments (www.cogstate.com).

[2] CANTAB assessments (www.cambridgecognition.com).

[a] Sensitivity estimates taken from the FOCUS study.

[b] Sensitivity estimates taken from the CONNECT study.

Computers are well-suited to the assessment of attention. Tests that feature mental chronometry, often referred to as 'reaction time tests', require precise timing of test stimuli delivery and study participant responses. This precision is best achieved with use of modern digital devices. The assessment of episodic visual memory is also more easily achieved using computerized testing. Computers are well-suited to efficiently delivering sequences of visual 'to-be-remembered-items' and capturing study participant responses. The use of a forced-choice paradigm in the recognition phase of visual memory tests allows for the capture of not just the study participant's accuracy, but also the speed of the response. In contrast, for measures such as tests of verbal fluency, computerized assessment currently confers no particular advantage beyond P&P assessment aided with stopwatches and recording devices. With improvements in machine learning and voice recognition technology, automatic assessment may yet prove useful for tasks that require verbal responses from study participants. It is our view that cognition tests should be selected according to best practice principles. Computerized and P&P assessments should not be seen as mutually exclusive possibilities. Reliability, sensitivity, and validity are the criteria by which tests must be judged. In the next section (see section on 'Best Practice Guidance for the Assessment of Cognition', we will consider these issues in greater detail.

Best Practice Guidance for the Assessment of Cognition

Recently, Harrison (6) has proposed a variety of selection criteria, building on advice offered by Harrison and Maruff (7), as well as earlier contributions from Ferris et al. (8). This latter paper was written to provide advice on the selection of objective cognitive measures for use in Alzheimer's disease. However, the advice is equally applicable to other neurological and psychiatric conditions, as well as therapeutic areas such as cardiology and oncology. Ferris et al. specified a number of ideal test characteristics, including acceptable, and ideally high, levels of reliability, validity, and sensitivity. In addition, they suggest the use of parallel test versions to mitigate content learning effects, the selection of culture-independent tests, and the use of computerized testing, where possible. In this latter context, the authors mandated the use of simple devices, such as external key pads and button boxes, to ensure that it was the cognitive skills of study participants that were being assessed, and not their computer literacy.

Recommendations have also included advice on the statistical characteristics exhibited by appropriate tests. These include the absence of range restrictions, such as floor and ceiling effects, appropriate data transformations, and the management of extreme values and statistical outliers (7). Advice has also been forthcoming regarding methods of analysis. The most obvious manifestation of this has been the use of a z-score transformation to correct for different methods of scaling (9, 10). This methodology allows for the comparison of, for example, measures of latency, reckoned in milliseconds, with word list learning, which can have a dynamic range of as little as 0–10. Simple addition of the two measures has the potential for latency changes to swamp those in word recall, whereas transforming individual change scores puts these metrics on a common scale.

A further source of helpful guidance for assessing cognition concerns the management of test administration and the testing environment. These precautions have been designed to reduce error variance introduced through experimenter effects and extraneous sources of distraction. The focus has been on environmental factors, test procedures, and managing internal sources of variable performance. Management of the testing environment extends to ensuring that the location at which testing will occur is quiet, well-lit, and comfortable. A full list of further precautions is beyond the remit of this chapter, but a basic list includes the following:

1. Telephones and pagers turned off and a 'Do not disturb' sign placed on the door.
2. A room that is well lit and set to a comfortable temperature.
3. Accessible seating with a table at which the patient can be sat comfortably.

Continuity is a key factor with respect to test management procedures. This precaution extends to the following issues:

1. Where possible the same rater, for the same patient, for all study visits.
2. Testing should be conducted in the same room.
3. Assessments should also be scheduled for approximately the same time of day.

With respect to the third point, diurnal variation in cognitive performance is a well-documented phenomenon in even typical controls and might, if anything, be exacerbated in patients with neurological and psychiatric disorders.

A further issue is the extent to which the patient is free of distractions that might disrupt their ability to concentrate. This is part of the rationale for conducting assessments in protected locations, which help to mitigate the impact of any possible stress or agitation. For many patients, the experience of being tested might be new and could induce some mild test anxiety. This can be managed by exposing the patient to study testing procedures on their screening visit. Other precautions include ensuring that the patient is not distracted by discomfort, such as the need to visit the toilet before testing. The impact of not being able to void a full bladder has a clear negative effect on cognition (11). Patients should also be given access to light refreshments before being tested and access to liquids during testing procedures. In this section, we have been concerned with good testing practice and test selection. In the next section (see section on 'Measuring Cognitive Impairments and Cognitive Change among MDD Patients in Clinical Trials'), we will describe how these needs have been met in the context of detecting and monitoring cognitive change in patients with MDD.

So far in this chapter we have been concerned with the procedure for ensuring that the assessment of cognition captures the study participant's true competence, i.e. their ideal level of test performance. All the precautions discussed optimize the assessment process to help ensure that test score change after an intervention has been made can be reliably attributed solely to the therapeutic agent. We, and others, have been critical of the measures used to capture treatment effect on cognition in clinical drug trials (12). When considering this issue, it is helpful to reflect on a recent example of a successful programme of development that has yielded label claims supporting the pharmacological remediation of cognitive deficits. Therefore, we will describe the approach employed in a successful recent treatment development programme.

Measuring Cognitive Impairments and Cognitive Change among MDD Patients in Clinical Trials

Patients with MDD often suffer cognitive difficulties. It has been supposed that these difficulties were due to changes in mood. The logic of this position is that alleviation of the patient's mood complaints will be accompanied by a restoration of their cognitive skills. However, research has shown that patients with MDD between depressive episodes complain that often their thinking is impaired (13). Residual difficulties have been a major challenge in restoring patients to full function. There has been a tendency to pigeonhole cognition and function as different constructs. However, it seems certain that deficits in various cognitive domains, but especially executive function, underlie functional difficulties. As well as remedying the issues with mood, addressing cognitive deficits would seem to be a useful co-strategy. It is presumably for this reason that the Food and Drug Administration (FDA) has recently extended the labelling for Brintellix (vortioxetine) to include its prescription for processing speed deficits.

The first evidence of a pro-cognitive effect of vortioxetine was reported in a study of elderly individuals with a history of MDD (14). In this study, cognitive effects of treatment with duloxetine and vortioxetine were assessed using the Rey Auditory Verbal Learning Test (RAVLT) and the Digit Symbol Substitution Test (DSST). The results showed that treatment with both compounds improved performance on the RAVLT. However, vortioxetine also showed beneficial treatment effects on the DSST. The DSST has a long history of use in clinical psychology and has been employed extensively in a variety of neurological and psychiatric disorders (15). The Committee for Medicinal Products for Human Use of the European Medicines Agency describes the DSST as a 'timed executive function test' (16) and, whilst true, the DSST in fact measures a good deal more than executive function. Analysis of the test content indicates that the functional integrity of cognitive resources, such as attention and working memory, are also required for successful completion of the measure. The test is relatively brief (around 2–3 minutes in duration) and reliable. However, the simplicity of the test belies its capacity to make keen demands on the cognitive skills listed. It is therefore unsurprising that it is a sensitive measure of dysfunction in a number of indications (including Alzheimer's disease [17]) and that DSST performance can be influenced by a number of psychopharmacological interventions. This makes the test a useful measure of both cognitive deficit and cognitive change, but one that is uninformative with respect to which domains have been impacted by treatment. Thus, a key question for later studies of vortioxetine was to establish which cognitive domains were positively benefitted by treatment. This study (18) is described next.

The follow-up study was designed primarily to be a replication of the Katona et al. study (14). Consequently, the chosen primary outcome was a composite measure of the RAVLT and DSST. The secondary question was which cognitive domains were positively impacted by treatment. It should be acknowledged that there are no entirely pure measures of specific cognitive domains. However, tests linked to individual domains tend to make robust demands on the associated domain. For example, measures of 'episodic verbal memory', such as the RAVLT, require the recollection of a 15 word list, which is sufficiently challenging to ensure that the measure is free of ceiling effects in the target population. Reaction time tests are demanding measures of 'attention' and indicate how attentive the study participant was when the 'go' signal arrived.

A number of measures have been employed to measure cognitive deficits in patients with MDD and the typical pattern of impairment is usually in the order of –0.8 SD in patients in the midst of a depressive episode (19). On average patients between episodes tend to exhibit deficits in the effect size range of –0.3 to –0.6 (20). However, detailed investigation of patient cohorts has revealed that the cognitive deficits are not necessary sequelae of MDD. In a recent analysis 52% of patients in full- or part-time work or study did not exhibit clear evidence of cognitive dysfunction (21). While the evaluation of cognitive deficits in patients with MDD has been commonly reported, changes in the signs and symptoms of the disease have usually been focused on measures of mood. However, this emphasis has shifted in recent trials of multimodal antidepressant treatments, including the FOCUS study of vortioxetine, which we will describe next.

The procedure for selecting cognitive tests for use in the FOCUS study was a two-stage process. First, the cognitive domains of interest were specified and then appropriate tests of these domains were selected. We chose to assess the domains of attention, episodic memory, working memory, and executive function. Test selection was informed by available best practice guidance and especially with reference to requirements for reliability, validity, and sensitivity. The selected assessments, together with the domains indexed, are listed in Table 6.4.

The CogState Detection and Identification tasks were selected as measures of attention on the assumption that mean latency for correct responses is an accurate proxy measure of attention. Computerized versions of the remaining tasks were unavailable and so were administered in their traditional P&P formats. The full assessment required just less than 30 minutes to administer. This was a deliberate policy to avoid fatiguing patients. Experience suggests that this is a sensible limitation for cognitive assessment in patients with neurological or psychiatric disorders. Assessments of this length avoid factors that impact performance such

Table 6.4 Cognitive measures selected for the FOCUS study

	Test	Domain
1	Rey Auditory Verbal Learning Test (RAVLT)	Episodic memory
2	Simple & Choice Reaction Time (SRT & CRT)	Attention
3a	Trail Making Test Part A (TMT A)	Attention
3b	Trail Making Test Part B (TMT B)	Executive function
4	Stroop test	Executive function
5	Digit Symbol Substitution Test (DSST)	Multiple skills

as fatigue and ennui. Significant precautions were taken to ensure that tests were well understood prior to testing. Further precautions included careful site selection, extensive data review, and thorough rater training.

The results of the FOCUS study showed significant improvements on the DSST and in performance across all the preselected cognitive domains after 8 weeks of treatment with vortioxetine (22). The DSST effect was further replicated in the later CONNECT study, which featured further cognitive tests (23). The time needed to administer the selected measures in the CONNECT study was extended well past our recommended 30-minute maximum, often taking as long as 1 hour. This extended administration time might account for the smaller effect sizes observed after vortioxetine treatment in CONNECT. For example, the positive treatment effect size observed on the DSST in the FOCUS study was slightly better than 0.5. A recent meta-analysis of the use of the DSST in vortioxetine studies reported a positive effect size of 0.35 (24).

The FOCUS study results showed that the selected measures are capable of detecting psychopharmacological treatment effects, a critical component of the validation process. We have recently been critical of studies reporting null treatment effects, but which have used cognitive measures we would consider to be not fit for purpose, particularly with regard to the important characteristic of assay sensitivity (25). As well as validating the responsiveness to treatment effects of the selected measures, the FOCUS study also permitted validation of the z-score methodology used in this study. Assessing and interpreting cognitive data by domain seems to us the most informative means of determining treatment effects. The domain approach avoids oversimplifying the assessment of cognition by analysing a single, composite measure, while also avoiding the need for harsh statistical correction for family-wise error. An important caveat to attach is that we do not consider that the assessment used in FOCUS should be a 'gold standard' for assessing cognition in patients with MDD. The FOCUS assessments have robustly demonstrated their capacity to detect treatment effects. However, we consider that the process outlined above represents a suitable and scientifically defendable approach when assessing cognition in trials of new chemical entities. We would further suggest that such an approach could be reasonably adopted for assessing cognition for any drug class and any indication.

Issues with screening for cognitive impairment in MDD

The use of appropriate measures of critical cognitive domains facilitates the process of population screening. This is particularly important in the detection of 'caseness' and, by extension, to the recruitment of appropriate patients for assessment in clinical drug trials. Recent studies have shown that cognitive deficits are not routinely tested for during healthcare visits for patients with MDD. On the rare occasions when assessments are conducted, this tends to be only when dementia might be an issue. Various groups have initiated programmes designed to raise awareness of the importance of cognitive issues in MDD. Among these has been the THINC Task Force, who have sought to raise awareness of cognitive issues in depression through educational programmes. The early work of this group identified that, while functional deficits and partial remission are well-known features of the condition, these problems were often not typically connected to the cognitive deficits. Dialogue with healthcare providers revealed a keenness to discuss these issues informally, as well as to evaluate the nature of the cognitive difficulties with subjective and objective assessments (26). In response to this expressed need, the task force developed and specified a combination of objective cognitive measures and a brief, five-item version of the Perceived Deficit Questionnaire (27). Interviews with potential users revealed the need for a brief, computerized screening assessment that can be administered by non-experts. Delivery of results was required to be presented in a rudimentary fashion and available in real time. In response to these specifications the THINC Task Force designed an assessment with the following attributes:

1. Brevity—less than 15 minutes' administration time.
2. Non-expert administration—tests delivered by available staff.
3. Simple interpretation—basic reporting using a traffic light system.
4. Gamified tests—the use of visually engaging measures.

The objective cognitive measures for THINC-it were drawn from paradigms that have previously shown sensitivity to impairment, but that might also function successfully as measures of change. The following paradigms were selected:

1. Choice Reaction Time.
2. One Back Test.
3. Repeatable Trails B test.
4. Symbol coding test.

The selected measures were chosen as assessments of attention, working memory, executive function, and as a broad measure of cognitive function, analogous to the use of the DSST. Thus, three of the four measures mirrored the use of paradigms included in the FOCUS study. All the THINC-it measures were validated in a study of n=100 typical controls so that key psychometric data could be obtained and reported (28). Two facets of this data were the collection of temporal (also known as 'test–retest') reliability and stability. Individuals were tested after a 1-week interval to estimate temporal reliability correlations (test–retest reliability). Study participants were assessed at three 'back-to-back' assessments on their first study visit to assess stability based on a within-subject SD value. These two metrics are required for the calculation of Reliable Change Index (RCI) scores, which are the smallest differences that can be considered a 'real' change in performance.

Various methods of calculating RCI have been incorporated into the THINC-it system to facilitate decisions about individual changes in performance.

Conclusions and Recommendations

We began this chapter by reviewing many of the measures previously used to assess cognition in patients with depression. The focus of our initial assessment was on the P&P measures reviewed in recent meta-analyses. In the second part of the review we considered the use of computerized assessment. Cognition testing using either traditional or digital technologies has proven capable of detecting deficits. The cognitive measures in the Douglas et al. study (19) are amongst the largest effect size deficits represented in the literature. It is of note that this study featured both P&P and computer-based measures, suggesting that the detection of impairment is independent of the assessment technology employed. However, from a practical perspective it is efficient to match technology to the required task. For example, tests such as the previously described verbal fluency measures do not benefit from the use of digital technology, though improved speech recognition may make digital administration a possibility. Technological developments of this kind would also facilitate the assessment of verbal memory. In contrast, for the assessment of certain skills digital technology facilitates testing and yields precise data. For example, reaction time paradigms such as those described in the earlier section offer a brief and precise means of assessing attention. Similarly, the few available P&P visual memory paradigms are lengthy and require specialist paraphernalia and expert administration. In contrast, visual memory is readily assessed using digital technology.

In this chapter, we have offered a methodology for selecting cognitive measures for use in patients with MDD. This approach also provides statistical methods for detecting cases, measuring cognitive change, and providing data upon which evidenced-based decisions about healthcare can be based. This methodology relies on the initial selection of the appropriate cognitive domains of interest. We have further suggested that test selection must be made via the application of best practice guidance based on empirical data. Using the experience of assessing cognition in patients with MDD we have provided an example of how this approach can be applied, not just in this indication, but in any central nervous system disorder.

References

1. Randolph C, Tierney MC, Mohr E, Chase TN. The Repeatable Battery for the Assessment of Neuropsychological Status (RBANS): preliminary clinical validity. J Clin Exp Neuropsychol 1998;20(3): 310–19.

2. Sahakian BJ Morris RG Evenden JL, et al. A comparative study of visuospatial memory and learning in Alzheimer-type dementia and Parkinson's disease. Brain 1988;111:695–718.

3. Gualtieri CT, Johnson LG. Reliability and validity of a computerized neurocognitive test battery CNS Vital Signs. Arch Clin Neuropsychol 2006;21(7):623–43.

4. Simpson PM, Surmon DJ, Wesnes KA, Wilcock GK. The cognitive drug research computerized assessment system for demented patients: a validated study. Int J Geriatr Psychiatry 1991;6(2):95–102.

5. Cysique LA, Maruff PA, Darby D, Brew BJ. The assessment of cognitive function in advanced HIV-1 infection and AIDS dementia complex using a new computerised cognitive test battery. Arch Clin Neuropsychol 2006;21(2):185–94.

6. Harrison JE. Measuring the mind: detecting cognitive deficits and measuring cognitive change in patients with depression. In: McIntyre RS, Cha D. (eds). *Cognitive Impairment in Major Depressive Disorder.* Cambridge: Cambridge University Press, 2016; pp. 229–41.

7. Harrison JE, Maruff P. Measuring the mind: assessing cognitive change in clinical drug trials. Expert Rev Clin Pharmacol 2008;1(4):471–3.

8. Ferris SH, Lucca U, Mohs R, et al. Objective psychometric tests in clinical trials of dementia drugs. Position paper from the International Working Group on Harmonization of Dementia Drug Guidelines. Alzheimer's Dis Assoc Disord 1997;11(S3): 34–8.

9. Harrison J, Minassian SL, Jenkins L, Black RS, Koller M, Grundman M. A neuropsychological test battery for use in Alzheimer disease clinical trials. Arch Neurol 2007;64:1323–9.

10. Harrison JE, Rentz DM, McLaughlin T, et al. Cognition in MCI & Alzheimer's disease: baseline data from a longitudinal study of the NTB. Clin Neuropsychol 2014;28(2):252–68.

11. Lewis MS, Snyder PJ, Pietrzak RH, Darby D, Feldman RA, Maruff P. The effect of acute increase in urge to void on cognitive function in healthy adults. Neurourol Urodynamics 2011;30(1):183–7.

12. Harrison JE, Hendrix S. The assessment of cognition in translational medicine: a contrast between the approaches used in Alzheimer's disease and major depressive disorder. In: Nomikos G, Feltner D. (eds). *Translational Medicine in CNS Drug Development*, Volume 27, 2018. Cambridge MA: Academic Press.

13. Conradi CK, Ormel J, De Jonge P. Presence of individual (residual) symptoms during depressive episodes and peridos of remission: a 3-year prospective study. Psychol Med 2011;41(6):1165–74.

14. Katona C, Hansen T, Olsen CK. A randomized double-blind placebo-controlled duloxetine-referenced fixed-dose study comparing the efficacy and safety of Lu AA21004 in elderly patients with major depressive disorder. Int Clin Psychopharmacol 2012;27(4):215–23.

15. Lezak MD. *Neuropsychological Assessment.* Oxford: Oxford University Press, 1995.

16. CHMP. Discussion paper on the clinical investigation of medicines for the treatment of Alzheimer's disease and other dementias. EMA/CHMP/539931/2014, 2014.

17. Winblad B, Gauthier S, Scinto L, et al. Safety and efficacy of galantamine in subjects with mild cognitive impairment. Neurology 2008;70(22):2024–35.

18. McIntyre RS, Lophaven S, Olsen CK. A randomized double-blind placebo-controlled study of vortioxetine on cognitive function in depressed adults. Int J Neuropsychopharmacol 2014;30:1–11.

19. Douglas KM, Porter RJ, Knight RG, Maruff P. Neuropsychological changes and treatment response in severe depression. Br J Psychiatry 2011;198(2):115–22.

20. Rock PL, Roiser JP, Riedel WJ, Blackwell AD. Cognitive impairment in depression: a systematic review and meta-analysis. Psychol Med 2014;44(10):2029–40.

21. Maruff P, Jaeger J. Understanding the importance of cognitive dysfunction and cognitive change in major depresssive disorder. In: McIntyre RS, Cha D. (eds). *Cognitive Impairment in Major Depressive Disorder.* Cambridge: Cambridge University Press, 2016; pp. 15–29.

22. Harrison JE, Lophaven S, Olsen CK. Which cognitive domains are improved by treatment with vortioxetine? Int J Neuropsychopharmacol 2016;pii:pyw054.

23. Mahableshwarkar AR, Zajecka J, Jacobson W, Chen Y, Keefe R. A randomized placebo-controlled active-reference double-blind flexible-dose study of the efficacy of vortioxetine on cognitive function in major depressive disorder. Neuropsychopharmacology 2015;40:2015–37.

24. McIntyre RS, Harrison JE, Loft H, Jacobson W, Olsen CK. The effects of vortioxetine on cognitive function in patients with major depressive disorder (MDD): a meta-analysis of three randomized controlled trials. Int J Neuropsychopharmacol 2016;ug 24 pii: pyw055 http://dxdoiorg/101093/ijnp/pyw055.

25. Harrison JE, Lam RW, Baune BT, McIntyre RS. Selection of cognitive tests for trials of therapeutic agents. The Lancet Psychiatry 2016;8(8):1–13.

26. McAllister-Williams RH, Bones K, Goodwin GM, et al. Analysing UK clinicians' understanding of cognitive symptoms in major depression: a survey of primary care physicians and psychiatrists. J Affective Disor 2017;207:346–52.

27. McIntyre RS, Barry H, Baune BT, et al. The THINC-integrated tool (THINC-it) screening assessment for cognitive dysfunction: validation in patients with major depressive disorder. J Clin Psychiatry 2017;78(7):873–81.

28. Harrison JE, Barry H, Baune BT, et al. Stability, reliability, and validity of the THINC-it screening tool for cognitive impairment in depression: A psychometric exploration in healthy volunteers. Int J Methods Psychiatr Res 2018:27(3):e1736.

29. Ahern E, Semkovska M. Cognitive functioning in the first-episode of major depressive disorder: a systematic review and meta-analysis. Neuropsychol 2017;31(1):52–72.

30. Lee RSC, Hermens DF, Porter MA, Redoblado-Hodge MA. A meta-analysis of cognitive deficits in first-episode major depressive disorder. J Affective Disor 2012;140:113–24.

31. Rock PL, Roiser JP, Riedel WJ, Blackwell AD. Cognitive impairment in depression: a systematic review and meta-analysis. Psychol Med 2014;44:2029–40.

32. Snyder HR. Major depressive disorder is associated with broad impairments on neuropsychological measures of executive function: a meta-analysis and review. Psychol Bull 2013;139(1):81–132.

7

Molecular Neurobiology of Cognitive Dysfunction in Major Depressive Disorder

Natalie T. Mills and Bernhard T. Baune

Introduction

Cognitive changes observed in major depressive disorder (MDD) include changes in memory, executive function, and attention (1). Neurobiological theories of depression, such as the monoamine hypothesis, and the macrophage theory of depression, can assist in providing an understanding of the molecular underpinnings of this cognitive dysfunction. It is important to note that these biological systems closely interact, e.g. the broadly reported interactions between neurotransmitters such as serotonin and proinflammatory markers (2). Furthermore, molecules of the immune system, e.g. proinflammatory cytokines, exert effects on the neural systems by modulating synaptic plasticity and neurogenesis (2, 3). This chapter first discusses neurotransmitters and their receptors and then the role of inflammation in cognitive dysfunction observed in MDD. Genetic polymorphisms, changes in gene expression, and epigenetic pathways are reviewed for their role in the neurobiological underpinnings of cognitive dysfunction in MDD.

Neurotransmitter Receptors
Serotonin

Tryptophan, an essential amino acid needed for protein synthesis, is a precursor for serotonin (4). Individuals in remission from MDD, who also use antidepressant medication, have demonstrated lowering of mood in the setting of acute tryptophan depletion (4). Furthermore, in studies that have examined effects of acute tryptophan depletion, a consistent outcome is impaired delayed recall of episodic memory (5). Low extracellular serotonin levels have also been found to be associated with impaired memory consolidation (6).

Different subtypes of serotonin receptors exist in the brain and have a role in depression and the cognitive changes seen in this disorder (6). Serotonin also modulates neuroplasticity characteristics via these receptors (7). The serotonin 1A ($5\text{-}HT_{1A}$) receptor has a particularly complex signalling system, with conflicting results in pharmacological studies (8). A small study found an improvement in verbal memory in patients with MDD, but not controls, with the use of the partial $5\text{-}HT_{1A}$ receptor agonist ipsapirone (9). However, when healthy individuals were administered the $5\text{-}HT_{1A}$ receptor agonist tandospirone, an impairment in verbal memory was observed (10).

Other serotonin receptor subtypes are also thought to have a role in MDD and the cognitive changes seen in this disorder. The role of the $5\text{-}HT_{1B}$ receptor includes modulating learning and memory through a glutamatergic mechanism (11). Antagonism of $5\text{-}HT_3$ receptors and $5\text{-}HT_7$ receptors has been shown to increase cognitive function and antidepressant activity in preclinical studies (12–16).

The finding of an effect on memory through action on different serotonin receptor subtypes is consistent with the distribution of these receptors in the brain, with most serotonin receptors found in areas associated with learning and memory, such as the prefrontal cortex and hippocampus (6, 17).

Dopamine

The monoamine dopamine also has a role in cognition and depression (18). Dopamine regulates domains of cognition affected in depression, such as attention and memory (19, 20). With regard to memory, the antidepressant reboxetine has been observed to improve memory in animal models of depression, likely through stimulating the dopaminergic system in the prefrontal cortex (20).

Both dopamine D1 and dopamine D2 receptors are thought to have a role in cognition (21). Dopamine D1 receptors are located in the hippocampus and prefrontal cortex (21). Furthermore, D1 receptor knockout mice have been found to have deficits in spatial learning (21). Dopamine D2 receptor knockout mice have been found to show impaired hippocampal learning and memory (22).

Changes in psychomotor speed, also seen in MDD, are thought to involve dysfunction in dopamine-containing areas of the basal ganglia (23, 24). Specifically, reduced dopamine receptor occupancy in the basal ganglia is thought to reflect reduced dopamine function and has been correlated with reduced motor function and reduced verbal fluency and reaction time in patients with MDD (24).

Glutamate

Glutamate is an essential neurotransmitter for cognitive processing and also has a role in MDD (11). However, increased glutamate can lead to neurotoxicity through activation of N-methyl-D-aspartate (NMDA) receptors, which activate microglia (25). The activation of microglia then leads to release of inflammatory mediators, such as quinolinic acid and tumour necrosis factor-alpha (TNF-α) (25). Increased levels of TNF-α lead to further release of glutamate (26). This is compounded by decreased numbers of astrocytes in MDD, resulting in decreased clearance of glutamate, thereby impairing neuroplasticity (25).

Of the three main glutamate receptor classes involved in learning and memory, the metabotropic glutamate receptor (mGluR) subtypes appear to be involved in memory consolidation and long-term memory (27). Glutamate transmission is also modulated by serotonin through serotonin receptor subtypes (11). Therefore, glutamatergic neurotransmission is complex, with interactions occurring between serotonin receptors and proinflammatory markers.

Inflammation and Cognitive Dysfunction in Depression

Elevated levels of the proinflammatory cytokines TNF-α and IL-6 have been associated with MDD in adults (28). Furthermore, proinflammatory cytokines or other agents that induce inflammation have been found to not only induce symptoms of depression but also cognitive changes seen in MDD (29, 30).

In healthy individuals, acute experimental inflammation can lead to the negative biases in emotional processing and social cognition seen in MDD (31). These changes consist of reduced ability to recall emotional faces (32), subjective experiences of social disconnectedness (33), and reduced selection of high-probability reward/increased avoidance of high-probability loss (34). However, not all studies have found changes in behavioural measures of emotional and social processing in response to an endotoxin challenge (35). Furthermore, conflicting effects of acute experimental inflammation on attention, executive function, and memory have been observed, possibly owing to different inflammatory challenges and different doses of endotoxin between studies (31).

The relationship between inflammatory markers and psychomotor performance has also been investigated in healthy individuals, in patients receiving interferon for medical illnesses, and in MDD. In elderly females with Mini-Mental State Examination scores ≥24 at baseline, higher levels of IL-6 have been associated with greater declines in psychomotor speed (36). Reduced psychomotor speed has also been observed in patients receiving interferon therapy (37). In individuals with MDD, both proinflammatory and anti-inflammatory markers have been found to be associated with psychomotor performance, with increased levels of the proinflammatory cytokine IL-6 found to be associated with slower simple and choice movement times, and the anti-inflammatory cytokine IL-10 associated with better performance on the Digit Symbol Substitution Task (DSST) (38).

The relationship between memory and inflammatory markers is complex, with physiological levels of proinflammatory cytokines required for normal cognitive function (39, 40). Decreases in memory have been associated with intrahippocampal TNF-α administration (41). However, TNF-α deficiency has also been associated with reduced memory in animal models (39). Figure 7.1 shows pathways where inflammatory markers and neurotransmitters involved in cognitive dysfunction in MDD interact.

Inflammation, Neuronal Plasticity and Neurogenesis

The proinflammatory cytokines TNF-α, IL-6, and IL-1β play an important role in synaptic plasticity, long-term potentiation (LTP), and learning and memory processes (26, 29, 42). LTP is a form of synaptic plasticity, where synaptic connections are strengthened through repeated stimulation (43, 44). LTP is thought to be important in learning and the formation of memory (43). Furthermore, LTP has been found to be impaired in depression and has also been proposed as leading to the cognitive biases seen in this illness (45).

High concentrations of IL-1β have been shown to inhibit LTP in the hippocampus, thus affecting memory (46, 47). However, physiological levels of IL-1β are required for normal memory function (40). TNF-α has also been found to inhibit LTP; however, TNF-α is also thought to be important in synaptic scaling (46, 48).

Neurogenesis is involved in memory processes, with a role for hippocampal neurogenesis proposed in spatial memory as well as the formation of long-term memories (49, 50). In adults, decreased hippocampal neurogenesis has been proposed as a factor in the cognitive changes observed in depression (51).

Both IL-1 and IL-6 have been found to have a role in neurogenesis, with a reduction of hippocampal neurogenesis observed in animal models (42). Specifically, decreased hippocampal neurogenesis was observed in mice administered exogenous IL-1β (52). With regard to IL-6, a reduction in hippocampal neurogenesis was observed in transgenic mice chronically expressing IL-6 in astroglia (53). In humans, elevated levels of both TNF-α and IL-6 have been found to be associated with smaller hippocampus volumes in older adults (54).

The Hypothalamic–Pituitary–Adrenal Axis

The hypothalamic–pituitary–adrenal (HPA) axis is thought to have a role in MDD and the cognitive dysfunction observed in this disorder (55). Compared to healthy controls and patients with MDD without psychotic features, patients with

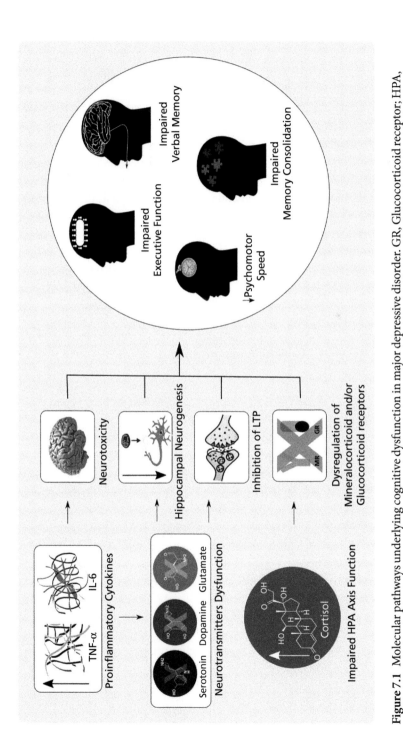

Figure 7.1 Molecular pathways underlying cognitive dysfunction in major depressive disorder. GR, Glucocorticoid receptor; HPA, hypothalamic–pituitary–adrenal; IL-6, interleukin-6; LTP, long-term potentiation; MR, mineralocorticoid receptor; TNF-α, tumour necrosis factor-alpha.

MDD with psychotic features have been found to have higher evening cortisol levels and poorer cognitive performance (55, 56).

Interestingly, higher cortisol levels have also been associated with decreased working memory in healthy adults with no history of MDD (57). Impaired auto-biographical memory retrieval has also been observed in healthy controls following acute cortisol administration (58).

In humans, the role of the HPA axis in MDD hypothesizes a dysregulation of the mineralocorticoid and/or glucocorticoid receptor (59, 60). Specifically, increased cortisol levels lead to disruption of the mineralocorticoid/glucocorticoid receptor ratio, with increased glucocorticoid receptor occupation (60). This is in contrast to the usual mineralocorticoid/glucocorticoid receptor balance, where cortisol binds with high affinity to mineralocorticoid receptors in the brain and with less affinity to glucocorticoid receptors (55). Consistent with this, stimulation of the mineralocorticoid receptor with fludrocortisone inhibits cortisol secretion and has been found to improve verbal memory and executive function in depressed patients (61). In contrast, blocking the mineralocorticoid receptor in healthy controls has been found to impair memory and executive function (62).

Genetics
Genetic Polymorphisms

A range of genetic variants has been associated with aspects of cognition, both in animals and humans. These include polymorphisms of the serotonin transporter gene (*SLC6A4*), including 5-HTTLPR and STin2, the catechol-O-methyl transferase (*COMT*) gene, inflammatory marker genes, and corticosteroid receptor genes.

In healthy females, the *S/S* 5-HTTLPR genotype has been associated with reduced performance on difficult n-Back tasks (63), a measure of working memory. Other groups have found an association between the *S/S* 5-HTTLPR genotype and reduced verbal memory (64), with some only finding a nominal association in the context of increased depressive symptoms (65), and some studies not finding an association between 5-HTTLPR genotype and verbal memory (66, 67). Individuals carrying the *S/S* 5-HTTLPR genotype who also have a history of MDD, when compared to those with no MDD history, have also been found to have lower levels of specific autobiographical memory (68).

With regard to the STin2 polymorphism of the serotonin transporter gene, the STin2.12 allele has been associated with higher expression of the serotonin transporter (69). The availability of the serotonin transporter is thought to be important in learning and memory, consistent with a finding of individuals homozygous for the STin2.10 allele not performing as well in tests of verbal learning and memory (69).

Variants of the *COMT* gene, including interactions with other genes, have also been investigated in regard to neuropsychological aspects of depression (18). Specifically, an interaction between the *COMT* (Met/Met) polymorphism and the *NR3C1* single nucleotide polymorphism (SNP) rs41423247 on working memory has been observed (70).

Genetic variants of TNF-α and TNF receptors TNFR1 and TNFR2 are also important for normal cognition. Mice deficient in TNF-α (TNF-/-) and TNF receptors (TNF-R1-/- and TNF-R2-/-) have been found to have poorer learning and memory, with TNF-/- mice showing greater deficits in cognitive function compared to TNF-R1-/- and TNF-R2-/- mice (39). In humans, genetic variants of TNF-α have been associated with processing speed, with better processing speed observed with the GA/AA genotype of the TNF-α 308G → A polymorphism in elderly individuals (71). Polymorphisms of other proinflammatory cytokine genes have also been associated with domains of cognition. Specifically, the IL-1β-1418C → T polymorphism has been associated with memory in elderly individuals, with the CT/TT genotype associated with poorer memory (71).

Variation of the glucocorticoid receptor (GR) gene (*NR3C1*) and mineralocorticoid receptor (MR) gene (*NR3C2*) has also been found to predict aspects of cognitive function (55). Specifically, genetic variation of the GR *NR3C1* gene has been found to have a role in attention and executive function (55). Whereas the *NR3C1* SNP's rs10052957 and rs41423247 have been found to predict attention, variation of the MR *NR3C2* gene has been observed to predict verbal memory (55). It has been proposed that these areas of cognition are consistent with the distribution of GR and MR in the primate brain (72). Figure 7.2 shows the main genetic polymorphisms in humans that have been associated with the cognitive changes found in MDD.

Gene Expression

Altered gene expression is a pathway to be considered when examining cognitive dysfunction in MDD. Increased expression of TNF-α, TNFRSF1A, and TNFRSF1B has been found to correlate negatively with working memory and executive function (73). Specifically, when compared to healthy controls, the expression of these genes, both through protein and mRNA, has been found to be higher in those with recurrent MDD (73). Changes in hippocampal MR mRNA expression have also been observed in MDD, with a decrease in MR mRNA expression found in the anterior hippocampus of patients with MDD compared to controls (74).

Changes in peripheral blood gene expression have also been observed in remitted MDD. Specifically, when whole blood transcriptomic data were

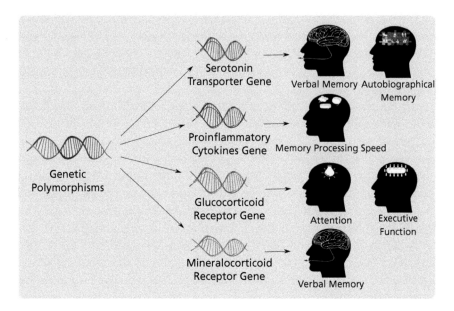

Figure 7.2 Genetic polymorphisms associated with changes in cognitive domains in Major Depressive Disorder.

analysed, transcripts encoding ribosome S40 component S26, and promoting B-lymphocyte proliferation were found to be associated with cognitive dysfunction (75).

Epigenetics

Epigenetics have an important role in synaptic plasticity and memory (76). Epigenetic pathways are thought to modulate neurogenesis, with changes in cognitive domains and depression-like activities (77). Methyl-CpG binding domain (MBD) proteins , including MBD1, have a role in repression of transcription and epigenetic gene regulation (78, 79). Furthermore, *Mbd1*-deficient mice have been observed to show increased depression-like behaviours and cognitive deficits (80).

Histone deacetylases (HDACs) also have a role in regulating neurogenesis through epigenetic pathways (77). HDAC inhibitors have a role in the regulation of epigenetic changes associated with regulation of cognition and behaviour (81). An example of the importance of this regulation is in HDAC2-overexpressing mice, where reduced learning and memory formation have been observed (82). Further research should provide more understanding of this complex area.

Conclusion

Neurotransmitters, neurotransmitter receptors, inflammatory markers, genetic polymorphisms and changes in gene expression all have a role in cognitive dysfunction in MDD. Preclinical models suggest potential targets for antidepressant medication, such as serotonin receptor subtypes, for improving this cognitive dysfunction. Targeting inflammation/immune system dysregulation, which would need to be tailored to those individuals with raised inflammatory markers, may improve mood and cognitive symptoms in depression. Future research should investigate whether augmenting the treatment of MDD with other neurobiological interventions such as immune-active agents would also improve cognitive function. Further research on the role of changes in gene expression and epigenetic mechanisms could also improve the understanding of the molecular neurobiology of cognitive dysfunction in MDD.

References

1. Beblo T, Sinnamon G, Baune BT. Specifying the neuropsychology of affective disorders: clinical, demographic and neurobiological factors. Neuropsychol Rev 2011;21(4):337–59.

2. Maes M, Yirmiya R, Noraberg J, et al. The inflammatory & neurodegenerative (I&ND) hypothesis of depression: leads for future research and new drug developments in depression. Metabol Brain Dis 2009;24(1):27–53.

3. Khairova RA, Machado-Vieira R, Du J, Manji HK. A potential role for proinflammatory cytokines in regulating synaptic plasticity in major depressive disorder. Int J Neuropsychopharmacol 2009;12(4):561–78.

4. Ruhe HG, Mason NS, Schene AH. Mood is indirectly related to serotonin, norepinephrine, and dopamine levels in humans: a meta-analysis of monoamine depletion studies. Mol Psychiatry 2007;12(4):331–59.

5. Mendelsohn D, Riedel WJ, Sambeth A. Effects of acute tryptophan depletion on memory, attention and executive functions: a systematic review. Neurosci Biobehavior Rev 2009;33(6):926–52.

6. Cowen P, Sherwood AC. The role of serotonin in cognitive function: evidence from recent studies and implications for understanding depression. Journal of Psychopharmacology. 2013;27(7):575–83.

7. Kraus C, Castren E, Kasper S, Lanzenberger R. Serotonin and neuroplasticity—links between molecular, functional and structural pathophysiology in depression. Neurosci Biobehavior Rev 2017;77:317–26.

8. Savitz J, Lucki I, Drevets WC. 5-HT1A receptor function in major depressive disorder. Prog Neurobiol 2009;88(1):17–31.

9. Riedel WJ, Klaassen T, Griez E, Honig A, Menheere P, van Praag HM. Dissociable hormonal, cognitive and mood responses to neuroendocrine challenge: evidence for receptor-specific serotonergic dysregulation in depressed mood. Neuropsychopharmacol 2002;26(3):358–67.

10. Yasuno F, Suhara T, Nakayama T, et al. Inhibitory effect of hippocampal 5-HT1A receptors on human explicit memory. Am J Psychiatry 2003;160(2):334–40.

11. Pehrson AL, Sanchez C. Serotonergic modulation of glutamate neurotransmission as a strategy for treating depression and cognitive dysfunction. Cns Spectrums 2014;19(2):121–33.

12. Staubli U, Xu FB. Effects of 5-HT3 receptor antagonism on hippocampal theta-rhythm, memory, and LTP induction in the freely moving rat. J Neurosci 1995;15(3):2445–52.

13. Roychoudhury M, Kulkarni SK. Effects of ondansetron on short-term memory retrieval in mice. Methods Findings Exp Clin Pharmacol 1997;19(1):43–6.

14. Martin P, Gozlan H, Puech AJ. 5-HT3 receptor antagonists reverse helpless behavior in rats. Eur J Pharmacol 1992;212(1):73–8.

15. Bonaventure P, Kelly L, Aluisio L, et al. Selective blockade of 5-hydroxytryptamine (5-HT)(7) receptors enhances 5-HT transmission, antidepressant-like behavior, and rapid eye movement sleep suppression induced by citalopram in rodents. J Pharmacol Exp Therapeut 2007;321(2):690–8.

16. Bonaventure P, Aluisio L, Shoblock J, et al. Pharmacological blockade of serotonin 5-HT7 receptor reverses working memory deficits in rats by normalizing cortical glutamate neurotransmission. Plos One 2011;6(6):PMC3119073.

17. Puig MV, Gulledge AT. Serotonin and prefrontal cortex function: neurons, networks, and circuits. Mol Neurobiol 2011;44(3):449–64.

18. Antypa N, Drago A, Serretti A. The role of COMT gene variants in depression: bridging neuropsychological, behavioral and clinical phenotypes. Neurosci Biobehavior Rev 2013;37(8):1597–610.

19. Nieoullon A. Dopamine and the regulation of cognition and attention. Prog Neurobiol 2002;67(1):53–83.

20. De Bundel D, Femenia T, DuPont CM, et al. Hippocampal and prefrontal dopamine D-1/5 receptor involvement in the memory-enhancing effect of reboxetine. Int J Neuropsychopharmacol 2013;16(9):2041–51.

21. El-Ghundi M, Fletcher PJ, Drago J, Sibley DR, O'Dowd BF, George SR. Spatial learning deficit in dopamine D-1 receptor knockout mice. Eur J Pharmacol 1999;383(2):95–106.

22. Rocchetti J, Isingrini E, Dal Bo G, et al. Presynaptic D-2 dopamine receptors control long-term depression expression and memory processes in the temporal hippocampus. Biol Psychiatry 2015;77(6):513–25.

23. Martinot MLP, Bragulat V, Artiges E, et al. Decreased presynaptic dopamine function in the left caudate of depressed patients with affective flattening and psychomotor retardation. Am J Psychiatry 2001;158(2):314–16.

24. Shah PJ, Ogilvie AD, Goodwin GM, Ebmeier KP. Clinical and psychometric correlates of dopamine D-2 binding in depression. Psychol Med 1997;27(6):1247–56.

25. McNally L, Bhagwagar Z, Hannestad J. Inflammation, glutamate, and glia in depression: a literature review. Cns Spectrums 2008;13(6):501–10.

26. Bortolato B, Carvalho AF, Soczynska JK, Perini GI, McIntyre RS. The involvement of TNF-alpha in cognitive dysfunction associated with major depressive disorder: an opportunity for domain specific treatments. Curr Neuropharmacol 2015;13(5):558–76.

27. Riedel G, Platt B, Micheau J. Glutamate receptor function in learning and memory. Behavioural Brain Res 2003;140(1–2):1–47.

28. Dowlati Y, Herrman N, Swardfager W, et al. A meta-analysis of cytokines in major depression. Biol Psychiatry 2010;67:446–57.

29. McAfoose J, Baune BT. Evidence for a cytokine model of cognitive function. Neurosci Biobehav Rev 2009;33(3):355–66.

30. Krogh J, Benros ME, Jorgensen MB, Vesterager L, Elfving B, Nordentoft M. The association between depressive symptoms, cognitive function, and inflammation in major depression. Brain Behavior Immunity 2014;35:70–6.

31. Bollen J, Trick L, Llewellyn D, Dickens C. The effects of acute inflammation on cognitive functioning and emotional processing in humans: a systematic review of experimental studies. J Psychosomatic Res 2017;94:47–55.

32. Grigoleit JS, Kullmann JS, Wolf OT, et al. Dose-dependent effects of endotoxin on neurobehavioral functions in humans. Plos One 2011;6(12):e28330.

33. Moieni M, Irwin MR, Jevtic I, Breen EC, Eisenberger NI. Inflammation impairs social cognitive processing: a randomized controlled trial of endotoxin. Brain Behavior Immunity 2015;48:132–8.

34. Harrison NA, Voon V, Cercignani M, Cooper EA, Pessiglione M, Critchley HD. A neurocomputational account of how inflammation enhances sensitivity to punishments versus rewards. Biol Psychiatry 2016;80(1):73–81.

35. Kullmann JS, Grigoleit JS, Wolf OT, et al. Experimental human endotoxemia enhances brain activity during social cognition. Social Cognitive Affective Neurosci 2014;9(6):786–93.

36. Palta P, Xue QL, Deal JA, Fried LP, Walston JD, Carlson MC. Interleukin-6 and C-reactive protein levels and 9-year cognitive decline in community-dwelling older women: The Women's Health and Aging Study II. J Gerontology Series A–Biological Sciences and Medical Sciences 2015;70(7):873–8.

37. Haroon E, Felger JC, Woolwine BJ, et al. Age-related increases in basal ganglia glutamate are associated with TNF, reduced motivation and decreased psychomotor speed during IFN-alpha treatment: preliminary findings. Brain Behavior Immunity 2015;46:17–22.

38. Goldsmith DR, Haroon E, Woolwine BJ, et al. Inflammatory markers are associated with decreased psychomotor speed in patients with major depressive disorder. Brain Behavior Immunity 2016;56:281–8.

39. Baune BT, Wiede F, Braun A, Golledge J, Arolt V, Koerner H. Cognitive dysfunction in mice deficient for TNF and its receptors. Am J Med Gen Part B—Neuropsychiatric Gen 2008;147B(7):1056–64.

40. Avital A, Goshen I, Kamsler A, et al. Impaired interleukin-1 signaling is associated with deficits in hippocampal memory processes and neural plasticity. Hippocampus 2003;13(7):826–34.

41. Matsumoto Y, Watanabe S, Suh YH, Yamamoto T. Effects of intrahippocampal CT105, a carboxyl terminal fragment of beta-amyloid precursor protein, alone/ with inflammatory cytokines on working memory in rats. J Neurochem 2002;82(2): 234–9.

42. Eyre H, Baune BT. Neuroplastic changes in depression: a role for the immune system. Psychoneuroendocrinology 2012;37:1397–416.

43. Lynch MA. Long-term potentiation and memory. Physiol Rev 2004;84(1):87–136.

44. Lynch MA. Age-related impairment in long-term potentiation in hippocampus: a role for the cytokine, interleukin-1 beta? Prog Neurobiol 1998;56(5):571–89.

45. Drago A, Crisafulli C, Sidoti A, Serretti A. The molecular interaction between the glutamatergic, noradrenergic, dopaminergic and serotoninergic systems informs a detailed genetic perspective on depressive phenotypes. Prog Neurobiol 2011;94(4):418–60.

46. Pickering M, O'Connor JJ. Pro-inflammatory cytokines and their effects in the dentate gyrus. Dentate Gyrus: A Comprehensive Guide to Structure, Function, and Clinical Implications. 2007;163:339–54.

47. Coogan AN, O'Neill LAJ, O'Connor JJ. The p38 mitogen-activated protein kinase in-hibitor SB203580 antagonizes the inhibitory effects of interleukin-1 beta on longterm potentiation in the rat dentate gyrus in vitro. Neuroscience 1999;93(1):57–69.

48. Turrigiano GG, Nelson SB. Homeostatic plasticity in the developing nervous system. Nature Rev Neurosci 2004;5(2):97–107.

49. Drapeau E, Mayo W, Aurousseau C, Le Moal M, Piazza PV, Abrous DN. Spatial memory performances of aged rats in the water maze predict levels of hippocampal neurogenesis. Proc Natl Acad Sci U S A 2003;100(24):14385–90.

50. Snyder JS, Hong NS, McDonald RJ, Wojtowicz JM. A role for adult neurogenesis in spatial long-term memory. Neuroscience 2005;130(4):843–52.

51. Sahay A, Hen R. Adult hippocampal neurogenesis in depression. Nature Neurosci 2007;10(9):1110–15.

52. Koo JW, Duman RS. IL-1 beta is an essential mediator of the antineurogenic and an-hedonic effects of stress. Proc Natl Acad Sci U S A 2008;105(2):751–6.

53. Vallieres L, Campbell IL, Gage FH, Sawchenko PE. Reduced hippocampal neurogen-esis in adult transgenic mice with chronic astrocytic production of interleukin-6. J Neurosci 2002;22(2):486–92.

54. Sudheimer KD, O'Hara R, Spiegel D, et al. Cortisol, cytokines, and hippocampal volume interactions in the elderly. Front Aging Neurosci 2014;6:153.

55. Keller J, Gomez R, Williams G, et al. HPA axis in major depression: cortisol, clinical symptomatology and genetic variation predict cognition. Mol Psychiatry 2017;22(4):527–36.

56. Gomez RG, Fleming SH, Keller J, et al. The neuropsychological profile of psychotic major depression and its relation to cortisol. Biol Psychiatry 2006;60(5):472–8.

57. Lupien SJ, Gillin CJ, Hauger RL. Working memory is more sensitive than declarative memory to the acute effects of corticosteroids: a dose-response study in humans. Behavior Neurosci 1999;113(3):420–30.

58. Schlosser N, Wolf OT, Fernando SC, et al. Effects of acute cortisol administration on autobiographical memory in patients with major depression and healthy controls. Psychoneuroendocrinol 2010;35(2):316–20.

59. Young EA, Lopez JF, Murphy-Weinberg V, Watson SJ, Akil H. Mineralocorticoid receptor function in major depression. Arch Gen Psychiatry 2003;60(1):24–8.

60. Holsboer F. The corticosteroid receptor hypothesis of depression. Neuropsychopharmacology 2000;23(5):477–501.

61. Otte C, Wingenfeld K, Kuehl LK, et al. Mineralocorticoid receptor stimulation improves cognitive function and decreases cortisol secretion in depressed patients and healthy individuals. Neuropsychopharmacology 2015;40(2):386–93.

62. Rimmele U, Besedovsky L, Lange T, Born J. Blocking mineralocorticoid receptors impairs, blocking glucocorticoid receptors enhances memory retrieval in humans. Neuropsychopharmacology 2013;38(5):884–94.

63. Jonassen R, Endestad T, Neumeister A, Haug KBF, Berg JP, Landro NI. Serotonin transporter polymorphism modulates N-back task performance and fMRI BOLD signal intensity in healthy women. Plos One. 2012;7(1):e30564.

64. Zilles D, Meyer J, Schneider-Axmann T, et al. Genetic polymorphisms of 5-HTT and DAT but not COMT differentially affect verbal and visuospatial working memory functioning. Eur Arch Psychiatry Clin Neurosci 2012;262(8):667–76.

65. Price JS, Strong J, Eliassen J, et al. Serotonin transporter gene moderates associations between mood, memory and hippocampal volume. Behav Brain Res 2013;242:158–65.

66. Mannie ZN, Barnes J, Bristow GC, Harmer CJ, Cowen PJ. Memory impairment in young women at increased risk of depression: influence of cortisol and 5-HTT genotype. Psychol Med 2009;39(5):757–62.

67. Reneman L, Schilt T, de Win MM, et al. Memory function and serotonin transporter promoter gene polymorphism in ecstasy (MDMA) users. J Psychopharmacol 2006;20(3):389–99.

68. Sumner JA, Vrshek-Schallhorn S, Mineka S, et al. Effects of the serotonin transporter polymorphism and history of major depression on overgeneral autobiographical memory. Cognition Emotion 2014;28(5):947–58.

69. Sarosi A, Gonda X, Balogh G, et al. Association of the STin2 polymorphism of the serotonin transporter gene with a neurocognitive endophenotype in major depressive disorder. Prog Neuro-Psychopharmacol Biol Psychiatry 2008;32(7):1667–72.

70. El-Hage W, Phillips ML, Radua J, et al. Genetic modulation of neural response during working memory in healthy individuals: interaction of glucocorticoid receptor and dopaminergic genes. Mol Psychiatry 2013;18(2):174–82.

71. Baune BT, Ponath G, Rothermundt M, Riess O, Funke H, Berger K. Association between genetic variants of IL-1 beta, IL-6 and TNF-alpha cytokines and cognitive performance in the elderly general population of the MEMO-study. Psychoneuroendocrinology 2008;33(1):68–76.

72. Patel PD, Lopez JF, Lyons DM, Burke S, Wallace M, Schatzberg AF. Glucocorticoid and mineralocorticoid receptor mRNA expression in squirrel monkey brain. J Psychiatric Res 2000;34(6):383–92.

73. Bobinska K, Galecka E, Szemraj J, Galecki P, Talarowska M. Is there a link between TNF gene expression and cognitive deficits in depression? Acta Biochimica Polonica 2017;64(1):65–73.

74. Medina A, Seasholtz AF, Sharma V, et al. Glucocorticoid and mineralocorticoid receptor expression in the human hippocampus in major depressive disorder. J Psychiatric Res 2013;47(3):307–14.

75. Schubert KO, Stacey D, Air T, Baune BT. Peripheral blood gene expression analysis implicates B lymphocyte proliferation and ribosomal S26 transcripts in cognitive dysfunction in people with remitted major depression. J Affective Dis 2016;190:754–6.

76. Levenson JM, Sweatt JD. Epigenetic mechanisms in memory formation. Nature Rev Neurosci 2005;6(2):108–18.

77. Mateus-Pinheiro A, Pinto L, Sousa N. Epigenetic (de)regulation of adult hippocampal neurogenesis: implications for depression. Clin Epigen 2011;3:5.

78. Fujita N, Watanabe S, Ichimura T, et al. MCAF mediates MBDI-dependent transcriptional repression. Mol Cell Biol 2003;23(8):2834–43.

79. Fujita N, Watanabe S, Ichimura T, et al. Methyl-CpG binding domain 1 (MBD1) interacts with the Suv39h1-HP1 heterochromatic complex for DNA methylation-based transcriptional repression. J Biol Chem 2003;278(26):24132–8.

80. Allan AM, Liang XM, Luo YP, et al. The loss of methyl-CpG binding protein 1 leads to autism-like behavioral deficits. Human Mol Gen 2008;17(13):2047–57.

81. Machado-Vieira R, Ibrahim L, Zarate CA. Histone deacetylases and mood disorders: epigenetic programming in gene–environment interactions. Cns Neurosci Therapeutics 2011;17(6):699–704.

82. Guan JS, Haggarty SJ, Giacometti E, et al. HDAC2 negatively regulates memory formation and synaptic plasticity. Nature 2009;459(7243):55–60.

8

Clinical Characteristics of Emotional-Cognitive Dysfunction in Major Depressive Disorder

Thomas Beblo and Lorenz B. Dehn

Introduction

The main symptoms of major depressive disorder (MDD) affect patients' emotions (1, 2). Typically, patients experience excessive negative emotions such as depressed mood, sadness, anxiety, and anger. In addition, patients show diminished positive emotions (anhedonia) as well as decreased interest in and motivation for activities they formerly enjoyed (1, 2). Emotional dysfunctions in MDD are closely related to information processing and cognition. In agreement with increased negative emotions, cognitive theories of depression such as the model of Beck (3) suggest that depressed patients show biased processing of emotional information favouring negative content. Furthermore, depressive patients are hypersensitive to negative feedback and tend to ruminate; that is, they focus repetitively on dysphoric symptoms, their causes, and their consequences (4). It is known that these emotional dysfunctions have a negative impact on MDD patients' cognitive performance.

Emotional-Cognitive Dysfunctions

Reduced Motivation

According to Pizzagalli (5), several findings suggest that anhedonia is not only a main MDD symptom. Anhedonia also often precedes MDD and, thus, might be relevant for identifying individuals at risk. In the *Diagnostic and Statistical Manual of Mental Disorders,* 5th edn (DSM-5), anhedonia is defined as 'decreased interest and pleasure in most activities most of the day'. This definition indicates that, apart from the inability to feel pleasure, anhedonia also includes motivational deficits (6, 7).

The close relationship between anhedonia and motivation is also stressed by Barch et al. (8), linking hedonic experience and motivated behavioural response. The authors discuss six mechanisms with possible relevance for motivational deficits in depressed patients: 1) responsiveness to positive stimuli (reward); 2) reward prediction and wanting; 3) reward and reinforcement learning; 4) represent and update information about the hedonic properties and related information; 5) effort allocation; and 6) planning and goal-directed action. With respect to depression, most studies indicate reduced responsiveness to positive stimuli (mechanism 1), including primary rewards (e.g. food) and secondary rewards (money). A reduced responsiveness to positive stimuli was shown to be predictive for the future onset of depression (9). Once depression has developed, reduced responsiveness to positive stimuli is—as expected—closely related to symptoms of anhedonia (10).

Motivation also implies the anticipation and wanting of reward (mechanism 2). A study by Sherdell et al. (11) showed that in MDD this 'wanting' is even more reduced than 'liking' (mechanism 1). However, this seems only to be true if wanting is related to anticipated rewards ('approach motivation') but not to anticipated punishment or avoidance of punishment ('avoidance motivation') (12). Also, Trew (13) emphasized the importance of distinguishing between approach and avoidance motivation and summarized evidence for a disruption in approach motivation in depression. Approach motivation deficits predict depressive symptoms, episode duration, general functioning, average weekly depression, and time to recovery. That is, approach motivation deficits may contribute to the onset, experience, and maintenance of depression. Pizzagalli (5) summarized evidence that depressed patients generally expect less positive outcomes, which may explain reduced approach motivation. With respect to avoidance motivation, however, Trew (13) reviewed studies indicating an increased avoidance activity in depression. While it is clear that decreased approach motivation is dysfunctional and contributes to anhedonia in depression, dysfunctional implications of increased avoidance motivation are less obvious. Trew pointed out that avoidance may lead to short-term relief but also to an exacerbation of the avoided (but not solved or accepted) problem that has originally led to depression. In addition, avoidance may direct attention away from positive stimuli and makes positive reinforcement for adaptive behaviour more unlikely. More generally, Hayes et al. (14) reviewed research demonstrating that many forms of psychopathology can be conceptualized as unhealthy efforts to escape and avoid emotions, thoughts, memories, and other experiences. Finally, Trew (13) suggested that approach and avoidance motivation are not independent but in an opposing relationship; that is, underactivation of one of these motivation systems strengthens the other system and vice versa.

Motivational deficits of depressed patients were not only found with respect to the ability to experience pleasure and the anticipation and wanting of pleasure but also with respect to the other motivational mechanisms described by Barch et al. (8). Barch et al. and Pizzagalli (5) summarized evidence for impaired reinforcement learning (mechanism 3) in depressed patients. That is, patients have problems in establishing functional behaviour that is related to positive consequences. Interestingly, this deficit appears primarily to affect implicit learning processes while explicit reinforcement learning seems to be intact. Depressed patients are also less willing to spend physical effort to receive rewards (mechanism 5). However, their willingness to spend cognitive effort has not been sufficiently investigated. In addition, depressed patients show impairments with respect to cognitive processes that are related to the update of information about hedonic properties of a stimulus (mechanism 4). With regard to cognitive processes that are related to planning and goal-directed action (mechanism 6), evidence of an impairment is less clear.

Negative Processing Bias

Negative Cognitive Bias

Cognitive models of depression suggest that the onset, maintenance, and recurrence of depressive episodes are related to a negative cognitive bias (15, 16). The influential model of Beck (3) claims that information processing in depression is biased by negative cognitive schemata. Schemata are typically characterized by negative and dysfunctional beliefs, e.g. to be convinced of one's own failure. These schemata serve as filters of contradicting information and facilitate the processing of consistent information and thus determine the depressive individual's interpretation of the environment. According to these schemata, patients with MDD consistently appraise themselves, the world, and their future with a negative view (17). In line with this approach, network models of mood and memory (18) posit that there are associations between 'mental nodes' which typically represent cognitive concepts, memories, or emotions. Nodes can be activated by internal or external stimuli, and this activation spreads to related nodes. In the case of depressed patients, a 'sadness node' might be linked to other nodes representing concepts such as 'failure' or 'being incompetent'. Thus, triggered sadness leads to spreading activation across the associative network and an increased activation of each of these related nodes, which then might cause biased processing congruent with the prevailing depressive emotion (19). Further cognitive frameworks have been proposed for depression (see 20, 21), suggesting enhanced elaboration of negative information (22, 23), negatively biased self-referential information (24), and impairments in cognitive control of negative contents (25). In agreement with these models, there is clearly evidence for a mood-congruent negative bias in depression involving all domains of information processing, such as attention, memory, interpretation, and feedback response.

Attention Bias

Research findings consistently indicate that patients with MDD selectively attend to negatively valenced emotional information. Such an attention bias has been observed toward mood-congruent cues, including socially threating words, negative and depression-related words, faces, and pictures (26, 27). Researchers found attention biases both in children at risk for depression and in currently depressed and remitted individuals, demonstrating their considerable relevance for depression (13). The attention bias disappears with shorter or masked stimulus presentations, pointing to a biased processing at later stages of the processing process (15). However, some studies suggest that depressed individuals do not more frequently attend to negative stimuli than do control participants. Instead, they exhibit difficulties in disengaging from negative stimuli once they capture their attention, possibly indicating the involvement of cognitive control processes (28). Difficulties in disengaging from negative material might lead to a maintained attention on mood-congruent information, causing recurrent ruminative thoughts (29). There are also studies suggesting that individuals with MDD do not only show greater difficulty in shifting attention away from negative stimuli; they may have general difficulties in shifting their attention from emotional to non-emotional stimuli, indicating a more general dysfunction of the attentional control network with a general bias toward emotionally relevant stimuli (30). However, these data are in conflict with studies demonstrating an attentional bias away from positively valenced stimuli (31).

Memory Bias

Memory performance depends on attention. Therefore, findings of an attentional bias in MDD suggest that depressed patients also exhibit a memory bias for emotionally negative stimuli. Indeed, Koster et al. (32) found that an attention bias for negative words predicted free recall of negative words in dysphoric subjects. A depression-related memory bias has been identified for the recognition of sad faces, the recall of negative self-referantial information, and negative or depressed words (13). The memory bias is more evident for explicit than for implicit memory and may only occur at later stages of processing—similar to the domain of attention (33, 34). However, severely impaired patients also show an implicit processing bias, indicating that depression-related information may even automatically be activated (35). In addition, research has shown that the mood-congruent memory bias in depression might be exacerbated by self-focused attention, such as rumination (36).

Autobiographical memory functioning in depression is not only biased by an enhanced recall of negative information but also by an enhanced recall of overgeneralized information (37): when depressed patients are asked to recall memories of specific autobiographical events, they are more likely than healthy controls to retrieve overgeneral memories that summarize a category of similar events. It was suggested that low recall specificity might function as a way of regulating affect, as it might help depressed individuals to avoid or minimize aversive emotions by recalling events in a less concrete way (37). Besides the involvement of functional avoidance, rumination processes and impaired executive control performance may also underlie and contribute to overgeneral memory in depression (38). It has been shown that overgeneralized autobiographical memory predicts longer durations of depressive episodes (16).

Interpretation Bias

Depressive patients also tend to interpret (ambiguous) information more negatively than non-depressed individuals (39). For instance, they have been found to evaluate ambiguous or neutral facial expressions as more sad and happy faces as neutral (27). This bias primarily appears to occur at later stages of processing and is less verifiable when quick and superficial appraisal is required (33). In addition, patients with MDD also demonstrate a moderate deficit in identifying and discriminating facial emotion in general (40).

Feedback Bias

In accordance with cognitive theories of depression, depressed individuals do not only judge their performance more negatively but also perceive and recall environmental feedback excessively negatively (41). For example, after cognitive testing, depressed individuals are more likely to remember the experience of failure and are less likely to recall success than non-depressed individuals (33). They also show a decreased task performance after error feedback, indicating a greater sensitivity to negative feedback (42). This sensitivity might be related to an impaired mechanism of top-down control of the prefrontal cortex over the amygdala (43). However, depressed patients reactions to failure may depend on the accuracy of feedback: a study by Murphy et al. (19) reported that patients show normal performance when negative feedback was accurate and informative while performance was impaired when feedback was misleading or ambiguous. Consistent with these studies, several studies also indicate that depressed patients are hyposensitive to positive feedback (44). In line with these and the abovementioned findings, Rottenberg and Hindash (45) conclude that there is substantial evidence for a lack of appropriate reactivity to all kind of emotional information in depression, regardless of its valence.

Rumination

Over the past three decades of research, rumination has evolved as an influential cognitive mechanism of depression. Among the many different definitions and models of rumination, possibly the most influential theory of rumination

(46) is Nolen-Hoeksema's response style theory (RST; 4, 36). In RST, rumination implies repetitively thinking about the causes, consequences, and symptoms of one's negative feelings. In contrast to worries, which are typically related to future events and anticipated threats, rumination is rather past- or present-orientated and focuses on issues of self-worth, meaning, and loss (36). Findings suggest that rumination can be conceptualized as a trait factor of MDD patients, being present even in the absence of dysphoria (47).

Ciesla and Roberts (48) suggest, in their interactive rumination model, separating the repetitive process of thinking (rumination) from its typically negative contents (negative cognitions) such as negative beliefs (3) and internal attributions for negative events (49). It is suggested that the reciprocal relationship between depressive affect and negative cognition is amplified by ruminating (repetitive thinking) about both the depressive affect itself and negative cognitions. The authors showed that the coexistence of rumination and negative cognitions are particularly associated with depression.

In their attentional scope model (ASM), Whitmer and Gotlib (50) explained why the incidence of rumination is increased when mood is negative. According to the ASM, mood changes the scope of attentional selection. Whereas positive mood appears to widen the attentional scope, negative mood narrows it; that is, less information from the environment and long-term memory is available and a more limited array of information is maintained in working memory. If less information is available, the likelihood increases that thoughts become repetitive (rumination). This ruminative cognitive style may be favourable in emotionally challenging situations because it allows individuals to maintain focus on the same important issue without being distracted by relatively irrelevant information. Similarly, Andrews and Thomson Jr. (51) summarized research indicating that rumination supports the cognitive analysis of complex problems; that is, breaking a problem into smaller components that are more manageable than the problem as a whole (although, however, rumination has deleterious effects on the implementation of problem solutions; 36). Thus, rumination may provide cognitive benefits, especially in trait-ruminators who are not depressed and individuals who do not have negative cognitions. However, once negative mood becomes stronger and negative cognitions occur, rumination leads to a downward spiral (48, 50); negative mood emphasizes attentional narrowing on negative cognitions, which in turn will further worsen mood. That is, under these conditions a ruminative (repetitive) thinking style becomes increasingly maladaptive.

Another (maladaptive) function of rumination might be that it implies the avoidance of negative mood (46). As already outlined, the avoidance of experiences has negative effects, especially in the long term (52). It can be assumed that ruminators may experience spontaneous relief as a result of rumination, but continuously worsen their general condition.

Given these mechanisms, it is not surprising that rumination was found pro-spectively to have a negative impact on depression severity, depression dur-ation, recovery from depression, and onset of (new) episodes of depression (48). Although originally it was assumed that rumination predicts duration of depres-sion more than depression onset (4), the opposite seems to be true in the light of recent studies (36). Nolen-Hoeksema et al. (36) speculate that, once depression has developed, other autonomous self-perpetuating processes may be dominant and determine depression duration, particularly state-dependent neurobiological processes (e.g. hypercortisolism).

Implications for Cognitive Performance

Emotional dysfunction in MDD is not only related to cognitive contents (e.g. negative memories) and cognitive style (e.g. rumination) but also to cognitive performance. Of note, apart from cognitive performance that is related to emo-tional stimuli (e.g. learning of positively valenced words), cognitive performance in general is also affected.

Rumination has a negative effect on cognitive performance in general, possibly by distracting the attention during cognitive tasks (53, 54). Accordingly, several studies show that rumination has a negative impact on the specificity of auto-biographical memory (55), inhibition (56), cognitive flexibility (57), problem-solving (53), and working memory (58). More specifically, the ASM (50) suggests rumination to be associated with a narrowed attentional scope, with difficulties in flexibly switching strategies if needed. Nolen-Hoeksema et al. (36) summar-ized evidence that ruminators (independent of mood) show more perseveration errors, stereotypical responses, and inhibition of previously useful strategies. That is, depressed ruminators have a double disadvantage for tasks that require a wide attentional scope; first, they are generally distracted by the negative contents of their ruminative thoughts and, second, their narrowed attentional scope inter-feres with these types of tasks.

However, according to the ASM, the narrowed attentional scope of ruminators may be preferable in some situations and tasks when a clear focus is required and distraction needs to be minimized. Based on empirical evidence, Andrews and Thomson Jr. (51) suggest that rumination particularly helps depressed patients to analyse complex problems that may have caused depression. According to the au-thors, depressed patients show a more realistic estimate of their situational con-trol (judgement of control tasks), they are less likely to be deceived by the external expression of an individual (e.g. diminished fundamental attribution error), and they often behave more rationally in decision-making situations. However, this advantage of rumination processing holds only true if rumination is related to the task but not to issues other than the task. Thus, ruminative thinking may improve cognitive performance if, first, the ruminative thinking style is directed to the task (and not to task-irrelevant contents) and, second, if the task primarily requires the application of analytical strategies (but not other cognitive functions such as flexibility) (51).

As described above, biased processing primarily appears to influence cognitive performance if emotional stimuli are involved. There is substantial evidence to suggest that depressive patients show decreased attention to information other than that which is negative (13). As attention is closely related to memory, it is not surprising that depressed patients predominantly recall negatively valenced stimuli (32) and that their memory performance is particularly impaired if distracting negative stimuli are present (59). In addition, depressed patients show a decreased recall of specific autobiographical memories (37). Generally, the depression-related impairment of information processing primarily occurs at later stages of processing (33). The negative processing bias also implies a less functional coping of failure (or assumed failure) during neuropsychological testing with negative effects on subsequent test performance (e.g. 42).

With respect to motivation, it is still unclear whether depressed patients show reduced motivation to accomplish neuropsychological tasks and—if yes—whether these motivational deficits account for cognitive impairment in depression. Research has provided conflicting results (60–62). In a neuropsychological study, Moritz et al. (63) found clear evidence of increased fears and concerns about the assessment of depressed patients compared to healthy control subjects but mixed results with respect to motivation. Possibly, motivational deficits seem to be more relevant for cognitive function in everyday situations rather than in an artificial neuropsychological testing environment (64). More research is clearly needed to estimate the impact of motivation on cognitive performance in depressed patients.

Conclusions

Increased negative affect, diminished positive emotions, and decreased approach motivation are cardinal symptoms of patients with MDD. These challenging emotional states are closely related to dysfunctional cognitive processes. In particular, there is evidence for a mood-congruent negative processing bias in MDD, including an elevated sensitivity to negative feedback. Depressive patients also show rumination; that is, they think intensively about the causes, consequences, and symptoms of their negative feelings. It is noteworthy that altered cognition in MDD is not only characterized by different thought contents and a modified way of thinking. Often, the challenging emotional states of patients with MDD are closely related to an impaired cognitive performance.

In our model of 'Depression-associated Cognitive Deficits' ('DECODE'; 65) we summarize several relationships between: (a) negative cognitive contents, motivational deficits, and dysfunctional cognitive style ('emotional cognition'); (b) emotion-related cognitive performance; and (c) cognitive performance in general ('cold cognition') in MDD (Figure 8.1) that were presented above. The depressed patients' fundamentally negatively biased view about themselves is related to modified reactions with respect to emotionally relevant information, e.g. a diminished executive control of negative information (arrow 1). The bias may also imply that depressive patients are more sensitive to negative feedback and less sensitive to positive feedback (arrow 2). This is also relevant for patients' motivation as motivation depends on the expectation of reward. Negative and stressful events in general and negative feedback in particular are known to trigger rumination (arrow 3). Rumination is harder to control for those patients who show a diminished executive control of negative thoughts (arrow 4). Further, altered processing of feedback and reduced motivation can negatively affect cognitive performance in general (arrow 5). Rumination also has a negative impact on cognitive performance in general (arrow 7) and autobiographical memory in particular ('overgeneralized memory', arrow 6). In addition, overgeneralized memory may also be a more direct consequence of diminished executive control (arrow 8). Finally, cognitive performance in general (e.g. executive functions) influences emotion-related cognitive performance (arrow 9). Further reverse causal

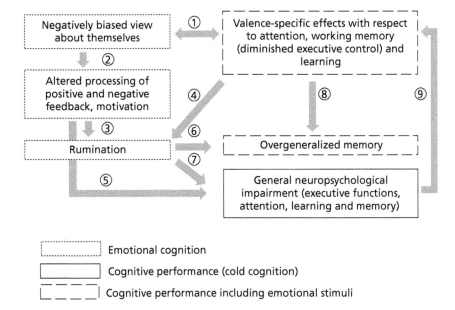

Figure 8.1 Model of Depression-associated Cognitive Deficits ('DECODE').

relations can be assumed as well, e.g. rumination may also emphasize the negative processing bias.

The massive relevance of the emotional-cognitive dysfunctions described in this chapter is also reflected by studies indicating that these dysfunctions are not just correlates of MDD but contribute to the onset, maintenance, and recurrence of MDD. Consequently, emotional-cognitive dysfunctions should be considered in psychotherapeutic MDD treatment programmes. As described in chapters 19–21, several existing programmes have incorporated the treatment of emotional-cognitive dysfunctions with different emphases.

References

1. American Psychiatric Association. *Diagnostic and Statistical Manual of Mental Disorders, Fifth Edition (DSM-5)*. Washington D.C.: American Psychiatric Association; 2013.

2. WHO. *The ICD-10 Classification of Mental and Behavioural Disorders. Clinical descriptions and diagnostic guidelines*. Geneva: WHO; 1992.

3. Beck AT. *Depression: Clinical, experimental and theoretical aspects*. New York: Harper and Row, 1967.

4. Nolen-Hoeksema S. Responses to depression and their effects on the duration of depressive episodes. J Abnorm Psychol 1991;100(4):569–82.

5. Pizzagalli DA. Depression, stress, and anhedonia: toward a synthesis and integrated model. Annu Rev Clin Psychol 2014;10:393–423.

6. Thomsen KR. Measuring anhedonia: impaired ability to pursue, experience, and learn about reward. Front Psychol 2015;6:1409.

7. Treadway MT, Zald DH. Reconsidering anhedonia in depression: lessons from translational neuroscience. Neurosci Biobehav Rev 2011;35(3):537–55.

8. Barch DM, Pagliaccio D, Luking K. Mechanisms underlying motivational deficits in psychopathology: similarities and differences in depression and schizophrenia. Curr Top Behav Neurosci 2016;27:411–49.

9. Bress JN, Foti D, Kotov R, Klein DN, Hajcak G. Blunted neural response to rewards prospectively predicts depression in adolescent girls. Psychophysiol 2013;50(1):74–81.

10. Liu WH, Wang LZ, Shang HR, et al. The influence of anhedonia on feedback negativity in major depressive disorder. Neuropsychologia 2014;53:213–20.

11. Sherdell L, Waugh CE, Gotlib IH. Anticipatory pleasure predicts motivation for reward in major depression. J Abnorm Psychol 2012;121(1):51–60.

12. McFarland BR, Klein DN. Emotional reactivity in depression: diminished responsiveness to anticipated reward but not to anticipated punishment or to nonreward or avoidance. Depress Anxiety 2009;26(2):117–22.

13. Trew JL. Exploring the roles of approach and avoidance in depression: an integrative model. Clin Psychol Rev 2011;31(7):1156–68.

14. Hayes SC, Wilson KG, Gifford EV, Follette VM, Strosahl K. Experimental avoidance and behavioral disorders: a functional dimensional approach to diagnosis and treatment. J Consult Clin Psychol 1996;64(6):1152–68.

15. Mathews A, MacLeod C. Cognitive vulnerability to emotional disorders. Annu Rev Clin Psychol 2005;1:167–95.

16. Gotlib IH, Joormann J. Cognition and depression: current status and future directions. Annu Rev Clin Psychol 2010;6;285–312.

17. Beck AT. The evolution of the cognitive model of depression and its neurobiological correlates. Am J Psychiatry 2008;165(8):969–77.

18. Bower GH. Mood and memory. Am Psychol 1981;36(2);129.

19. Murphy FC, Michael A, Robbins TW, Sahakian BJ. Neuropsychological impairment in patients with major depressive disorder: the effects of feedback on task performance. Psychol Med 2003;33(3):455–67.

20. Power M, Dalgleish T. *Cognition and Emotion*. New York: Psychology Press; 2008.

21. Everaert J, Koster EH, Derakshan N. The combined cognitive bias hypothesis in depression. Clin Psychol Rev 2012;32(5):413–24.

22. Ingram RE. Toward an information-processing analysis of depression. Cognit Ther Res 1984;8(5):443–77.

23. Williams JMG, Watts FN, MacLeod C, Mathews A. *Cognitive Psychology and Emotional Disorders* (2nd ed.). Chichester, UK: Wiley; 1997.

24. Teasdale JD. Cognitive vulnerability to persistent depression. Cogn Emot 1988;2(3): 247–74.

25. Joormann J, Yoon KL, Zetsche U. Cognitive inhibition in depression. Appl Prev Psychol 2007;12(3):128–39.

26. Peckham AD, McHugh RK, Otto MW. A meta-analysis of the magnitude of biased attention in depression. Depress Anxiety 2010;27(12):1135–42.

27. Bourke C, Douglas K, Porter R. Processing of facial emotion expression in major depression: a review. Aust NZ J Psychiatry 2010;44(8):681–96.

28. Joormann J. Cognitive inhibition and emotion regulation in depression. Curr Dir Psychol Sci 2010;19(3):161–6.

29. Joormann J, Siemer M. Emotion regulation in mood disorders. In: Gross JJ (ed.). *Handbook of Emotion Regulation*. 2nd ed. New York, NY: Guilford Press New York; 2014; pp. 413–27.

30. Malhi GS, Byrow Y, Fritz K, et al. Mood disorders: neurocognitive models. Bipolar Disord 2015;17(S2):3–20.

31. Leppänen JM. Emotional information processing in mood disorders: a review of behavioral and neuroimaging findings. Curr Opin Psychiatry 2006;19(1): 34–9.

32. Koster EH, De Raedt R, Leyman L, De Lissnyder E. Mood-congruent attention and memory bias in dysphoria: exploring the coherence among information-processing biases. Behav Res Ther 2010;48(3):219–25.

33. Wisco BE. Depressive cognition: self-reference and depth of processing. Clin Psychol Rev 2009;29(4):382–92.

34. Kircanski K, Joormann J, Gotlib IH. Cognitive aspects of depression. Wiley Interdiscip Rev Cogn Sci 2012;3(3):301–13.

35. Ellwart T, Rinck M, Becker ES. Selective memory and memory deficits in depressed inpatients. Depress Anxiety 2003;17(4):197–206.

36. Nolen-Hoeksema S, Wisco BE, Lyubomirsky S. Rethinking rumination. Perspect Psychol Sci 2008;3(5):400–24.

37. Williams JMG, Barnhofer T, Crane C, et al. Autobiographical memory specificity and emotional disorder. Psychol Bull 2007;133(1):122.

38. Williams JMG. Capture and rumination, functional avoidance, and executive control (CaRFAX): three processes that underlie overgeneral memory, cognition and emotion. Cognition Emotion 2006;20:3–4, 548–68.

39. Dearing KF, Gotlib IH. Interpretation of ambiguous information in girls at risk for depression. J Abnorm Child Psychol 2007;37(1):79–91.

40. Kohler CG, Hoffman LJ, Eastman LB, Healey K, Moberg PJ. Facial emotion perception in depression and bipolar disorder: a quantitative review. Psychiatry Res 2011;188(3):303–9.

41. Murphy FC, Sahakian BJ, O'Carroll RE. Cognitive impairment in depression: psychological models and clinical issues. In: Ebert D, Ebmeier KP (eds). *New Models for Depression*. Basel: Karger Publishers; 1998: pp. 1–33.

42. Elliott R, Sahakian BJ, Herrod JJ, Robbins TW, Paykel ES. Abnormal response to negative feedback in unipolar depression: evidence for a diagnosis specific impairment. J Neurol Neurosurg Psychiatry 1997;63(1):74–82.

43. Tavares JVT, Clark L, Furey ML, Williams GB, Sahakian BJ, Drevets WC. Neural basis of abnormal response to negative feedback in unmedicated mood disorders. Neuroimage 2008;42(3):1118–26.

44. Roiser JP, Sahakian BJ. Hot and cold cognition in depression. CNS Spec 2013;18(3):139–49.

45. Rottenberg J, Hindash AC. Emerging evidence for emotion context insensitivity in depression. Curr Opin Psychol 2015;4:1–5.

46. Smith JM, Alloy LB. A roadmap to rumination: a review of the definition, assessment, and conceptualization of this multifaceted construct. Clin Psychol Rev 2009;29(2):116–28.

47. Roberts JE, Gilboa E, Gotlib IH. Ruminative response style and vulnerability to episodes of dysphoria: gender, neurotizism, and episode duration. Cognit Ther Res 1998;22(4):401–23.

48. Ciesla JA, Roberts JE. Rumination, negative cognition, and their interactive effects on depressed mood. Emotion 2007;7(3):555–65.

49. Abramson LY, Seligman MEP, Teasdale JD. Learned helplessness in humans: critique and reformulation. J Abnorm Psychol 1978;87:49–74.

50. Whitmer AJ, Gotlib IH. An attentional scope model of rumination. Psychol Bull 2013;139(5):1036–61.

51. Andrews PW, Thomson JA Jr. The bright side of being blue: depression as an adaptation for analyzing complex problems. Psychol Rev 2009;116(3):620–54.

52. Campbell-Sills L, Barlow DH, Brown TA, Hofmann SG. Effects of suppression and acceptance on emotional responses of individuals with anxiety and mood disorders. Behav Res Ther 2006;44(9):1251–63.

53. Donaldson C, Lam D. Rumination, mood and social problem-solving in major depression. Psychol Med 2004;34(7):1309–18.

54. Young KD, Erickson K, Drevets WC. Differential effects of emotionally versus neutrally cued autobiographical memories on performance of a subsequent cognitive task: effects of task difficulty. Front Psychol 2012;3:299.

55. Crane C, Barnhofer T, Visser C, Nightingale H, Williams JM. The effects of analytical and experiential rumination on autobiographical memory specificity in individuals with a history of major depression. Behav Res Ther 2007;45(12):3077–87.

56. Philippot P, Brutoux F. Induced rumination dampens executive processes in dysphoric young adults. J Behav Ther Exp Psychiatry 2008;39(3):219–27.

57. Watkins E, Brown RG. Rumination and executive function in depression: an experimental study. J Neurol Neurosurg Psychiatry 2002;72(3):400–2.

58. Joormann J, Gotlib IH. Updating the contents of working memory in depression: interference from irrelevant negative material. J Abnorm Psychol 2008;117(1):182–92.

59. Beblo T, Mensebach C, Wingenfeld K, et al. The impact of neutral and emotionally negative distraction on memory performance and its relation to memory complaints in major depression. Psychiatry Res 2010;178:106–11.

60. Benitez A, Horner MD, Bachman D. Intact cognition in depressed elderly veterans providing adequate effort. Arch Clin Neuropsychol 2011;26(3):184–93.

61. Richards PM, Ruff RM. Motivational effects on neuropsychological functioning: comparison of depressed versus nondepressed individuals. J Consult Clin Psychol 1989;57:396–402.

62. Scheurich A, Fellgiebel A, Schermuly I, Bauer S, Wolfges R, Muller MJ. Experimental evidence for a motivational origin of cognitive impairment in major depression. Psychol Med 2008;38(2):237–46.

63. Moritz S, Stockert K, Hauschildt M, et al. Are we exaggerating neuropsychological impairment in depression? Reopening a closed chapter. Expert Rev Neurother 2017;17(8):839–46.

64. Lahr D, Beblo T, Hartje W. Cognitive performance and subjective complaints before and after remission of major depression. Cogn Neuropsychiatry 2007;12(1):25–45.

65. Beblo T. Neuropsychological impairment of patients with depression. In: Baune BT, Tully P. (eds). *Cardiovascular Diseases and Depression—Treatment and Prevention in Psychocardiology*. Heidelberg: Springer; 2016: pp. 123–44.

9

Neurocircuitries of Emotion Processing Affected in Major Depressive Disorder

Anjali Sankar and Cynthia H.Y. Fu

Introduction

Affect and cognition had been considered to be mutually exclusive constructs and their neural correlates had been independently examined in depression. The interaction between affect and cognition has become increasingly recognized as essential in the pathophysiology and in understanding the mechanisms of treatments.

Impairments in processing emotions are a core feature of major depressive disorder (MDD), which is generally characterized by maladaptive responses to negative emotional stimuli coupled with difficulty in sustaining positive emotional experiences. Although biases during emotion recognition in MDD are most evident when stimuli are presented for longer duration, allowing for extensive processing, emotion recognition difficulties can also be observed when emotions are processed subliminally using masked or brief presentations (<30 ms) of stimuli. In addition to maladaptive emotion recognition, individuals with MDD also tend to pay more attention to and show greater recollection of negative stimuli such as words (1, 2), images (3), and facial expressions (4). Such hyperresponsivity to emotional stimuli has also been shown to interfere with their cognitive processing (5). The negative emotional bias has been observed even during the recovery period (6, 7) and the presence of such biases at recovery is known to be a risk factor for relapse (8).

Affective cognition, or the response to affective stimuli during cognitive evaluation, involves many subprocesses, which include perception, recognition, and, in some instances, categorization and suppression of different emotions. Models have sought to delineate the neural correlates linked with the components of emotion processing: automatic recognition of the emotion, integration of somatic responses, and monitoring of the affective state (9–11). To describe the neurocircuitries of emotion processing affected in MDD, we will focus on paradigms designed to measure neural responses to emotionally valenced stimuli.

Emotion Processing Paradigms

Functional magnetic resonance imaging (fMRI) studies have typically used standardized series of facial expressions (Ekman series [12]), or pictures (International Affective Picture System (IAPS) (13) to examine the neural correlates of emotion processing. Facial emotion processing tasks are considered to involve non-conscious (subliminal, or implicit) or conscious (explicit) processes predominantly. Subliminal emotion processing tasks typically involve extremely short presentations of emotional faces masked with a neutral stimulus, such that the visual stimulus does not elicit a conscious, voluntary perception of emotion. In an implicit facial expression task, the explicit instruction may be task-irrelevant, such as identifying the gender of the presented face while the emotional expression is processed unintentionally or implicitly. Explicit emotion processing tasks, on the other hand, would most likely have explicit instructions to identify the emotion expressed by the presented face. Explicit facial processing tasks involve active recognition and labelling of emotions, and therefore compete with attentional demands. The advantage of implicit and subliminal emotion processing tasks is that they are more reliable and consistent and may help tease out early, rapid, automatic processes from more elaborate conscious processes, albeit implicit tasks may also engage active suppression mechanisms (14, 15).

Similar to facial expressions paradigms, tasks that utilize affective images involve either covert or overt processing of emotions. Some paradigms entail passive viewing of affective pictures or require a task-irrelevant response, such as identifying whether the picture depicted a scene that was indoors or outdoors, while other tasks require active recognition and categorization of emotions. These paradigms, although developed to delineate the neurocircuitries involved in emotion processing, are likely to involve cognitive processes at least to some extent. Hence, the neural correlates of emotion processing are best understood when cognitive demands elicited by these tasks are considered, which in part are influenced by duration of the presented stimulus, level of task difficulty, and the task instructions.

Neural Models of Healthy Emotion Processing and Regulation

Neural networks involved in processing and regulating emotions are crucially implicated in the pathophysiology of MDD. Phillips and colleagues (10) proposed a model identifying the neural correlates of emotion processing. The model describes two different neural systems: the ventral and the dorsal systems. The ventral system comprises the amygdala, insula, ventral striatum, and ventral anterior cingulate (ACC) gyrus, ventrolateral and orbitofrontal cortex (OFC), important for identifying emotionally salient stimuli and producing an affective state. The dorsal system is where affective input can be influenced by cognitive processes and includes the hippocampus, dorsal ACC gyrus, dorsolateral prefrontal cortex (PFC) and dorsomedial PFC, important for voluntary regulation of the affective states.

Ochsner and Gross (16) proposed a neural basis of emotion regulation, based on cognitive and affective neuroscience models. Emotion regulation, or the cognitive control of emotion, is posited to involve interaction between top-down control of emotions as well as bottom-up emotion appraisal (16, 17). The bottom-up emotion appraisal component involves the amygdala and the basal ganglia, while the top-down system centres around the ACC, ventral, or dorsal prefrontal cortices (17).

Phillips and colleagues (10) revised their model to investigate the neural systems involved in both automatic and more voluntary emotion regulatory systems. They proposed that a ventromedial system consisting of the OFC, ACC, and dorsomedial PFC are involved in automatic aspects of emotion regulation, while the lateral prefrontal system (dorsolateral PFC and ventrolateral PFC) may subserve voluntary aspects of emotional regulation. These neural models have provided a theoretical framework to examine neural abnormalities associated with disorders characterized by emotional dysfunctions such as MDD.

Neurocircuitries of Emotion Processing Affected in Major Depressive Disorder: Evidence from Negative Face Processing Tasks

The amygdala plays a key role in processing emotions, and is important in emotion recognition, categorization, and emotion memory (18). Since optimal amygdala response is critical for healthy regulation of emotions, a substantial number of neuroimaging studies have sought to examine amygdalar responses in MDD in response to mood-congruent affective stimuli using whole brain and region-of-interest (ROI) approaches. Although the amygdala had been postulated to be primarily involved in processing threat-related stimuli, it is engaged by salient emotions of all valences (19). As a result, cross-sectional neuroimaging studies in MDD have utilized varied task stimuli, ranging from sad and angry facial expressions to unpleasant pictures and negative words, and varied presentation modes whereby instructions called for either unconscious or more explicit processing of emotions.

Findings from whole brain and ROI-based studies using facial expressions as cues showed heightened activations in the amygdala in response to subliminally processed sad (20) and threat-related (21) faces, as well as during implicit or unconscious processing of sad (14, 22, 23) and fearful/angry faces (24), and less consistently during explicit processing of negative facial expressions (25). There is limited evidence of differences between MDD and healthy participants have been reported in response to explicit facial recognition (26–29).

A region considered important in face processing is the fusiform gyrus (30). In MDD, greater fusiform activity is seen relative to controls in response to increasing the intensity of sad facial expressions that were subliminally (23) and implicitly (22) processed, indicating mood-congruent affective biases in MDD, albeit the reverse (that is, decreased activations in MDD relative to controls) were also observed during implicit processing of sad facial expressions (31) and angry and fearful faces (32). Activations in the fusiform gyrus may be modulated by emotional expressions as enhanced activations have been observed in response to increasing intensities of facial expressions, especially fearful ones (33). The enhanced sensitivity to emotional expressions may be through direct feedback signals from the amygdala to the visual cortex (33). The findings described above support behavioural evidence which shows that patients are more likely to attend to faces of increasing sadness compared to healthy controls (6, 19).

The ACC is an important component of the limbic system, but it is also engaged by tasks of cognitive demands, such as those involved in decision-making and reward-processing (34). Implicit processing of sad facial expressions was associated with enhanced activations in the ACC in MDD relative to healthy participants (14). The part of the ACC that is ventral to the genu of the corpus callosum (i.e. subgenual cingulate) is hyperactive in MDD in response to sad facial expressions (35). The findings of increased activity in the subgenual cingulate are consistent with resting state studies that show greater subgenual cingulate functional connectivity from this region (36), hinting at an underlying abnormality associated with depression that is independent of the nature of the tasks.

The posterior cingulate is an important region in the default mode network (DMN) (37, 38) and has functional connections with the limbic system (for a review, see [38]). It is also associated with episodic memory (40), shows activation in response to affective stimuli, both negative and positive (41), and plays a key role in regulating attention (39). Increased activation in the posterior cingulate has been found in patients with MDD relative to controls during implicit processing of sad facial expressions (14, 42). Increases in posterior cingulate activity may be more likely in response to treatment that potentiates the noradrenergic system. In support, studies have shown that, in patients with MDD who received either mirtazapine or venlafaxine, increased pretreatment activity in the posterior cingulate during sad facial processing was associated with better response to treatment (43). In our recent study, we found that a course of treatment with duloxetine, a dual-acting antidepressant that modulates noradrenergic and serotonergic systems, was associated with increases in posterior cingulate activity in patients with MDD (44). Even in healthy controls, acute administration of a noradrenergic receptor inhibitor (NRI) was associated with increased posterior cingulate activity during processing of emotional pictures (45). A comparison of selective serotonin reuptake inhibitor (SSRI) and NRI classes of antidepressants in healthy controls showed that acute administration of reboxetine (an NRI) led to increases in the posterior cingulate, a finding not seen with citalopram (an SSRI), which was more associated with prefrontal modulations (46).

The neural abnormalities seen in the amygdala in MDD are also observed in other limbic and paralimbic structures, including the insula, hippocampus, and parahippocampal gyrus during subliminal presentations as well as implicit processing of sad facial expressions (23, 31), fearful and angry faces (32), and expressions of disgust (22).

There is some consensus that MDD may be associated with enhanced behavioural and striatal responses to negative stimuli (47), while anhedonia is likely to be associated with blunted response to negatively valenced feedback (48) as well as reduced activations in the ventral striatum in response to negative incentive stimuli (49). Whether anhedonia and depressed mood are distinct predictors of loss-related behaviour needs further investigation (50).

Studies in which facial expressions were used as cues have reported less consistent findings in the PFC. Processing of negative facial expressions was associated with decreased activations in the OFC, ventrolateral PFC, middle frontal/dorsolateral prefrontal and superior frontal gyrus (14, 32, 51–53). Decreased response in the lateral PFC suggests decreased capacity in MDD for regulating emotion-laden information, necessary for appropriate behavioural response. Yet sad facial processing has also been associated with increases in these regions (23, 27) as well as with no significant differences (54) in patients with MDD relative to controls.

Neurocircuitries of Emotion Processing Affected in Major Depressive Disorder: Evidence from Negative Non-Facial Processing Tasks

Abnormal corticolimbic activations observed in MDD during processing of negative facial cues are also seen in response to non-facial presentations. Patients with MDD not only show elevated amygdala activations in response to negative emotional stimuli (55) but the elevated amygdalar activations are also sustained over longer durations compared to healthy controls (56, 57). Moreover, participants with MDD do not show any sustained downregulation effect in the amygdala and their ability to downregulate amygdalar activations tends to decrease with increasing depression severity (58). Enhanced activations in MDD were also observed in other limbic regions, such as the hippocampus (55, 59) and insula, in response to negative pictures and sad mood induction (42) and dysfunctional attitudes (59). Additional increases were found in patients with MDD in the PFC, especially in the dorsolateral PFC (42, 55) and the medial PFC (55, 60). However, these results are far from consistent, as studies have also reported decreased pre-frontal activations in MDD in response to negative stimuli (31, 61).

There have also been some task-specific activations observed in MDD relative to healthy participants. A meta-analysis showed that the pregenual ACC showed increased activations in MDD during presentation of negative facial expressions, while negative non-facial stimuli were associated with reduced responses in this region in MDD, irrespective of emotional valence (47). Since the pregenual ACC is associated with integrating cognitive and emotional processes, these findings might suggest greater involvement of emotional and cognitive processes during presentations of facial expressions relative to pictorial stimuli (47).

Neurocircuitries of Emotion Processing Affected in Major Depressive Disorder: Evidence from Positive Emotion Processing Tasks

Although initial neuroimaging investigations in MDD focused on negative emotional stimuli, later studies extended this work to positive and rewarding stimuli to examine the preferential processing of negative emotions in relation to positive ones observed in MDD, as well as to understand anhedonia, another core feature of MDD characterized by blunted response to rewards. Although positive emotional stimuli are rewarding, reward responsivity and anhedonia are considered predominantly engaging cognitive processes. Hence, for the purposes of this chapter we examine anhedonia only if studies have used emotional stimuli to examine it.

In the processing of positive emotional stimuli, extant evidence, although with some notable exceptions (62, 63), suggests decreased activations in MDD relative to healthy participants in the amygdala, parahippocampal gyrus (53), ACC (31), fusiform gyrus (22), basal ganglia, and thalamus (62). Overall, the findings outline the functional network consistent with behavioural evidence that shows a preferential processing for negative over positive stimuli in MDD compared to healthy participants, who, in turn, attend more to positive stimuli (6).

It is postulated that depression is associated with impaired responses to positive or pleasurable stimuli in regions associated with reward and motivation, such as the ventral striatum, particularly the nucleus accumbens (NAcc), yet no group differences in NAcc activity in response to positive emotional stimuli have been reported (64, 65). These findings highlight that anhedonia may not be associated with reductions in hedonic capacity, but reduced ability to sustained positive feelings over time, which may reflect poor positive emotion regulation (66). In support, Heller and colleagues (67) showed that patients with MDD and healthy controls did not differ in NAcc activity while upregulating positive affect during the initial scan, but they were unable to sustain NAcc activity with time, unlike healthy controls, who showed constant engagement. This is in contrast with findings from negative emotional processing studies whereby patients with MDD rather than healthy controls show sustained amygdalar activity in MDD that continued even after task presentation. In other words, both groups showed amygdalar response, but individuals with MDD continued to show activations even in the presence of a non-emotion task (56).

Neurobiological Markers

Whether neural responses to emotional stimuli can be reliable markers of vulnerability to depression has been investigated in individuals at high risk for developing MDD. Individuals identified as at high risk based on their neuroticism scores showed linear increases in the fusiform gyrus and left middle temporal gyrus in response to increasing fearful expressions, while individuals in the low-risk group showed the opposite effect (68). Individuals at high risk also showed enhanced neural responses to other negative stimuli, such as negative words (68), coupled with impaired ACC modulation in response to both positive and negative emotional stimuli (69). These studies highlight that individuals at high risk show a pattern of neural dysfunction similar to that seen in MDD in an acute depressive episode, suggesting that neural responses to emotional stimuli may be putative biomarkers of vulnerability to MDD.

Although our understanding of the neurobiological correlates of depression has improved, one question is how to translate these findings to meaningful clinical applications. The current diagnostic system for depression is characterized by significant heterogeneity. There are multiple potential combinations of clinical features that do not necessarily represent biological subtypes. Diagnostic biomarkers could aid in the early identification in high-risk individuals.

For neuroimaging findings to be biomarkers, it is important that classification measures have high predictive accuracy and confidence levels that can be applied to individual subjects (70, 71). Multivariate pattern analysis integrates the subtle and spatially distributed alterations into models, learning to categorize the patterns and then to identify them in new data. It is possible to create such models using machine learning methods and to then identify the subtypes in MDD at the individual level based on patterns of brain alterations. It is likely that a number of biological subtypes comprise the current clinical diagnosis of major depression and others are potential predictors of clinical outcome, including models which incorporate cognitive impairments (72-74).

Conclusion

Interactions between affective processing and cognitive control are crucial for healthy functioning, and dysfunctions in these circuits might underlie emotion regulation difficulties evident in MDD. Neuroimaging studies have revealed impairments in widespread regions; these are evident in the first episode and are supported by neuropathological abnormalities. Models have sought to distinguish the neural circuitry associated with recognition of the emotion, integration of somatic responses, and monitoring of the affective state. Future research should consider inclusion of individualized stimuli as these could enhance the ecological value and salient engagement of emotion processing circuits. These offer the potential to develop biomarkers for the identification of MDD subtypes and predictors of clinical outcome.

References

1. Bradley BP, Mogg K, Williams R. Implicit and explicit memory for emotion-congruent information in clinical depression and anxiety. Behav Res Ther 1995;33(7):755–70.

2. Donaldson C, Lam D, Mathews A. Rumination and attention in major depression. Behav Res Ther 2007;45(11):2664–78.

3. Eizenman M, Lawrence HY, Grupp L, et al. A naturalistic visual scanning approach to assess selective attention in major depressive disorder. Psychiatry Res 2003;118(2):117–28.

4. Ridout N, Astell A, Reid I, Glen T, O'Carroll R. Memory bias for emotional facial expressions in major depression. Cognition Emotion 2003;17(1):101–22.

5. Joormann J, Gotlib IH. Updating the contents of working memory in depression: interference from irrelevant negative material. J Abnormal Psychol 2008;117(1):182.

6. Joormann J, Gotlib IH. Selective attention to emotional faces following recovery from depression. J Abnormal Psychol 2007;116(1):80.

7. Bhagwagar Z, Cowen PJ, Goodwin GM, Harmer CJ. Normalization of enhanced fear recognition by acute SSRI treatment in subjects with a previous history of depression. Am J Psychiatry 2004;161(1):166–8.

8. Bouhuys AL, Geerts E, Gordijn MC. Depressed patients' perceptions of facial emotions in depressed and remitted states are associated with relapse: a longitudinal study. J Nervous Mental Dis 1999;187(10):595–602.

9. Mayberg HS. Limbic-cortical dysregulation: a proposed model of depression. J Neuropsychiatry Clin Neurosci 1997;9(3):471–81.

10. Phillips ML. Understanding the neurobiology of emotion perception: implications for psychiatry. Br J Psychiatry 2003;182:190–2.

11. Leppänen JM. Emotional information processing in mood disorders: a review of behavioral and neuroimaging findings. Curr Opinion Psychiatry 2006;19(1):34-9.

12. Ekman P, Friesen W. *Pictures of Facial Affect*. Palo Alto, CA: Consulting Psychologists, 1976.

13. Lang PJ, Bradley MM, Cuthbert BN. *International Affective Picture System (IAPS): Instruction manual and affective ratings*. University of Florida: The center for research in psychophysiology, 1999.

14. Fu CH, Williams SC, Cleare AJ, et al. Attenuation of the neural response to sad faces in major depression by antidepressant treatment: a prospective, event-related functional magnetic resonance imagingstudy. Arch Gen Psychiatry 2004;61(9):877-89.

15. Elliott R, Zahn R, Deakin JW, Anderson IM. Affective cognition and its disruption in mood disorders. Neuropsychopharmacology 2011;36(1):153.

16. Ochsner KN, Gross JJ. The cognitive control of emotion. Trends Cognitive Sci 2005;9(5):242-9.

17. Ochsner KN, Gross JJ. Cognitive emotion regulation: insights from social cognitive and affective neuroscience. Curr Dir Psychol Sci 2008;17(2):153-8.

18. Berntson GG, Bechara A, Damasio H, Tranel D, Cacioppo JT. Amygdala contribution to selective dimensions of emotion. Social Cognitive Affective Neurosci 2007;2(2):123-9.

19. Costafreda SG, Brammer MJ, David AS, Fu CH. Predictors of amygdala activation during the processing of emotional stimuli: a meta-analysis of 385 PET and fMRI studies. Brain Res Rev 2008;58(1):57-70.

20. Victor TA, Furey ML, Fromm SJ, Öhman A, Drevets WC. Relationship between amygdala responses to masked faces and mood state and treatment in major depressive disorder. Arch Gen Psychiatry 2010;67(11):1128-38.

21. Sheline YI, Barch DM, Donnelly JM, Ollinger JM, Snyder AZ, Mintun MA. Increased amygdala response to masked emotional faces in depressed subjects resolves with antidepressant treatment: an fMRI study. Biol Psychiatry 2001;50(9):651-8.

22. Surguladze S, Brammer MJ, Keedwell P, et al. A differential pattern of neural response toward sad versus happy facial expressions in major depressive disorder. Biol Psychiatry 2005;57(3):201-9.

23. Suslow T, Konrad C, Kugel H, et al. Automatic mood-congruent amygdala responses to masked facial expressions in major depression. Biol Psychiatry 2010;67(2):155-60.

24. Zhong M, Wang X, Xiao J, et al. Amygdala hyperactivation and prefrontal hypoactivation in subjects with cognitive vulnerability to depression. Biol Psychol 2011;88(2-3):233-42.

25. Peluso MA, Glahn DC, Matsuo K, et al. Amygdala hyperactivation in untreated depressed individuals. Psychiatry Research: Neuroimaging 2009;173(2):158-61.

26. Frodl T, Scheuerecker J, Schoepf V, et al. Different effects of mirtazapine and venlafaxine on brain activation: an open randomized controlled fMRI study. J Clin Psychiatry 2011;72(4):448.

27. Scheuerecker J, Meisenzahl EM, Koutsouleris N, et al. Orbitofrontal volume reductions during emotion recognition in patients with major depression. J Psychiatry Neurosci: JPN 2010;35(5):311.

28. Almeida JR, Versace A, Hassel S, Kupfer DJ, Phillips ML. Elevated amygdala activity to sad facial expressions: a state marker of bipolar but not unipolar depression. Biol Psychiatry 2010;67(5):414–21.

29. Townsend JD, Eberhart NK, Bookheimer SY, et al. fMRI activation in the amygdala and the orbitofrontal cortex in unmedicated subjects with major depressive disorder. Psychiatry Research: Neuroimaging 2010;183(3):209–17.

30. Adolphs R. Neural systems for recognizing emotion. Curr Opinion Neurobiol 2002;12(2):169–77.

31. Fu CH, Williams SC, Cleare AJ, et al. Neural responses to sad facial expressions in major depression following cognitive behavioral therapy. Biol Psychiatry 2008;64(6):505–12.

32. Ruhé HG, Booij J, Veltman DJ, Michel MC, Schene AH. Successful pharmacological treatment of major depressive disorder attenuates amygdala activation to negative facial expressions. An fMRI study. Dose-escalation in the picture. Pharmacological and imaging studies in depression. 2005;46:195.

33. Vuilleumier P, Pourtois G. Distributed and interactive brain mechanisms during emotion face perception: evidence from functional neuroimaging. Neuropsychologia 2007;45(1):174–94.

34. Shidara M, Richmond BJ. Anterior cingulate: single neuronal signals related to degree of reward expectancy. Science 2002;296(5573):1709–11.

35. Gotlib IH, Sivers H, Gabrieli JD, et al. Subgenual anterior cingulate activation to valenced emotional stimuli in major depression. Neuroreport 2005;16(16):1731–4.

36. Greicius MD, Flores BH, Menon V, et al. Resting-state functional connectivity in major depression: abnormally increased contributions from subgenual cingulate cortex and thalamus. Biol Psychiatry 2007;62(5):429–37.

37. Fransson P, Marrelec G. The precuneus/posterior cingulate cortex plays a pivotal role in the default mode network: evidence from a partial correlation network analysis. Neuroimage 2008;42(3):1178–84.

38. Leech R, Kamourieh S, Beckmann CF, Sharp DJ. Fractionating the default mode network: distinct contributions of the ventral and dorsal posterior cingulate cortex to cognitive control. J Neurosci 2011;31(9):3217–24.

39. Leech R, Sharp D. The role of the posterior cingulate cortex in cognition and disease. Brain J Neurol 2014;137:12–32.

40. Wagner AD, Shannon BJ, Kahn I, Buckner RL. Parietal lobe contributions to episodic memory retrieval. Trends Cognitive Sci 2005;9(9):445–53.

41. Maddock RJ, Garrett AS, Buonocore MH. Posterior cingulate cortex activation by emotional words: fMRI evidence from a valence decision task. Human Brain Mapping 2003;18(1):30–41.

42. Keedwell PA, Andrew C, Williams SC, Brammer MJ, Phillips ML. A double dissociation of ventromedial prefrontal cortical responses to sad and happy stimuli in depressed and healthy individuals. Biol Psychiatry 2005;58(6):495–503.

43. Samson AC, Meisenzahl E, Scheuerecker J, et al. Brain activation predicts treatment improvement in patients with major depressive disorder. J Psychiatric Res 2011;45(9):1214–22.

44. Sankar A, Adams TM, Costafreda SG, Marangell LB, Fu CH. Effects of antidepressant therapy on neural components of verbal working memory in depression. J Psychopharmacol 2017;31(9):1176–83.

45. Outhred T, Hawkshead BE, Wager TD, Das P, Malhi GS, Kemp AH. Acute neural effects of selective serotonin reuptake inhibitors versus noradrenaline reuptake inhibitors on emotion processing: implications for differential treatment efficacy. Neuroscience Biobehav Rev 2013;37(8):1786–800.

46. Brühl AB, Jäncke L, Herwig U. Differential modulation of emotion processing brain regions by noradrenergic and serotonergic antidepressants. Psychopharmacology 2011;216(3):389–99.

47. Groenewold NA, Opmeer EM, de Jonge P, Aleman A, Costafreda SG. Emotional valence modulates brain functional abnormalities in depression: evidence from a meta-analysis of fMRI studies. Neuroscience Biobehav Rev 2013;37(2):152–63.

48. Steele J, Kumar P, Ebmeier KP. Blunted response to feedback information in depressive illness. Brain 2007;130(9):2367–74.

49. Stoy M, Schlagenhauf F, Sterzer P, et al. Hyporeactivity of ventral striatum towards incentive stimuli in unmedicated depressed patients normalizes after treatment with escitalopram. J Psychopharmacol 2012;26(5):677–88.

50. Luking KR, Neiman JS, Luby JL, Barch DM. Reduced hedonic capacity/approach motivation relates to blunted responsivity to gain and loss feedback in children. J Clin Child Adolescent Psychol 2017;46(3):450–62.

51. Frodl T, Scheuerecker J, Albrecht J, et al. Neuronal correlates of emotional processing in patients with major depression. World J Biol Psychiatry 2009;10(3):202–8.

52. Lee B-T, Seok J-H, Lee B-C, et al. Neural correlates of affective processing in response to sad and angry facial stimuli in patients with major depressive disorder. Prog Neuro-Psychopharmacol Biol Psychiatry 2008;32(3):778–85.

53. Lawrence NS, Williams AM, Surguladze S, et al. Subcortical and ventral prefrontal cortical neural responses to facial expressions distinguish patients with bipolar disorder and major depression. Biol Psychiatry 2004;55(6):578–87.

54. Fu CH, Costafreda SG, Sankar A, et al. Multimodal functional and structural neuroimaging investigation of major depressive disorder following treatment with duloxetine. BMC Psychiatry 2015;15(1):82.

55. Anand A, Li Y, Wang Y, et al. Activity and connectivity of brain mood regulating circuit in depression: a functional magnetic resonance study. Biol Psychiatry 2005;57(10):1079–88.

56. Siegle GJ, Steinhauer SR, Thase ME, Stenger VA, Carter CS. Can't shake that feeling: event-related fMRI assessment of sustained amygdala activity in response to emotional information in depressed individuals. Biol Psychiatry 2002;51(9):693–707.

57. Siegle GJ, Thompson W, Carter CS, Steinhauer SR, Thase ME. Increased amygdala and decreased dorsolateral prefrontal BOLD responses in unipolar depression: related and independent features. Biol Psychiatry 2007;61(2):198–209.

58. Erk S, Mikschl A, Stier S, et al. Acute and sustained effects of cognitive emotion regulation in major depression. J Neurosc 2010;30(47):15726–34.

59. Sankar A, Scott J, Paszkiewicz A, Giampietro V, Steiner H, Fu C. Neural effects of cognitive–behavioural therapy on dysfunctional attitudes in depression. Psychol Med 2015;45(7):1425–33.

60. Yoshimura S, Okamoto Y, Onoda K, Matsunaga M, Ueda K, Suzuki S-i. Rostral anterior cingulate cortex activity mediates the relationship between the depressive symptoms and the medial prefrontal cortex activity. J Affective Disord 2010;122(1):76–85.

61. Canli T, Sivers H, Thomason ME, Whitfield-Gabrieli S, Gabrieli JD, Gotlib IH. Brain activation to emotional words in depressed vs healthy subjects. Neuroreport 2004;15(17):2585–8.

62. Kumari V, Mitterschiffthaler MT, Teasdale JD, et al. Neural abnormalities during cognitive generation of affect in treatment-resistant depression. Biol Psychiatry 2003;54(8):777–91.

63. Beauregard M, Paquette V, Levesque J. Dysfunction in the neural circuitry of emotional self-regulation in major depressive disorder. Neuroreport 2006;17(8):843–6.

64. Epstein J, Pan H, Kocsis JH, et al. Lack of ventral striatal response to positive stimuli in depressed versus normal subjects. Am J Psychiatry 2006;163(10):1784–90.

65. Mitterschiffthaler M, Williams S, Walsh N, et al. Neural basis of the emotional Stroop interference effect in major depression. Psychol Med 2008;38(2):247–56.

66. Tomarkenand A, Keener AD. Frontal brain asymmetry and depression: a self-regulatory perspective. Cognition Emotion 1998;12(3):387–420.

67. Heller AS, Johnstone T, Shackman AJ, et al. Reduced capacity to sustain positive emotion in major depression reflects diminished maintenance of fronto-striatal brain activation. Proc Natl Acad Sci 2009;106(52):22445–50.

68. Chan SW, Norbury R, Goodwin GM, Harmer CJ. Risk for depression and neural responses to fearful facial expressions of emotion. Br J Psychiatry 2009;194(2):139–45.

69. Mannie ZN, Norbury R, Murphy SE, Inkster B, Harmer CJ, Cowen PJ. Affective modulation of anterior cingulate cortex in young people at increased familial risk of depression. Br J Psychiatry 2008;192(5):356–61.

70. Nouretdinov I, Costafreda SG, Gammerman A, et al. Machine learning classification with confidence: application of transductive conformal predictors to MRI-based diagnostic and prognostic markers in depression. Neuroimage 2011;56(2):809–13.

71. Fu CH, Steiner H, Costafreda SG. Predictive neural biomarkers of clinical response in depression: a meta-analysis of functional and structural neuroimaging studies of pharmacological and psychological therapies. Neurobiol Dis 2013;52:75–83.

72. Marquand AF, Mourão-Miranda J, Brammer MJ, Cleare AJ, Fu CH. Neuroanatomy of verbal working memory as a diagnostic biomarker for depression. Neuroreport 2008;19(15):1507–11.

73. Drysdale AT, Grosenick L, Downar J, et al. Resting-state connectivity biomarkers define neurophysiological subtypes of depression. Nat Med. 2017;23(1):28–38.

74. Fu CH, Costafreda SG. Neuroimaging-based biomarkers in psychiatry: clinical opportunities of a paradigm shift. Can J Psychiatry 2013;58(9):499–508.

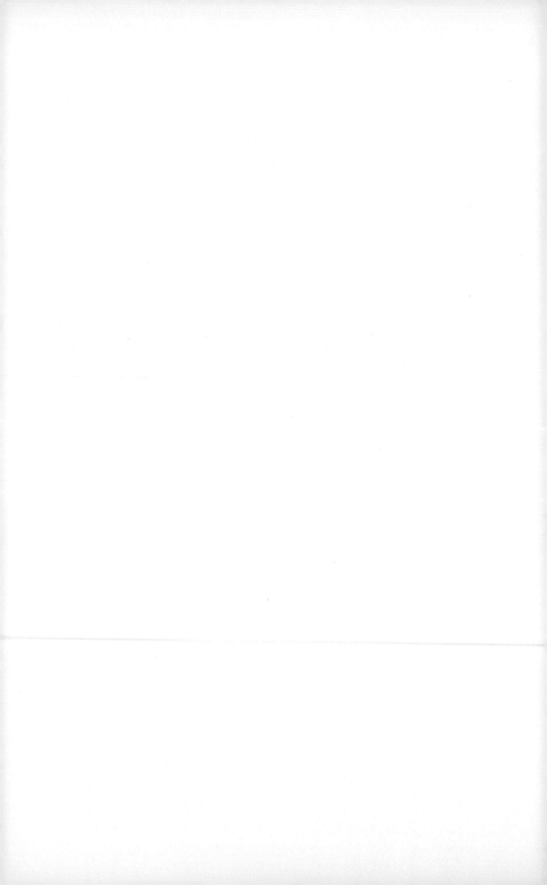

10

The Neural Circuitry of Negative Bias, Oversensitivity to Negative Feedback, and Hyposensitivity to Reward in Major Depressive Disorder

Oliver J. Robinson

Introduction

Major depressive disorder (MDD) is one of the most common causes of mental ill-health in the developed world. It carries substantial societal and economic costs but is, most importantly, exceptionally burdensome for individual sufferers (1). Contributing to this burden are disorder-related changes to the way that individuals process information; namely, the *cognitive symptoms* of MDD (2, 3). These symptoms include moderate impairments in executive function, memory, and attention (2), but also consistent alterations to emotional (i.e. affective) processing (3). Specifically, MDD is associated with increased sensitivity to negative information (and reduced sensitivity to rewards) across a range of cognitive processes. This sensitivity is referred to as *negative bias* and leads individuals to place disproportionate weight on negative life experiences (4).

The adverse impact of negative bias has been recognized for over half a century. Beck, the driving force behind modern psychological approaches to MDD treatment, referred to negative bias as 'negative schemata'. He argued that these schemata lead to cognitive distortions that he termed the 'negative cognitive triad'—a negative view of the self, the world, and the future (5). Decades of successful implementations of Beck's treatment—cognitive behavioural therapy (CBT)—which is built on this assumption, has borne out the importance of ameliorating negative bias in successful treatment of depression (4, 6). However, there are still many individuals who fail to respond to any of our current treatments, whether psychological or pharmacological. One of the reasons for this is that we still have a limited understanding of the biological underpinnings of negative affective bias and closing the treatment gap will likely require a better understanding of this underlying biology. In this chapter I provide a snapshot of

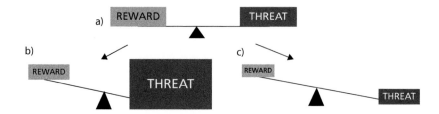

Figure 10.1 Two roads to negative bias. The scales of a) information processing can be tilted in favour of b) threats or away from c) rewards. In both cases this leads to a rightward—i.e. negative bias—tilt.

our current understanding of the neural circuitry of negative bias and where it might be heading in the future.

Measuring Cognitive Biases

Contemporary work extends Beck's self-report measures of negative bias into computerized cognitive tasks that measure implicit indices of negative affective bias (2, 3). Rather than asking patients with MDD to report whether they generally remember more negative experiences, for example, we can ask them to memorize affective information and then measure the accuracy of their recall. Alternatively, we can measure the speed at which they respond to negative stimuli on a reaction time task and thus attain a measure of their attentional biases. These systematic and less subjective measures of negative affective bias have also enabled exploration of the neural substrates of task performance.

Negative Affective Bias in Populations with Major Depressive Disorder

Affective processing describes the neural processing of environmental stimuli with survival value for the organism. We are attracted to positive, appetitive, rewarding stimuli (e.g. food, monetary gain, smiling faces) and repelled from negative, threatening, punishing stimuli (e.g. pain, monetary loss, angry faces) (4, 7). Negative affective bias therefore describes an increased focus on negative information relative to positive information across cognition: from perception, to attention, to memory. However, this bias can be driven from multiple directions; a bias toward threats can be driven by attenuated reward processing as well as oversensitive aversive processing (Figure 10.1) (8).

On the negative, threatening, side of the balance in Figure 10.1, a common observation is that patients with MDD show a 'catastrophic response to perceived failure'. That is to say, if they complete a cognitive task in which feedback is provided about correct/incorrect performance, their performance may be just as good as healthy controls up until the point at which they are informed that they have made a mistake. At this point their performance collapses. This is seen across a variety of cognitive tasks, even if the feedback is false (i.e. they are told they made a mistake even if they did not) (9–12) and it increases with symptom severity (10). Interestingly, it is also present in remitted individuals whose primary depressive mood symptoms have improved, suggesting that it could represent an underlying vulnerability (13). Ultimately, this suggests that negative feedback 'looms larger' in MDD and can even impair performance on unrelated cognitive tasks.

As highlighted in Figure 10.1, however, attenuated reward processing can also tip the scales of information processing toward negative affective bias. Individuals who have never been depressed generally demonstrate *positive* affective biases (3)—i.e. a bias *toward* rewarding information—which may serve to protect against environmental stress (5, 13, 14). However, this bias is generally absent in depressed individuals across cognition (15, 16). Perhaps the clearest demonstration of the balance between rewards and threats across never depressed and currently depressed individuals is the affective go–no-go reaction time task. Healthy individuals respond faster to positive relative to negative target words (a positive affective bias), whereas patients with MDD respond faster to negative relative to positive target words (a negative affective bias) (17, 18).

The advantage of measuring affective bias using cognitive tasks is that we can also ask patients and controls to complete the tasks in brain scanners and explore the neural activations associated with differential task performing. At the neuroimaging level, catastrophic response to perceived failure has been associated with attenuated subcortical caudate and ventromedial prefrontal cortical (PFC) responding in MDD (Figure 10.2a) (19), alongside increased subcortical amygdala response to aversive stimuli (20–22) (Figure 10.2b). A 2012 meta-analysis confirmed increased response to negative stimuli in the amygdala (Figure 10.2b), insula, and dorsal regions of the PFC (Figure 10.2a) alongside lower response in the dorsal striatum (Figure 10.2c) and dorsolateral prefrontal cortex in patients with MDD (23).

On the reward side, attenuation of appetitive processing in MDD is commonly associated with attenuations to subcortical striatal (Figure 10.2c) reward-based processing (24). In the Monetary Incentive Delay paradigm, for instance, participants are shown an expectancy cue, which informs them about how big a reward they will receive if they make a fast response. The task elicits reliable activation within the striatum in healthy individuals (25), but this activity is generally diminished in MDD (26). There is debate about whether attenuation is coupled

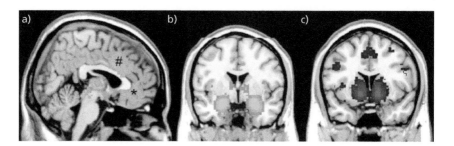

Figure 10.2 Functional localization of regions implicated in affective bias in major depressive disorder. The a) dorsal (#) and ventral (*) prefrontal regions and b) the amygdala are activated during the processing of negative stimuli (illustrated using the key word 'Fear' in neurosynth.org). In c) the striatum response to reward is shown (key word 'rewards' in neurosynth.org).

to anticipation of reward or receipt of reward, as well as which specific regions within the striatum are important (indeed, there are some prominent, well-powered null effects [27]), but currently published work together points to a role of the striatum in MDD neurobiology (26).

Moving beyond the localization studies highlighted above, however, recent work argues that ultimately it is the brain *circuits* that drive affective bias. In other words, the observed activity changes may actually reflect alterations to cortical–subcortical interactions. In particular, affective bias in MDD may be driven by a failure of ventral regions of the PFC (Figure 10.2a) to *dampen down* hyperactive subcortical amygdala (Figure 10.2b) responses to aversive stimuli (20, 28). This is in contrast with more dorsal (Figure 10.2a) regions of the PFC, which may be involved in the *excitation* of responses to aversive outcomes in subcortical regions such as the amygdala (28–30). As such, the balance between these competing circuits might drive the overall balance of aversive processing in MDD; more dorsal PFC regions promote hypersensitivity to punishment, while more ventral regions dampen punishment responding (31). This is supported by research in animal models (32) and will likely constitute an important avenue of research going forward.

Manipulating the Symptoms of Mood Disorders

There are nevertheless substantial discrepancies across studies in MDD (26). One reason for this is that the patient populations demonstrate high heterogeneity. Some individuals have comorbidities and some have non-overlapping symptoms within the broad MDD diagnostic checklist. To try to isolate the neural circuitry of affective bias in a more controlled manner we can turn to experimental manipulations in healthy control participants. This chapter focuses on two manipulations in particular: manipulating 1) the neuromodulator serotonin; and 2) psychological stress.

Serotonin manipulation

Serotonin (or 5-hydroxytryptamine [5-HT]) is the target of the most commonly used antidepressant medications—selective serotonin reuptake inhibitors (SSRIs) (14). The role that serotonin plays in the genesis of depressive symptoms remains unclear, but since the known cellular mechanism of SSRIs is to elevate availability of post-synaptic serotonin, it is plausible that *reduced* serotonin availability contributes to depression (33). Thus, experimentally reducing serotonin is thought to mimic, at least in part, the pharmacological environment of depression (34). One way to achieve serotonin reduction is through a dietary manipulation called *acute tryptophan depletion* (ATD). In this manipulation, participants consume a drink containing a balanced mix of amino acids, with the exception of tryptophan—the neurochemical precursor to serotonin. Following approximately 3–5 hours, tryptophan (and hence serotonin) levels are significantly depleted (34). On the flip side of the coin, participants can be provided with several weeks of SSRIs to study the impact of elevated serotonin (35) (for a comprehensive review of these effects see [14, 33]).

The earliest theories about the role of serotonin (36) highlighted its involvement in inhibitory control: in both rodents and non-human primates reduced serotonin can release (i.e. disinhibit) behavioural responding (36–38). In humans, early work showed that ATD could also result in inhibitory control failures (39, 40), but this was not borne out by later work in humans (41) and rodents (42). However, more recent studies adopted neutral tasks, i.e. they did not involve affective information. This is important because a large body of work also implicates serotonin in affective processing (43–47). ATD has been shown to *increase* aversive versus appetitive responding (48–52), whereas chronic SSRIs have been shown to *reduce* aversive versus appetitive responding (6, 53, 54). Moreover, in a task specifically designed to separate aversive and appetitive processing, it was shown that tryptophan depletion selectively increased aversive behavioural outputs while leaving reward behaviour intact (i.e. by tipping the aversive side of the scales in Figure 10.1) (44, 55).

Thus, serotonin is implicated in both inhibition and aversive processing. However, in practice these processes are rarely independent (7). This is because the prepotent (i.e. automatic) response to an aversive stimulus is inhibition (43). If I touch a hot pan and it burns my finger, it is adaptive to *inhibit* touching the pan again. Thus, reconciling the separate lines of evidence above, serotonin may be specifically involved in driving an adaptive inhibitory 'avoidance' bias, i.e. in-hibition of responses associated with aversive contexts (56, 57). Supporting this proposition, a task specifically designed to explore the impact of inhibiting aver-sive and appetitive responses used ATD to demonstrate that serotonin does not alter inhibition or aversive processing alone, but rather plays a key role in pro-moting inhibition in the context of aversive (and not appetitive) outcomes (58).

Serotonin manipulations can also be used to explore the neural circuitry of these effects. ATD during functional magnetic resonance imaging has shown in-creased amygdalar (59) and dorsal prefrontal responses (60) during aversive pro-cessing relative to placebo. Chronic SSRIs, on the other hand, lead to *decreased* amygdalar responses to negative stimuli (61, 62), as does greater 5-HT$_{1A}$ receptor availability (63, 64). These regions parallel the MDD studies highlighted above and suggest that serotonin function may play a role in the MDD pathophysiology. Indeed, as with the MDD literature, recent work has moved to explore cortical–subcortical circuitry. ATD in healthy controls has been shown to remove ventral PFC (Figure 10.2a*) putative inhibitory control over the amygdala (65) and in-crease dorsal PFC (Figure 10.2a#) putative excitatory control over the amygdala (66). Chronic SSRI treatment, on the other hand, may have the opposite effect; re-ducing dorsal prefrontal–amygdala excitatory control (67). Thus, the comparable patterns seen in MDD may be a result of altered serotonin systems in MDD; re-duced serotonin releases negative bias through *disinhibition of the neural circuits of aversive processing*, while SSRIs in MDD may serve to reverse this effect (14).

Stress Induction

An alternative way to mimic the symptoms of depression is to induce the emo-tional states that are found in these disorders. A common way to induce the state of stress associated with MDD is threat of unpredictable shock (68). This is a back-translated animal paradigm that reliably increases psychological, behav-ioural, and neurobiological indices of stress in humans (for a review see [68]). Behaviourally, as with MDD, this manipulation increases attention toward nega-tive outcomes (69–71) and increases the detection of negative information (29, 72, 73). Indeed, this is seen at very early stages of sensory processing (74–76), suggesting that stress serves to prioritize the downstream processing of negative information.

Threat of shock has also been consistently associated with *improved* inhibi-tory control. In particular, on a simple sustained attention task, where individuals are required to respond to frequent targets and inhibit this habitual response to infrequent targets, threat of shock reliably improves accuracy at withholding re-sponses (77–80). There is therefore a clear parallel with the serotonin literature reviewed above (see in the section on 'Serotonin manipulation'), where serotonin is thought to be involved in both inhibition and aversive processing. Recent work, therefore, tested whether threat of shock is also associated with aversive-linked inhibition. This work replicated the improved inhibition effect but extended it to demonstrate that threat of shock—as with the serotonin work reviewed in the section on 'Serotonin manipulation', above—selectively improves inhibition in aversive contexts (81). This leads to the proposal that stress—and perhaps, by extension, MDD and reduced serotonin—promotes 'Pavlovian' withdrawal biases. In other words, stress shifts decision-making toward more simple heuristics, i.e. *make an inhibitory response in the face of aversive outcomes* (81). Ultimately, this framework may help to reconcile many of the symptoms of MDD: it promotes a harm avoidance strategy that will be optimal under many natural (threatening) contexts (82) but which will be suboptimal in more complex or less threatening situations.

Work with threat of shock has also delineated some of the neural circuitry driving these effects. It has been shown to increase striatal response to aversive (rather than appetitive) stimuli (83), providing another mechanism by which striatal response can shift the balance from reward processing to aversive processing. Moreover, as with both the MDD and serotonin work, stress also appears to increase engagement of dorsal (Figure 10.2a) prefrontal–amygdala excitatory control circuits (29, 84, 85) while at the same time decreasing engagement of ventral (Figure 10.2a) prefrontal–amygdala inhibitory circuits (85). Thus, there is convergence across work with MDD and across the serotonin and stress manipulations. Ultimately, negative affective bias may be driven by the balance between excitatory and inhibitory cortical–subcortical circuits.

Future Work: Computational Approaches

Going forward, the computational approach to understanding negative affective bias—so-called *computational psychiatry*—is likely to grow in importance (86). In this approach, mathematical models of cognition are defined and tested (26, 86). These models can be constrained by biophysical plausibility, such that they are restricted to computations that can be generated by the underlying neurobiology. This approach may therefore help to bridge the neurobiological and behavioural levels of negative affective bias (26, 86). One influential model of serotonin function, for instance, is that it serves to 'prune the decision tree' (56, 57). This model uses Markov chains mathematically to formalize the idea that serotonin selectively inhibits chains of thoughts that lead to negative outcomes. Work supports the notion that healthy humans engage in this strategy (87) and that this may be impaired in MDD. Other computational work supports the proposition that MDD promotes basic Pavlovian heuristics (82). Specifically, individuals with mood and anxiety disorders show increased reliance on Pavlovian avoidance biases when subject to stress induced by threat of shock (82). This work used a reinforcement learning algorithm to provide mathematically defined predictions about how avoidance behaviours emerge (82). Work has also implicated reinforcement–learning processes in attenuated reward processing in MDD (68). Ongoing work will ultimately embed these computational accounts into the underlying neural circuitry, but such work is at present in its infancy.

Conclusion

Work across patients with MDD and selective manipulations implicate prefrontal–subcortical neural circuits in driving negative bias. Specifically, negative affective bias might be driven by *attenuated* striatal response to reward and *attenuated* ventral prefrontal control over negative processing in the amygdala. At the same time *elevated* dorsal prefrontal control over negative processing in the amygdala may *disinhibit* aversive processing. The ultimate balance of these neural circuits may therefore tip the balance of information processing away from rewards and toward threatening negative processing in MDD, and hence drive negative affective biases in cognition.

References

1. Fineberg NA, et al. The size, burden and cost of disorders of the brain in the UK. J Psychopharmacol 2013;27:761–70.

2. Rock P, Roiser J, Riedel W, Blackwell A. Cognitive impairment in depression: a systematic review and meta-analysis. Psychol Med 2014;44(10):2029–40.

3. Roiser JP, Elliott R, Sahakian BJ. Cognitive mechanisms of treatment in depression. Neuropsychopharmacology 2012;37(1):117–36.

4. Browning M, Holmes EA, Harmer CJ. The modification of attentional bias to emotional information: a review of the techniques, mechanisms, and relevance to emotional disorders. Cognitive, Affective, Behav Neurosci 2010;10(1):8–20.

5. Beck AT. *Depression: Clinical, experimental, and theoretical aspects.* Philadelphia: University of Pennsylvania Press, 1967.

6. Harmer CJ, Goodwin GM, Cowen PJ. Why do antidepressants take so long to work? A cognitive neuropsychological model of antidepressant drug action. Br J Psychiatry 2009;195(2):102–8.

7. Rangel A, Camerer C, Montague PR. A framework for studying the neurobiology of value-based decision making. Nature Reviews Neurosci 2008;9(7):545–56.

8. Eshel N, Roiser JP. Reward and punishment processing in depression. Biol Psychiatry 2010;68(2):118–24.

9. Beats B, Sahakian BJ, Levy R. Cognitive performance in tests sensitive to frontal lobe dysfunction in the elderly depressed. Psychol Med 1996;26(3):591–603.

10. Elliott R, et al. Neuropsychological impairments in unipolar depression: the influence of perceived failure on subsequent performance. Psychol Med 1996;26(5):975–89.

11. Elliott R, Sahakian B, Herrod J, Robbins T, Paykel E. Abnormal response to negative feedback in unipolar depression: evidence for a diagnosis specific impairment. J Neurol Neurosurg Psychiatry 1997;63(1):74–82.

12. Steffens DC, Wagner HR, Levy RM, Horn KA, Krishnan KRR. Performance feedback deficit in geriatric depression. Biol Psychiatry 2001;50(5):358–63.

13. Robinson O, Sahakian B. Recurrence in major depressive disorder: a neurocognitive perspective. Psychol Med 2008;38(3):315–18.

14. Robinson OJ, Roiser JP. The role of serotonin in aversive inhibition: behavioural, cognitive and neural perspectives. Psychopathology Rev 2015;3(1):29–40.

15. Joormann J, Gotlib IH. Is this happiness I see? Biases in the identification of emotional facial expressions in depression and social phobia. J Abnormal Psychol 2006;115(4):705.

16. Matt GE, Vázquez C, Campbell WK. Mood-congruent recall of affectively toned stimuli: a meta-analytic review. Clin Psychol Rev 1992;12(2):227–55.

17. Murphy F, Michael A, Robbins T, Sahakian B. Neuropsychological impairment in patients with major depressive disorder: the effects of feedback on task performance. Psychol Med 2003;33(3):455–67.

18. Erickson K, et al. Mood-congruent bias in affective go/no-go performance of unmedicated patients with major depressive disorder. Am J Psychiatry 2005;162(11):2171–3.

19. Elliott R, Sahakian B, Michael A, Paykel E, Dolan R. Abnormal neural response to feedback on planning and guessing tasks in patients with unipolar depression. Psychol Med 1998;28(3):559–71.

20. Tavares JVT, et al. Neural basis of abnormal response to negative feedback in unmedicated mood disorders. Neuroimage 2008;42(3):1118–26.

21. Victor TA, Furey ML, Fromm SJ, Öhman A, Drevets WC. Relationship between amygdala responses to masked faces and mood state and treatment in major depressive disorder. Arch Gen Psychiatry 2010;67(11):1128–38.

22. Victor TA, et al. The extended functional neuroanatomy of emotional processing biases for masked faces in major depressive disorder. PLoS One 2012;7(10):e46439.

23. Hamilton JP, et al. Functional neuroimaging of major depressive disorder: a meta-analysis and new integration of baseline activation and neural response data. Am J Psychiatry 2012;169(7):693–703.

24. Robinson OJ, Cools R, Carlisi CO, Sahakian BJ, Drevets WC. Ventral striatum response during reward and punishment reversal learning in unmedicated major depressive disorder. Am J Psychiatry 2012;169(2):152–9.

25. Wu CC, Samanez-Larkin GR, Katovich K, Knutson B. Affective traits link to reliable neural markers of incentive anticipation. Neuroimage 2014;84:279–89.

26. Robinson OJ, Chase H. Learning and choice in mood disorders: searching for the computational parameters of anhedonia. Comp Psychiatry 2017;1:208–33.

27. Rutledge RB, et al. Association of neural and emotional impacts of reward prediction errors with major depression. JAMA Psychiatry 2017;74(8):790–7.

28. Etkin A, Egner T, Kalisch R. Emotional processing in anterior cingulate and medial prefrontal cortex. Trends Cognitive Sci 2011;15(2):85–93.

29. Robinson OJ, Charney DR, Overstreet C, Vytal K, Grillon C. The adaptive threat bias in anxiety: amygdala–dorsomedial prefrontal cortex coupling and aversive amplification. Neuroimage 2012;60(1):523–9.

30. Robinson OJ, et al. The dorsal medial prefrontal (anterior cingulate) cortex–amygdala aversive amplification circuit in unmedicated generalised and social anxiety disorders: an observational study. Lancet Psychiatry 2014;1(4):294–302.

31. Kalisch R, Gerlicher AMV. Making a mountain out of a molehill: on the role of the rostral dorsal anterior cingulate and dorsomedial prefrontal cortex in conscious threat appraisal, catastrophizing, and worrying. Neurosci Biobehav Rev 2014;42:1–8.

32. Sierra-Mercado D, Padilla-Coreano N, Quirk GJ. Dissociable roles of prelimbic and infralimbic cortices, ventral hippocampus, and basolateral amygdala in the expression and extinction of conditioned fear. Neuropsychopharmacology 2011;36(2):529–38.

33. Harmer CJ. Serotonin and emotional processing: does it help explain antidepressant drug action? Neuropharmacology 2008;55(6):1023–8.

34. Crockett M, et al. Converging evidence for central 5-HT effects in acute tryptophan depletion. Mol Psychiatry 2012;17(2):121–4.

35. Harmer C, et al. Acute SSRI administration affects the processing of social cues in healthy volunteers. Neuropsychopharmacology 2003;28(1):148.

36. Soubrie P. Reconciling the role of central serotonin neurons in human and animal behavior. Behav Brain Sci 1986;9(2):319–35.

37. Evenden JL. Varieties of impulsivity. Psychopharmacology 1999;146(4):348–61.

38. Clarke HF, Dalley JW, Crofts HS, Robbins TW, Roberts AC. Cognitive inflexibility after prefrontal serotonin depletion. Science 2004;304(5672):878–80.

39. Crean J, Richards JB, de Wit H. Effect of tryptophan depletion on impulsive behavior in men with or without a family history of alcoholism. Behav Brain Res 2002;136(2):349–57.

40. LeMarquand DG, Benkelfat C, Pihl RO, Palmour RM, Young SN. Behavioral disinhibition induced by tryptophan depletion in nonalcoholic young men with multigenerational family histories of paternal alcoholism. Am J Psychiatry 1999;156(11):1771–9.

41. Clark L, Roiser J, Cools R, Sahakian B, Robbins T. Acute tryptophan depletion and the 5-HT transporter polymorphism do not modulate stop signal response inhibition. J Cognitive Neurosci 2005;88.

42. Eagle DM, et al. Serotonin depletion impairs waiting but not stop-signal reaction time in rats: implications for theories of the role of 5-HT in behavioral inhibition. Neuropsychopharmacology 2008;34(5):1311–21.

43. Robinson OJ, Overstreet C, Allen PS, Pine DS, Grillon C. Acute tryptophan depletion increases translational indices of anxiety but not fear: serotonergic modulation of the bed nucleus of the stria terminalis[quest]. Neuropsychopharmacology 2012;37(8):1963–71.

44. Robinson OJ, Cools R, Sahakian BJ. Tryptophan depletion disinhibits punishment but not reward prediction: implications for resilience. Psychopharmacology (Berl) 2012;219(2):599–605.

45. Cools R, Robinson OJ, Sahakian BJ. Acute tryptophan depletion in healthy volunteers enhances punishment prediction but does not affect reward prediction. Neuropsychopharmacology 2007;33:2291–9.

46. McCabe C, Mishor Z, Cowen PJ, Harmer CJ. Diminished neural processing of aversive and rewarding stimuli during selective serotonin reuptake inhibitor treatment. Biol Psychiatry 2010;67(5):439–45.

47. Harmer CJ. Serotonin and emotional processing: does it help explain antidepressant drug action? Neuropharmacology 2008;55:1023–8.

48. Murphy FC, Smith KA, Cowen PJ, Robbins TW, Sahakian BJ. The effects of tryptophan depletion on cognitive and affective processing in healthy volunteers. Psychopharmacology 2002;163(1):42–53.

49. Harrison AA, Everitt BJ, Robbins TW. Central serotonin depletion impairs both the acquisition and performance of a symmetrically reinforced go/no-go conditional visual discrimination. Behav Brain Res 1999;100(1–2):99–112.

50. Elliott R, Rubinsztein JS, Sahakian BJ, Dolan RJ. The neural basis of mood-congruent processing biases in depression. Arch Gen Psychiatry 2002;59(7):597–604.

51. Roiser JP, et al. Serotonin transporter polymorphism mediates vulnerability to loss of incentive motivation following acute tryptophan depletion. Neuropsychopharmacology 2006;31(10):2264–72.

52. O'Nions EJP, Dolan RJ, Roiser JP. Serotonin transporter genotype modulates subgenual response to fearful faces using an incidental task. J Cognitive Neurosci 2011;23(11):3681–93.

53. Harmer CJ, Hill SA, Taylor MJ, Cowen PJ, Goodwin GM. Toward a neuropsychological theory of antidepressant drug action: increase in positive emotional bias after potentiation of norepinephrine activity. Am J Psychiatry 2003;160(5):990–2.

54. Harmer CJ, Cowen PJ, Goodwin GM. Efficacy markers in depression. J Psychopharmacol 2011;25(9):1148–58.

55. Cools R, Robinson OJ, Sahakian B. Acute tryptophan depletion in healthy volunteers enhances punishment prediction but does not affect reward prediction. Neuropsychopharmacology 2007;33(9):2291–9.

56. Dayan P, Huys QJM. Serotonin in affective control. Annu Rev Neurosci 2009;32(1):95–126.

57. Dayan P, Huys QJM. Serotonin, inhibition, and negative mood. PLoS Computational Biology 2008;4(2):e4.

58. Crockett MJ, Clark L, Robbins TW. Reconciling the role of serotonin in behavioral inhibition and aversion: acute tryptophan depletion abolishes punishment-induced inhibition in humans. J Neurosci 2009;29(38):11993–9.

59. van der Veen FM, Evers EAT, Deutz NEP, Schmitt JAJ. Effects of acute tryptophan depletion on mood and facial emotion perception related brain activation and performance in healthy women with and without a family history of depression. Neuropsychopharmacology 2007;32(1):216–24.

60. Roiser JP, et al. Serotonin transporter genotype differentially modulates neural responses to emotional words following tryptophan depletion in patients recovered from depression and healthy volunteers. J Psychopharmacology 2012;26(11):1434–42.

61. Norbury R, Mackay CE, Cowen PJ, Goodwin GM, Harmer CJ. Short-term antidepressant treatment and facial processing: functional magnetic resonance imaging study. Br J Psychiatry 2007;190:531–2.

62. Harmer CJ, Mackay CE, Reid CB, Cowen PJ, Goodwin GM. Antidepressant drug treatment modifies the neural processing of nonconscious threat cues. Biol Psychiatry 2006;59(9):816–20.

63. Fakra E, Hyde LW, Gorka A, et al. Effects of htr1a c(−1019)g on amygdala reactivity and trait anxiety. Arch Gen Psychiatry 2009;66(1):33–40.

64. Fisher PM, Meltzer CC, Ziolko SK, Price JC, Hariri AR. Capacity for 5-HT1A-mediated autoregulation predicts amygdala reactivity. Nat Neurosci 2006;9(11):1362–3.

65. Passamonti L, et al. Effects of acute tryptophan depletion on prefrontal-amygdala connectivity while viewing facial signals of aggression. Biol Psychiatry 2012;71(1):36–43.

66. Robinson OJ, et al. The role of serotonin in the neurocircuitry of negative affective bias: serotonergic modulation of the dorsal medial prefrontal-amygdala 'aversive amplification' circuit. Neuroimage 2013;78:217–23.

67. McCabe C, et al. SSRI administration reduces resting state functional connectivity in dorso-medial prefrontal cortex. Mol Psychiatry 2011;16(6):592–4.

68. Robinson OJ, Vytal K, Cornwell BR, Grillon C. The impact of anxiety upon cognition: perspectives from human threat of shock studies. Frontiers in Human Neuroscience 2013;7:203.

69. Edwards MS, Burt JS, Lipp OV. Selective attention for masked and unmasked emotionally toned stimuli: effects of trait anxiety, state anxiety, and test order. Br J Psychol 2010;101(2):325–43.

70. Edwards MS, Burt JS, Lipp OV. Selective processing of masked and unmasked verbal threat material in anxiety: influence of an immediate acute stressor. Cognition Emotion 2006;20(6):812–35.

71. Cornwell BR, et al. Anxiety overrides the blocking effects of high perceptual load on amygdala reactivity to threat-related distractors. Neuropsychologia 2011;49(5):1363–8.

72. Grillon C, Charney DR. In the face of fear: anxiety sensitizes defensive responses to fearful faces. Psychophysiology 2011;48(12):1745–52.

73. Robinson OJ, Letkiewicz AM, Overstreet C, Ernst M, Grillon C. The effect of induced anxiety on cognition: threat of shock enhances aversive processing in healthy individuals. Cognitive, Affective, Behav Neurosci 2011;11(2):217.

74. Baas JM, Milstein J, Donlevy M, Grillon C. Brainstem correlates of defensive states in humans. Biol Psychiatry 2006;59(7):588–93.

75. Cornwell BR, et al. Neural responses to auditory stimulus deviance under threat of electric shock revealed by spatially-filtered magnetoencephalography. Neuroimage 2007;37(1):282–9.

76. Shackman AJ, Maxwell JS, McMenamin BW, Greischar LL, Davidson RJ. Stress potentiates early and attenuates late stages of visual processing. J Neurosci 2011;31(3):1156–61.

77. Robinson OJ, Krimsky M, Grillon C. The impact of induced anxiety on response inhibition. Front Human Neurosci 2013;7:69.

78. Grillon C, Robinson OJ, Mathur A, Ernst M. Effect of attention control on sustained attention during induced anxiety. Cognition Emotion 2016;30(4):700–12.

79. Wilson KM, Russell PN, Helton WS. Spider stimuli improve response inhibition. Consciousness Cognition 2015;33:406–13.

80. Torrisi S, et al. The neural basis of improved cognitive performance by threat of shock. Social Cog Affective Neurosci 2016;11(11):1677–86.

81. Mkrtchian A, Roiser JP, Robinson OJ. Threat of shock and aversive inhibition: induced anxiety modulates Pavlovian-instrumental interactions. J Exp Psychol: General 2017;146:1694–704.

82. Mkrtchian A, Aylward J, Dayan P, Roiser JP, Robinson OJ. Modeling avoidance in mood and anxiety disorders using reinforcement learning. Biol Psychiatry 2017;82:532–9.

83. Robinson OJ, Overstreet C, Charney DS, Vytal K, Grillon C. Stress increases aversive prediction-error signal in the ventral striatum. Proc Natl Acad Sci U S A 2013;110:4129–33.

84. Robinson OJ, et al. Anxiety-potentiated amygdala-medial frontal coupling and attentional control. Transl Psychiatry 2016;6:e833.

85. Vytal KE, Overstreet C, Charney DR, Robinson OJ, Grillon C. Sustained anxiety increases amygdala–dorsomedial prefrontal coupling: a mechanism for maintaining an anxious state in healthy adults. J Psychiatry Neurosci: JPN 2014;39(5):321–9.

86. Huys QJM, Maia TV, Frank MJ. Computational psychiatry as a bridge from neuroscience to clinical applications. Nat Neurosci 2016;19(3):404–13.

87. Huys QJ, et al. Bonsai trees in your head: how the Pavlovian system sculpts goal-directed choices by pruning decision trees. PLoS Comp Biol 2012;8(3):e1002410.

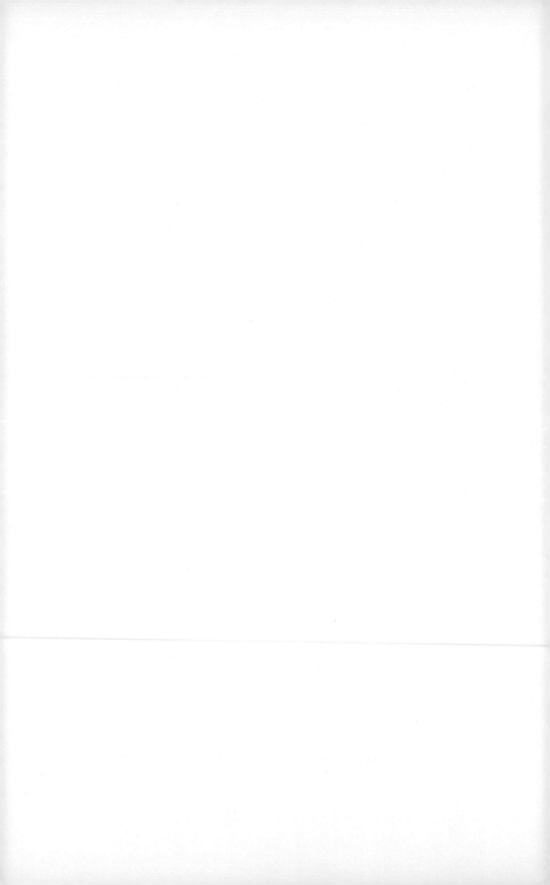

11

Reward Processing in Adolescents with Depression

Georgia O'Callaghan and Argyris Stringaris

Introduction

Depression has a high incidence in adolescence and is associated with impaired functioning in work and social and family life, as well as an increased risk of self-harm behaviour and suicide (1–3). Indeed, adolescent (15–19 years old) suicide rates increased to 14.2 per 100,000 population in 2015 (4), making it the second highest cause of death in 15–29-year-olds (5). Furthermore, while many adolescents achieve remission from their first depressive episode by adulthood, there is a high rate of recurrence throughout the lifespan, highlighting the need for more efficacious, targeted, treatments (6). A better appreciation of the causal mechanisms for the emergence of depression in adolescence may give rise to such treatments. One potential mechanism, which this review will focus on, is a model of reward dysfunction in the brain. We will outline the evidence for such a dysfunction in adolescent depression by summarizing evidence across neuroimaging modalities.

Reward Processing: Definitions and its Origins in the Brain

Rewards have been defined as stimuli (ranging from simple to complex objects, persons, or situations) for which organisms will expend effort in an attempt to approach or acquire (7). These may be necessary for survival, may induce a hedonic response, or may form part of a more complex sequence of goal-directed behaviours (8, 9). Reward processing involves an initial sensory detection, through the object's salience, followed by identification and valuation (7). Perceived value in the object results in the anticipation of the reward, or 'wanting', which facilitates motivational processes such as internal decisions and overt choices to expend effort to approach the object. If the reward is obtained this incurs a hedonic experience ('liking') and the value representation of the object is updated to inform future decision-making, reinforcing the approach behaviour (7, 10).

The ventral tegmental area (VTA), striatum, and features of the substantia nigra are considered to be at the centre of reward processing in the brain (8, 9). While the ventral striatum (VS; comprised of the nucleus accumbens [NAcc] and ventral aspects of the caudate and putamen) is most frequently implicated, there is increasing evidence of the role of dorsal caudal regions in reward processing (9, 11). These regions are part of a greater 'reward' circuit, which includes input from, and output to, frontal regions such as the orbital frontal cortex (OFC), ventromedial prefrontal cortex (VMPFC), anterior cingulate cortex (ACC), and dorsolateral prefrontal cortex (DLPFC), together with limbic structures such as the amygdala and hippocampus (9). Dopamine neurons within this reward circuit have received particular attention, as dopamine neuron firing has been shown to be associated with reward anticipation and consummation, motivation, and reward prediction (7, 9).

Evidence of a Causal Role of Reward Processing Aberrations in the Emergence of Depression in Adolescence

Reviews so far have not examined the causal involvement of reward processing in depression. Such an approach requires an assessment of the plausibility of the association between reward deficits and depression; the strength, consistency, and specificity of this relationship; whether its effects may be experimentally manipulated (for example, by examining the impact of treatments on reward processing); and its temporal properties, by reviewing longitudinal work. In this chapter we attempt to address each of these points, based on common criteria for establishing causality (12), to elucidate the potential causal role of reward processing deficits in the emergence of depression in adolescence.

Conceptual Links Between Reward Processing and Depression

Engaging with the environment leads to regular exposure to positive reinforcers, generating positive affect (13). Many features of depression, such as reduced energy, loss of appetite, social withdrawal, and a loss of enjoyment in activities, reduce engagement in the environment, leading to a reduction in positive affect (14). Anhedonia, a decreased interest in, or pleasure from, daily activities, is defined as one of the core diagnostic features of major depressive disorder (MDD), in addition to low mood (15). While not included in this definition, depression is often further conceptualized by deficits in volition and motivation (16). It has been suggested that such decreases are the result of aberrations in the brain's processing of rewarding stimuli (17, 18). Indeed, rodent models of depression suggest that impaired dopaminergic function in the NAcc may be causally related to the emergence (19) and severity (20) of anhedonic symptoms.

A meta-analysis by Keren, O'Callaghan, et al. (21) mapped clinical features of depression onto the phases of reward processing. During the first phase, 'prediction', the object is recognized as potentially rewarding, a process that involves existing knowledge about the value of objects. This prediction phase also encompasses the subjective experience of anticipation. The cost associated with obtaining the reward is then computed, leading to the decision to approach or avoid the reward ('decision' phase). Next is an 'action' phase, during which effort is expended, or a series of goal-directed behaviours are implemented, to acquire the reward. Once obtained, the reward is 'experienced', a phase that encompasses the consummation of a reward and the feelings that may be associated with it; it also entails the consolidation of this experience in memory, which may be accessed for future reward processing. These phases correspond to a clinical feature or symptom of depression and the role of reward processing deficits in each may be examined in translational research using behavioural and neuroimaging tasks, as seen in Figure 11.1.

The Strength and Consistency of Reward Processing Deficits in Adolescent Depression

In humans, there is strong evidence of striatal hypoactivation in unipolar depression during both anticipation and receipt of rewards (18). For example, a meta-analysis of functional magnetic resonance imaging (fMRI) studies of reward in depression (22) identified a reduced blood oxygen level-dependent (BOLD) response to monetary rewards in the caudate in participants with MDD relative to controls. This was present during both the anticipation and receipt of monetary rewards. Furthermore, this study noted relatively greater activity in frontal regions during reward anticipation, including the ACC and middle frontal gyrus.

However, as this meta-analysis (22) pooled the results of child/adolescent and adult samples, it is unclear how these effects may vary as a function of age. Indeed, studies of brain development from childhood to adulthood have revealed that reward processing regions undergo dramatic structural and functional changes throughout adolescence (23), with many suggesting that adolescents are more sensitive to rewards than children and adults (24, 25). As a result, it is useful to assess the extent to which a model of reward aberration may be applied to adolescent depression.

A subsequent review observed that reward processing deficits in youth MDD were primarily located in the bilateral caudate (both head and tail), whereas this hypoactivation was localized more ventrally, in the ventral caudate and NAcc, in adult MDD (26). Consistent with this, Olino et al. (27) reported greater

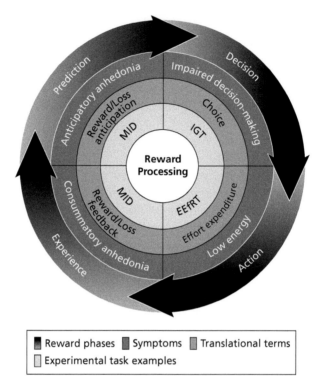

Figure 11.1 Phases of reward processing mapped onto clinical features of depression. EEfRT, Effort expenditure for rewards task; IGT, Iowa Gambling Task; MID, Monetary Incentive Delay.

activation of the caudate when anticipating a potential reward in healthy 8–16-year-olds compared to participants with MDD. Similarly, research has found reduced caudal activation in children and adolescents with MDD (aged 8–17 years) during both anticipation and outcome phases of reward processing compared to matched controls (28, 29). This pattern was determined to be stable across pre- to late-adolescence and to be linked to lower self-reported positive affect, collected daily throughout the study with ecological momentary assessment (EMA) (29). Decreased VS activity has been observed in healthy adolescents with increased risk for depression, most often characterized as the presence of a first-degree relative with MDD, such as a mother (30, 31). These findings are supported by Keren, O'Callaghan, et al. (21), who found reduced dorsal caudate activity in depression, which was further pronounced in youth samples.

Hypoactivation of the VS during reward tasks has also been reported in adolescent samples (32–34). The magnitude of these reductions in VS activity was also associated with greater depression severity (32) and may be specifically related to the presence and severity of anhedonia as a feature of depression (34). Stringaris et al. (34) observed that decreased VS activity was present in individuals with anhedonic symptoms, and anhedonia in conjunction with low mood, but not in those who reported low mood in the absence of anhedonia. Moreover, this reduction was most pronounced in individuals experiencing both symptoms.

While the analyses of many of the above studies were confined to striatal regions through a priori region-of-interest analyses (e.g. 27, 31)[1], broader examinations have implicated additional aberrations in regions associated with reward processing in adolescent depression. For instance, one study (30) reported reduced left insula and increased right insula recruitment in high-risk adolescent girls when anticipating rewards, and further reductions in the thalamus and anterior, middle, and posterior cingulate cortices upon reward receipt. There is evidence too of corresponding deficits in prefrontal recruitment during reward processing. Greater BOLD signal in adolescents with depression has been observed in prefrontal regions such as the DLPFC during reward outcome (29) and the medial prefrontal cortex when anticipating a potential reward (32).

Indeed, aberrant frontostriatal functional connectivity (FC) has been observed in depressed populations (35–37). At rest, ventral and dorsal aspects of the striatum appear to demonstrate dissociative patterns of FC with frontal regions in both adult and adolescent depression. Regions such as the VMPFC, subgenual ACC, and the dorsomedial prefrontal cortex (DMPFC) have been shown to have decreased FC with the ventral striatum at rest (35, 38). In contrast, depression severity has been associated with increased resting FC between prefrontal regions and the VS (37) and dorsal caudate across development (adolescents [35], youths 15–24 years [36], adults [38]).

An electroencephalogram (EEG)-derived signal, feedback-related negativity (FRN; also termed reward positivity [RewP]) has emerged as a powerful measure of reward processing (39, 40). These potentials may partially reflect striatal signals (41, 42) or the indirect influence of striatal signals on other neural regions (43, 44). Within adolescents, an association between depression and blunting of the FRN/RewP is reported (45–47), with the exception of one study that observed the opposite trend (48). This resulted in a significant combined effect size ($d=0.5$; see Figure 11.2) for a blunting of the FRN in adolescent depression in a meta-analysis by Keren, O'Callaghan, et al. (21). This is indicative of a reduced differentiation between frontal responses to gain and loss feedback, typically owing to a weaker response to gain feedback.

---

[1]Sharp et al. (31) reported no significant effects of familial risk on activation in a secondary whole-brain analysis at their a priori significance threshold.

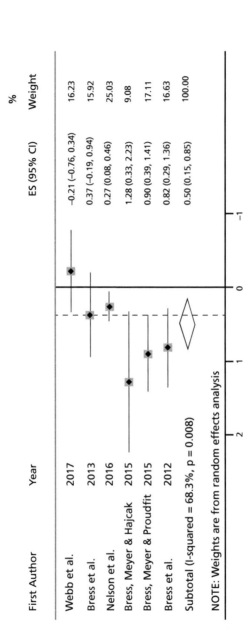

First Author	Year	ES (95% CI)	% Weight
Webb et al.	2017	−0.21 (−0.76, 0.34)	16.23
Bress et al.	2013	0.37 (−0.19, 0.94)	15.92
Nelson et al.	2016	0.27 (0.08, 0.46)	25.03
Bress, Meyer & Hajcak	2015	1.28 (0.33, 2.23)	9.08
Bress, Meyer & Proudfit	2015	0.90 (0.39, 1.41)	17.11
Bress et al.	2012	0.82 (0.29, 1.36)	16.63
Subtotal (I-squared = 68.3%, p = 0.008)		0.50 (0.15, 0.85)	100.00

NOTE: Weights are from random effects analysis

Figure 11.2 Meta-analysis of the feedback-related negativity and depression in adolescence. CI, Confidence interval; ES, Effect size.

Reproduced from *American Journal of Psychiatry*, 175, 11, Keren H, O'Callaghan G, Vidal-Ribas P et al, Reward Processing in depression: a conceptual and meta-analytic review across fMRI and EEG studies, pp. 1111–20. Copyright (2018) American Psychiatric Association.

Reward Processing Features as Precursors to Depression in Adolescence

Aberrant reward processing in the brain may be considered more than a scar of a depressive episode, as evidenced by longitudinal research. Longitudinal fMRI work in community-based samples suggests that striatal dysfunction in adolescence may be predictive of the emergence of depression. Morgan et al. (33) demonstrated that lower levels of baseline right caudate activity during reward anticipation in healthy adolescents were related to greater increases in depression symptomatology at a 2-year follow-up. In a large community sample of 1576 adolescents, Stringaris et al. (34) found that lower baseline VS activity predicted transition to subclinical or full depression in previously healthy adolescents after 2 years. Similarly, using a network-based FC approach, Pan and colleagues (37) found that left VS node strength to reward regions[2] at rest predicted depressive symptoms 3 years later in a community-based sample of over 600 adolescents, even when controlling for baseline depression.

Longitudinal EEG work by Nelson and colleagues found that blunting of reward feedback at baseline was associated with, and predictive of, greater dysphoria at follow-up in a community-based sample of 444 adolescent girls (49). Similarly, EEG recordings across two timepoints 2 years apart showed a stable association between blunted FRN and increased depression scores in children and young adolescents (46, 47). Reduced FRN has also been recorded in adolescents with high familial risk for MDD post sadness induction (50), which was predictive of a greater number of depressive symptoms at 2-year follow-up, even after controlling for baseline symptoms (51). In addition, baseline FRN has been reported to differentiate between individuals who subsequently experienced their first major depressive episode within the follow-up period from those who remained healthy (51). These studies may be considered further evidence of depression-related aberrations in the frontostriatal network employed during reward processing in adolescence and demonstrate how deficits may precede depression onset.

Reward Processing Aberrations in Other Disorders

Deficits in reward processing are held by many to be a mechanism that may cut across psychiatric disorders. Despite this, few studies have rigorously tested how features of reward aberrations may vary across disorders, and fewer have done so in adolescent populations. Given its high comorbidity with depression (52), we

---

[2]Left VS as the hub connecting the ACC, pre-supplementary motor area, right VS, bilateral thalamus, bilateral insula, VMPFC, VTA, and posterior cingulate cortex.

present here a selective overview of anxiety literature to examine whether these disorders demonstrate similar deficits.

Both similarities (reduced caudate activity) and differences (increased OFC activity in anxious individuals) have been found between adolescents with depression and anxiety, the latter of which was interpreted as an increased sensitivity to rewards (28). Further studies of adolescents with a developmental history of behavioural inhibition (a phenotype close to anxiety) showed increased striatal responses upon reward receipt compared to healthy controls, a pattern distinct from that seen in depression (53, 54). A study comparing depressed and socially anxious participants on a risk-adjustment task observed distinct patterns of behaviour between the two disorders: depression was associated with reductions in reward-seeking only at favourable reward probability levels, while social anxiety led to reductions in reward-seeking at low reward probabilities (55). Stringaris and colleagues (34) directly compared the association of depression and anxiety in a multivariate model with BOLD signal during the Monetary Incentive Delay task in adolescents. Only depression, but not anxiety, was associated with reduced activity in the VS during reward anticipation. Similarly, heightened left VS node strength was found to be specific to depression by Pan et al. (37), as no significant association with anxiety symptoms were observed. Finally, the FRN is thought to have a specific relationship to depressive symptoms, over the error-related negativity potential, which is increased in anxiety (45, 46).

Targeting Reward Mechanisms as Treatment for Depression

If deficits in reward processing are causally linked to the emergence or presence of depression, then treatments that target these may have particular clinical success. While some pharmacological (56–58) or psychological (59) interventions show promise in probing reward signal, they do not yet demonstrate that affecting reward modulates depressive symptoms. Furthermore, the majority of research in this area, with the exception of some therapeutic work, has been in adult depression, making the generalization of these findings to adolescent depression problematic.

An approach in pharmacological research is to probe reward mechanisms with compounds that influence dopamine, a key neurotransmitter involved in reward processing. Preclinical studies of the effects of antidepressants, such as desipramine, mianserin, imipramine, citalopram, and fluvoxamine, have observed enhanced dopamine functioning as a result of treatment, providing evidence to support the role of dopamine in depression (60). Work with pharmacological interventions in adult humans has demonstrated both efficacy at treating depressive symptoms and related changes in striatal functioning.

For example, a normalization effect of a 6-week, open-label treatment with escitalopram has been reported (58). Baseline hypoactivation of the VS when anticipating potential gains and losses in depressed participants, compared to healthy controls, was no longer present post-treatment (58). Similarly, depressed participants receiving amisulpride (believed to increase dopamine signalling through presynaptic autoreceptor blockade), exhibited increased striatal activation in response to monetary rewards, in addition to increased connectivity between the NAcc and middle cingulate (56). Finally, single infusions of ketamine have also been found to significantly, and rapidly, reduce anhedonic symptoms in depressed patients, an effect that was maintained for 3 days post infusion (57). Positron emission tomography scans of these participants revealed a significant association between anhedonic symptom decrease and increases in glucose metabolism in the hippocampus and dorsal ACC and decreases in the OFC and inferior frontal gyrus.

While these treatments suggest that targeting of aberrant reward processes may have antidepressant effects, further randomized, placebo-controlled trials are needed to establish the potential causal relationship between normalization of reward function and depressive symptom reduction. These studies should be conducted in conjunction with longitudinal follow-ups to track the progression of treatment as it relates to both changes in symptom profiles and alterations in neural reward processing.

Conclusion

Overall, the results summarized herein suggest a decreased sensitivity to anticipating and consuming reward in adolescent depression. For example, findings from the meta-analysis by Keren, O'Callaghan, et al. (21) provide strong support for the blunting of both fMRI and EEG measures of reward processing. Most informatively, though, longitudinal work appears to demonstrate that healthy adolescents with blunted neural responses to rewards may be at increased risk of developing MDD. This deviation from normative development, which is marked by increased sensitivity to rewards in healthy adolescents, may result in at-risk youths failing to pursue certain rewarding experiences, contributing to the development of depression (14, 33).

This result is attractively simple: decreased neural activity could underlie typical depressive symptoms such as diminished motivation, low energy levels, and reduced pleasure. However, more research in this area, such as whole-brain fMRI analyses to accompany region-of-interest work, is needed to establish the reliability of these findings and further test this hypothesis. It would also suggest that upregulating neural activity in these areas, through pharmacological or other interventions, could improve depressive symptoms. Early intervention research points to alterations in the function of frontal and striatal regions implicated in reward processing post treatment, coinciding with a reduction in depressive symptoms. Future randomized, placebo-controlled trials are needed to attempt to replicate these preliminary efforts. Furthermore, postulating depression to be a generalized inability to anticipate or perceive pleasure may be overly simplistic. There is surprisingly little work differentiating how deficits in reward processing may present between psychiatric disorders in adolescence, and even less using reward processing to parse the heterogeneity of adolescent depression.

Longitudinal and intervention-based studies have the greatest potential to establish whether reward processing deficits may play a causal role in the emergence of depression in adolescence. Such studies may also be used to establish whether normalization of aberrations result in depression remission and whether targeting these with treatment may prove more efficacious than current approaches.

References

1. Weissman MM, Wolk S, Goldstein RB, et al. Depressed adolescents grown up. J Am Med Assoc 1999;281(18):1707–13.

2. Birmaher B, Ryan ND, Williamson DE, et al. Childhood and adolescent depression: a review of the past 10 years. Part I. J Am Acad Child Adol Psychiatry 1996;35(11):1427–39.

3. Dunn V, Goodyer IM. Longitudinal investigation into childhood- and adolescence-onset depression: psychiatric outcome in early adulthood. Br J Psychiatry 2006;188:216–22.

4. CDC. QuickStats: Suicide Rates for Teens Aged 15–19 Years, by Sex—United States, 1975–2015 MMWR. Morb Mortal Wkly Rep 2017;66:8162017.

5. WHO. Mental health: Suicide data 2017. http://www.who.int/mental_health/prevention/suicide/suicideprevent/en/

6. Kovacs M, Obrosky S, George C. The course of major depressive disorder from childhood to young adulthood: recovery and recurrence in a longitudinal observational study. J Affective Disord 2016;203:374–81.

7. Schultz W. Dopamine reward prediction-error signalling: a two-component response. Nature Rev Neurosci 2016;17(3):183–95.

8. Schultz W. Multiple reward signals in the brain. Nature Rev Neurosci 2000;1(3):199–207.

9. Haber SN, Knutson B. The reward circuit: linking primate anatomy and human imaging. Neuropsychopharmacology 2010;35(1):4–26.

10. Berridge KC, Robinson TE, Aldridge JW. Dissecting components of reward: 'liking', 'wanting', and learning. Curr Opin Pharmacol 2009;9(1):65–73.

11. Haruno M, Kuroda T, Doya K, et al. A neural correlate of reward-based behavioral learning in caudate nucleus: a functional magnetic resonance imaging study of a stochastic decision task. J Neurosci 2004;24(7):1660–5.

12. Hill AB. The environment and disease: association or causation? Proc R Soc Med 1965;58(5):295–300.

13. Davidson RJ. Affective style, mood, and anxiety disorders: an affective neuroscience approach. In: Davidson RJ (ed.). *Anxiety, Depression, and Emotion.* Oxford; New York: Oxford University Press, 2000; pp. 88–108.

14. Davey CG, Yücel M, Allen NB. The emergence of depression in adolescence: development of the prefrontal cortex and the representation of reward. Neurosci Biobehav Rev 2008;32(1):1–19.

15. DSM-5. *Diagnostic and Statistical Manual of Mental Disorders,* Fifth Edition. Arlington, VA: American Psychiatric Association; 2013.

16. Kendler KS. The phenomenology of major depression and the representativeness and nature of DSM criteria. Am J Psychiatry 2016;173(8):771–80.

17. Kessel EM, Klein DN. Depressivity and anhedonia. In: Ziegler-Hill V, Marcus DK. (eds). *The Dark Side of Personality: Science and practice in social, personality, and clinical psychology.* Washington, DC: American Psychological Association; 2016.

18. Barch DM, Pagliaccio D, Luking K. Mechanisms underlying motivational deficits in psychopathology: similarities and differences in depression and schizophrenia. Curr Top Behav Neurosci 2016;27:411–49.

19. Di Chiara G, Loddo P, Tanda G. Reciprocal changes in prefrontal and limbic dopamine responsiveness to aversive and rewarding stimuli after chronic mild stress: implications for the psychobiology of depression. Biol Psychiatry 1999;46(12): 1624–33.

20. Gorwood P. Neurobiological mechanisms of anhedonia. Dialogues Clin Neurosci 2008;10(3):291–9.

21. Keren H, O'Callaghan G, Vidal-Ribas P, et al. Reward processing in depression: a conceptual and meta-analytic review across electrophysiological and fMRI studies. Am J Psychiatry 2018;175(11):1111–20.

22. Zhang WN, Chang SH, Guo LY, Zhang KL, Wang J. The neural correlates of reward-related processing in major depressive disorder: a meta-analysis of functional magnetic resonance imaging studies. J Affective Disord 2013;151(2):531–9.

23. Casey BJ, Getz S, Galvan A. The adolescent brain. Dev Rev 2008;28(1):62–77.

24. Ernst M, Pine DS, Hardin M. Triadic model of the neurobiology of motivated behavior in adolescence. Psychol Med 2006;36(3):299–312.

25. Braams BR, van Duijvenvoorde ACK, Peper JS, Crone EA. Longitudinal changes in adolescent risk-taking: a comprehensive study of neural responses to rewards, pubertal development, and risk-taking behavior. J Neurosci 2015;35(18):7226–38.

26. Kerestes R, Davey CG, Stephanou K, Whittle S, Harrison BJ. Functional brain imaging studies of youth depression: a systematic review. NeuroImage: Clinical 2014;4:209–31.

27. Olino TM, McMakin DL, Dahl RE, et al. 'I won, but I'm not getting my hopes up': depression moderates the relationship of outcomes and reward anticipation. Psychiatry Res 2011;194(3):393–5.

28. Forbes EE, Christopher May J, Siegle GJ, et al. Reward-related decision-making in pediatric major depressive disorder: an fMRI study. J Child Psychol Psychiatry 2006;47(10):1031–40.

29. Forbes EE, Hariri A, Martin S, et al. Altered striatal activation predicting real-world positive affect in adolescent major depressive disorder. Am J Psychiatry 2009;166(1):64–73.

30. Gotlib IH, Hamilton JP, Cooney RE, Singh MK, Henry ML, Joormann J. Neural processing of reward and loss in girls at risk for major depression. Arch Gen Psychiatry 2010;67(4):380–7.

31. Sharp C, Kim S, Herman L, Pane H, Reuter T, Strathearn L. Major depression in mothers predicts reduced ventral striatum activation in adolescent female offspring with and without depression. J Abnorm Psychol 2014;123(2):298–309.

32. Forbes EE, Ryan ND, Phillips ML, et al. Healthy adolescents' neural response to reward: associations with puberty, positive affect, and depressive symptoms. J Am Acad Child Adolesc Psychiatry 2010;49(2):162–72; e1–5.

33. Morgan JK, Olino TM, McMakin DL, Ryan ND, Forbes EE. Neural response to reward as a predictor of increases in depressive symptoms in adolescence. Neurobiol Dis 2013;52:66–74.

34. Stringaris A, Belil PVR, Artiges E, et al. The brain's response to reward anticipation and depression in adolescence: dimensionality, specificity, and longitudinal predictions in a community-based sample. Am J Psychiatry 2015;172(12):1215–23.

35. Gabbay V, Ely BA, Li Q, et al. Striatum-based circuitry of adolescent depression and anhedonia. J Am Acad Child Adolescent Psychiatry 2013;52(6):628–41.

36. Kerestes R, Harrison BJ, Dandash O, et al. Specific functional connectivity alterations of the dorsal striatum in young people with depression. NeuroImage: Clin 2015;7:266–72.

37. Pan PM, Sato JR, Salum GA, et al. Ventral striatum functional connectivity as a predictor of adolescent depressive disorder in a longitudinal community-based sample. Am J Psychiatry 2017;174(11):1112–19.

38. Furman DJ, Hamilton JP, Gotlib IH. Frontostriatal functional connectivity in major depressive disorder. Biol Mood Anxiety Disord 2011;1:11.

39. Hajcak G. The reward positivity: from basic research on reward to a biomarker for depression. Psychophysiology 2015;52(4):449–59.

40. Hajcak G, Moser JS, Holroyd CB, Simons RF. It's worse than you thought: the feedback negativity and violations of reward prediction in gambling tasks. Psychophysiology 2007;44(6):905–12.

41. Carlson JM, Foti D, Mujica-Parodi LR, Harmon-Jones E, Hajcak G. Ventral striatal and medial prefrontal BOLD activation is correlated with reward-related electrocortical activity: a combined ERP and fMRI study. NeuroImage 2011;57(4):1608–16.

42. Foti D, Weinberg A, Dien J, Hajcak G. Event-related potential activity in the basal ganglia differentiates rewards from nonrewards: temporospatial principal components analysis and source localization of the feedback negativity. Human Brain Mapping 2011;32(12):2207–16.

43. Holroyd CB, Coles MGH. The neural basis of human error processing: reinforcement learning, dopamine, and the error-related negativity. Psychol Rev 2002;109(4):679–709.

44. Luu P, Tucker DM, Derryberry D, Reed M, Poulsen C. Electrophysiological responses to errors and feedback in the process of action regulation. Psychol Sci 2003;14(1):47–53.

45. Bress JN, Meyer A, Hajcak G. Differentiating anxiety and depression in children and adolescents: evidence from event-related brain potentials. J Clin Child Adolescent Psychol 2015;44(2):238–49.

46. Bress JN, Meyer A, Proudfit GH. The stability of the feedback negativity and its relationship with depression during childhood and adolescence. Dev Psychopathol 2015;27(4 Pt 1):1285–94.

47. Bress JN, Smith E, Foti D, Klein DN, Hajcak G. Neural response to reward and depressive symptoms in late childhood to early adolescence. Biol Psychol 2012; 89(1):156–62.

48. Webb CA, Auerbach RP, Bondy E, Stanton CH, Foti D, Pizzagalli DA. Abnormal neural responses to feedback in depressed adolescents. J Abnorm Psychol 2017;126(1):19–31.

49. Nelson BD, Perlman G, Klein DN, Kotov R, Hajcak G. Blunted neural response to rewards as a prospective predictor of the development of depression in adolescent girls. Am J Psychiatry 2016;173(12):1223–30.

50. Foti D, Kotov R, Klein DN, Hajcak G. Abnormal neural sensitivity to monetary gains versus losses among adolescents at risk for depression. J Abnorm Child Psychol 2011;39(7):913–24.

51. Bress JN, Foti D, Kotov R, Klein DN, Hajcak G. Blunted neural response to rewards prospectively predicts depression in adolescent girls. Psychophysiology 2013;50(1):74–81.

52. Kendler KS. Major depression and generalised anxiety disorder. Same genes, (partly) different environments—revisited. Br J Psychiatry Suppl 1996;30:68–75.

53. Bar-Haim Y, Fox NA, Benson B, et al. Neural correlates of reward processing in adolescents with a history of inhibited temperament. Psychol Sci 2009;20(8):1009–18.

54. Casement MD, Guyer AE, Hipwell AE, et al. Girls' challenging social experiences in early adolescence predict neural response to rewards and depressive symptoms. Dev Cogn Neurosci 2014;8:18–27.

55. Rawal A, Riglin L, Ng-Knight T, Collishaw S, Thapar A, Rice F. A longitudinal high-risk study of adolescent anxiety, depression and parent-severity on

the developmental course of risk-adjustment. J Child Psychol Psychiatry Allied Disciplines 2014;55(11):1270–8.

56. Admon R, Kaiser RH, Dillon DG, et al. Dopaminergic enhancement of striatal response to reward in major depression. Am J Psychiatry 2017:174:378–86.

57. Lally N, Nugent AC, Luckenbaugh DA, Niciu MJ, Roiser JP, Zarate CA, Jr. Neural correlates of change in major depressive disorder anhedonia following open-label ketamine. J Psychopharmacol 2015;29(5):596–607.

58. Stoy M, Schlagenhauf F, Sterzer P, et al. Hyporeactivity of ventral striatum towards incentive stimuli in unmedicated depressed patients normalizes after treatment with escitalopram. J Psychopharmacol 2012;26(5):677–88.

59. Rice F, Rawal A, Riglin L, Lewis G, Lewis G, Dunsmuir S. Examining reward-seeking, negative self-beliefs and over-general autobiographical memory as mechanisms of change in classroom prevention programs for adolescent depression. J Affect Disord 2015;186:320–7.

60. Durlach-Misteli C, Van Res JM. Dopamine and melatonin in the nucleus accumbens may be implicated in the mode of action of antidepressant drugs. Eur J Pharmacol 1992;217(1):15–21.

12

Cognition-Related Brain Networks Underpin Cognitive, Emotional, and Somatic Symptom Dimensions of Depression

Genevieve Rayner

Introduction

Misery. Self-loathing. Bodily complaints. Difficulty concentrating. Anhedonia. A wish to die. These symptoms have been regarded as defining features of depression for millennia, and encapsulate three broad symptom dimensions that form the basis of current diagnostic criteria (1, 2). *Emotional symptoms* of dysphoria and anhedonia comprise the cardinal diagnostic features of the disorder. *Somatic symptoms* refer to the corporeal manifestations of depression, such as disturbed sleep and appetite, psychomotor changes, and excessive fatigue. Finally, *cognitive symptoms* take the form of maladaptive or distorted ways of thinking about the world, as well as issues with reduced attention, inhibition, and problem-solving that can manifest as symptoms such as intrusive thoughts, forgetfulness, and indecisiveness (see Chapters 4–7).

The emotional, somatic, and cognitive symptom dimensions of depression are currently framed as the product of abnormal function of large-scale brain networks (3–5), with different depressive symptom dimensions reflecting disturbance to different neurocognitive network substrates (5) (Box 12.1). These network abnormalities can stem from neurochemical-, structural-, or genetic-level mechanisms (5).

Growing evidence also points to the fundamental role played by abnormal *interactions* between cognition-related networks in depression. Systematic review of the functional neuroimaging literature indicates that different depression symptom dimensions are linked to a pathological imbalance between two major cognition-related networks, the autobiographic memory network (AMN) and the cognitive control network (CCN) (6). The aim of this chapter is to provide a model of depressive symptoms framed in terms of dysfunction between these two

---

Box 12.1 Side note: the Zeitgeist of brain networks

Brain networks are typically visualized using neuroimaging methodologies capable of mapping the brain's neural activity rather than its anatomical structure, such as functional magnetic resonance imaging (fMRI), positron emission tomography (PET), and magnetoencephalography (MEG). Their function can also be inferred indirectly through clinical methodologies, whereby abnormal behaviours or psychometric test performances index dysfunction in relevant networks.

'Brain networks' are stationary snapshots of fluctuating neural processing, typically derived by averaging the brain's connectivity or activation across a time series of data (5). This stationarity can be captured during a predefined cognitive or motor task, or while the participant is resting in the scanner (the so-called 'resting state').

Independent component analysis reveals at least half a dozen resting-state networks, some of which seem to be involved in cognitive domains such as sensorimotor planning, executive control, language, and memory (7). In contrast, when participants are asked to do an 'active' task in the scanner, patterns of regional coactivation emerge that are linked together to form a network whose function underpins the performance of that task, e.g. the 'autobiographic memory network', or the 'reading network'. This capacity is currently thought to arise from static neuronal architecture in conjunction with flexible connectivity. The static images produced by functional neuroimaging are therefore a heuristic. In reality, networks dynamically reconfigure moment-to-moment in response to changing internal and external demands (5).

---

neurocognitive networks. Specifically, it outlines: (i) the nature of altered AMN and CCN functioning in adults with depression; (ii) the abnormal dynamics between the AMN and CCN in depression; (iii) how abnormal AMN–CCN interrelationships have downstream effects on the regulation of emotion- and somatic-related brain networks; and (iv) how these altered network dynamics relate to the cognitive, emotional, and somatic symptom dimensions of depression.

A Neurocognitive Network Model of Depressive Symptoms
Cognitive Symptom Dimension

In essence, the neurocognitive network model links depressive symptoms to two brain networks. The AMN focuses on internal mental states but in depression is overactive, leading to pathological self-focus and symptoms such as rumination.

In contrast, the goal-directed CCN is underengaged in people with depression, leading to characteristic difficulties in efficiently attending and responding to environmental demands. The composition of these two networks can change between individuals and over time, plausibly accounting for both the idiosyncratic symptom presentation of depressive disorders and their fluctuating course.

Autobiographic Memory Network

The AMN is the most comprehensively described functional network (8). Commonly known in its resting-state form as the *default mode network*, it can be activated in a targeted manner by tasks requiring self-referential processing, including autobiographic memory, autonoetic consciousness, daydreaming, social cognition, and introspection (8–10). In the current chapter this network is referred to as the AMN rather than the default mode network for two reasons: (i) to more precisely reflect its best-documented function; and (ii) to avoid conflation of the default mode network with other resting-state networks (for expert commentary on this topic, see [9]). The research synthesized here examines the AMN in both its task-state and resting state forms.

In terms of its neuroanatomy[1], the AMN is a bilateral, widely distributed network with key nodes in (Figure 12.1 [10]):

- *The midline*: orbitomedial prefrontal cortex (PFC), dorsomedial PFC/rostral anterior cingulate cortex (ACC), hippocampus, posterior cingulate and retrosplenial cortex, precuneus.
- *Lateral cortical regions*: ventral PFC, anterior temporal cortex, temporoparietal junction.
- *Cerebellar* and *parietal* regions important for mental imagery.

A hyperactive AMN is characteristic of depression. Compared to healthy controls, individuals with depression show significantly increased activation of the AMN during self-referential cogitation, emotional processing, and at rest (see [6] for a review). Reduced deactivation is evident in the same regions when depressed patients attempt to perform externally focused tasks (see [6] for a review), giving the impression that the self-focused AMN is chronically overactive in depression. AMN hyperactivity is correlated with the severity of depression (13) and is accentuated during tasks designed to invoke sadness (14), providing a neurobiological substrate for the clinical impression that depressed patients have a bias for processing sad information. AMN hyperactivation is likely to be a marker of the morbid state of being depressed, given that antidepressant pharmacotherapy

---

[1] The anatomy of the networks described in this chapter was defined using the commonest consensus of seminal papers in the field (i.e. those cited >300 times, such as [7–9, 11, 12]).

restores normal attenuation of the AMN (15). This is true for selective serotonin reuptake inhibitors, serotonin–norepinephrine reuptake inhibitors, and atypical antidepressants such as bupropion (15), revealing that there may be multiple neurochemical modulators of AMN function.

Abnormal connectivity of AMN in depression. In addition to hyperactivity of the AMN in depression, connectivity within the AMN is also abnormal. Specifically, there is intensified intranetwork connectivity between anterior nodes of the AMN (PFC–ACC) as well as between the posterior nodes (see [6] for a review), with the dense AMN intraconnection associated with increased disease severity and duration (15). AMN hyperconnectivity is evident in first-episode, drug-naïve people with depression as well as in unmedicated individuals with dysthymic disorder (16, 17), indicating that AMN hyperconnectivity is evident at the onset of a spectrum of depressive diseases and is not iatrogenic. Moreover, AMN hyperconnectivity normalizes after treatment with serotonin–norepinephrine reuptake inhibitors (16) and, together with hyperactivation, may comprise an objective, neurobiological marker of disease remission or treatment response.

Clinical features of AMN dysfunction. Hyperactivity and hyperconnectivity of the AMN have been linked to a characteristic feature of depression: failure to downregulate self-critical introspective thinking. For instance, meta-analytic findings show hyperconnectivity between the AMN and subgenual PFC in people with depression that is associated with increasing levels of depressive rumination (18). These features are evident even at the first episode of depression, prior to the commencement of antidepressant treatment (19), providing potential neurobiological substrates for features of depression such as increased self-focus, brooding, inner conflict, suicidal ideation, less self-serving attribution styles, and rumination (20–22).

Altered AMN functioning may also undermine the formation of an autobiography in people with depression. Impoverished recall of events from one's own life is a robust behavioural vulnerability factor for depression and its recurrence (23), and altered AMN activation is evident during autobiographical memory processing in patients with first-episode, unmedicated, and remitted depression (see [6] for a review). Consistent with cognitive models of depression (24), the hypothesized function of this diminished specificity for past events is to blunt the emotional experience of the memory, or to passively avoid it.

In sum, functional neuroimaging findings suggest that the AMN of people with depression is hyperactive and shows altered internal connectivity from the onset of the disorder. AMN dysfunction is associated with disordered thinking styles characteristic of depression and is seemingly reversible with antidepressant pharmacotherapy.

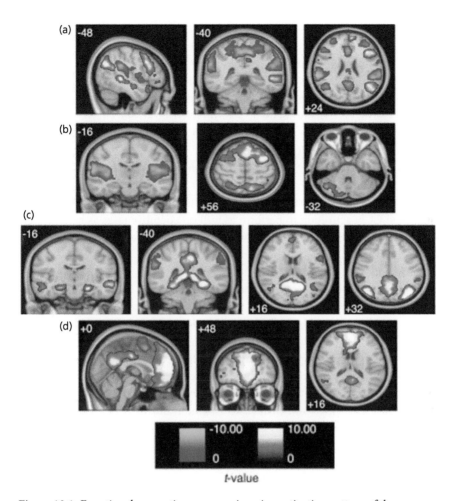

Figure 12.1 Functional magnetic resonance imaging activation pattern of the autobiographic memory network (AMN) in healthy controls during a task-based paradigm. Stemming from event-related independent component analysis, spatial weighting maps are shown for components of the AMN in which there is a significant main effect (*P*<0.00036). Component A is somewhat left-lateralized and is language-looking, occurring in the context of deactivation in bilateral supramarginal gyrus and precuneus. Component B shows deactivation in auditory and opercular somatosensory cortices in the context of activation in an attention-like network involving bilateral superior and middle frontal gyri plus right cerebellum; this can be interpreted as withdrawal from the processing of 'irrelevant' sensory- and movement-related information during internally focused processing. Component C shows a network of areas, including retrosplenial cortex extending bilaterally down through lingual and parahippocampal gyri into hippocampus. Component D shows medial prefrontal cortex, suggesting that self-reflection increases as you get deeper into a recollection. Spatial maps have been thresholded via dual regression at feature threshold: *P*<0.001, False Discovery Rate corrected (FDRc)<0.00036.

Adapted from *NeuroImage*, 152, Tailby C, Rayner G, Wilson S, Jackson G, The spatiotemporal substrates of autobiographical recollection: using event-related ICA to study cognitive networks in action, pp. 237–48. © 2017 Elsevier Inc. All rights reserved.

Cognitive Control Network

The CCN recruits the dorsolateral PFC and dorsal ACC (dACC), with auxiliary regions in the medial temporal lobe and intraparietal sulci (7, 11, 25). The CCN activates during externally focused, goal-directed behaviours (26), supporting working memory, selective attention to relevant tasks, flexible switching between tasks, and sustained attention.

Weak engagement of the CCN is characteristic of depression. People with depression exhibit decreased task-related activity throughout the CCN that is related to poorer task performances. Moreover, individuals with depression need intensified CCN activation to perform as well on cognitive tasks as healthy controls (see [6] for a review). Connectivity of the CCN in depression is abnormal, with some studies reporting within-network *hyper*connectivity (27) and others *hypo*connectivity (28).

Cognitive difficulties associated with reduced CCN activation in depression include poor attention, reduced inhibition of irrelevant negatively valenced stimuli, insufficiency in planning novel strategies, and working memory deficits (see [6] for a review). These difficulties are thought to account for clinical features such as indecisiveness, impulsive thinking, mental rigidity, and poor concentration. Poor cognitive control occurring in the context of depressive core beliefs about the self/world leads to systematic biases in information processing; namely, difficulties disengaging from maladaptive stimuli and increased elaboration of negative material typical of guilt and self-worthlessness (24). For instance, functional magnetic resonance imaging (fMRI) shows that, relative to healthy controls, people with depression show anomalous activation of the CCN during a task requiring them to expel negative material from their working memory, providing a putative neural basis for cognitive distortions typical of depression, such as selective abstraction (29).

Findings regarding the persistence of CCN abnormalities when the disease has clinically remitted are mixed. Positron emission tomography and fMRI studies show that underactivation of the CCN can broadly normalize after psychological, pharmacological, or transcranial magnetic stimulation treatment, and is associated with clinical improvement of symptoms (see [6] for a review). However, CCN normalization does not occur in every remission, with persistently attenuated CCN connectivity linked to subclinical cognitive features of depression such as brooding, pessimistic attributional style, and negative automatic thoughts (30). Together these findings give rise to a view that weak CCN function may be a trait-like neurobiological marker of vulnerability to depression that persists even when the individual no longer meets criteria for the disorder (6).

Altered AMN-CCN Dynamics in Depression: AMN Dominance

In depression, the anticorrelated relationship between the CCN and AMN appears to become pathologically imbalanced, with the AMN becoming 'stuck on'.

Box 12.2 Normal AMN–CCN Dynamics: Flexible Anticorrelation

In the healthy population, AMN and CCN have an anticorrelated relationship. In attentionally demanding tasks, the CCN is activated to marshal the necessary cognitive resources. To focus, self-referential processing is suppressed via AMN deactivation. This fits with the common experience that, in situations requiring intense concentration and thinking, daydreaming is replaced by increased alertness to the task at hand. Conversely, an activated AMN inhibits the CCN and depletes cognitive resources (7, 25), suggesting that self-focused thinking limits our ability to engage in goal-directed tasks. The anticorrelated relationship between the AMN and CCN appears to be part of the intrinsic organization of the human brain, with spontaneous anticorrelation observable at resting state.

Source data from Proceedings of the National Academy of Sciences of the United States of America, 102, Fox MD, Snyder AZ, Vincent JL, et al, *The human brain is intrinsically organized into dynamic, anticorrelated functional networks*, pp. 9673–9678, 2005, The National Academy of Sciences.

Specifically, during cognitively and emotionally demanding tasks people with depression show *hypo*activation of the CCN and *hyper*activation of the AMN (see [6] for a review; Box 12.2). That is, they are unable to disengage the self-focused AMN and successfully recruit the CCN during tasks (11, 31, 32). Imbalance between AMN and CCN in recurrent depression is evident during rest (33) and is underscored by evidence of abnormal functional connectivity between anterior nodes of the AMN and CCN (see [6] for a review). This model of dysfunctional AMN–CCN dynamics fits with the research showing AMN overactivation and CCN underactivation in depression.

It has been hypothesized that the impaired ability of people with depression to deactivate the AMN and successfully engage the CCN correlates with clinical features of the disorder like a dysfunctionally self-focused cognitive style co-occurring with a failure to attenuate self-focused thought when a task needs performing (11, 18, 33). It has been proposed that the persistence of this pattern during remission of depression may confer a cognitive risk for recurrence (33), with a selective focus on the negative aspects of life resulting in cognitive distortions thought to form the basis of depression.

Emotional and Somatic Symptom Dimensions

Disturbed AMN–CCN dynamics have the secondary effect of destabilizing the 'top-down' or cognitive regulation of emotion in people with depression.

Affective Network

The affective network (AN) overlaps with nodes of the AMN and CCN, as well as reward circuits and the hypothalamic–pituitary–adrenal (HPA) axis. Overactivation of the HPA axis in depression is a highly reliable finding (34), with clinical correlates consistent with its somatic symptom dimension. The AN includes subgenual and pregenual cingulate, ventromedial PFC, nucleus accumbens, amygdala, entorhinal cortex, striatum, hypothalamus, and midbrain (6). These cortico–subcortical nodes are interconnected in a way that supports reward processing and visceral monitoring, namely arousal, appetite, libido, sleep, etc., disturbances to which are thought to underpin vegetative, dysphoric, and anhedonic symptoms of depression (11).

Decoupling of the CCN and AN. Regulation of mood depends on the successful modulation of negative emotions using cognitive strategies (24), and, as such, is reliant on the CCN providing top-down regulation of the AN. In depression, current data suggest that chronically weak CCN engagement is associated with dysregulation of the AN. Decreased CCN activity occurring simultaneously with increased AN activity is linked to negative affect regulation, biased processing of emotionally valanced information, and poor attention-modulated reward processing in people with depression (35). Tao et al. (36) speculate that this decoupling of the CCN from the AN reflects reduced control over negative feelings toward the self, possibly accounting for the self-loathing common to depressed individuals. CCN–AN decoupling may also give rise to negative symptoms of depression characterized by poor reward processing and somatic changes (25), with single photon emission computed tomography showing hypofrontality in the CCN of depressed inpatients in conjunction with altered perfusion in the AN that relate to worse anergia, anhedonia, and psychomotor retardation (37). Successful psychological treatment of depressive symptoms has been associated with normalized AN function during emotionally valanced cognitive control tasks in an fMRI study (38), perhaps indicating that psychological therapies restore the normal top-down control of the CCN over emotional processing.

Strengthened coupling of the AMN and the AN. Altered regulation of AN function in depression has also been linked to abnormal AMN function. Functional connectivity techniques show that, in people with depression, the AMN has stronger coupling with anterior nodes of the AN, with enhanced connectivity linked to a longer length of current depressive episode and more severe symptomatology. Since similar hyperconnectivity is not evident in unmedicated patients in the early stages of treatment this may be a signature of more refractory or severe depression, perhaps suggesting that overrecruitment of emotion-processing regions into the AMN accumulates over the course of ongoing depressive disorder (6).

Clinically, exaggerated AMN–AN connectivity in people with depression has been linked to elevated rumination and brooding (see [6] for a review). Hamilton and colleagues (18) propose that the self-referential processes served by the AMN are abnormally influenced by emotionally valenced behavioural withdrawal processes controlled by the AN, producing a state of mind primed for maladaptive rumination. Although speculative, this might be conceptualized as the AN 'hijacking' the AMN and disrupting its function (11). Increased AN connectivity in depression can normalize with selective serotonin reuptake inhibitor treatment (39), suggesting that poor downregulation of the AN by the CCN and its overintegration with the AMN might form a pathogenic mechanism of depressed mood.

Salience Network

Highly integrated with both the AN and CCN, the salience network (SN) is thought to be important for detecting stimuli relevant to current goals, introspection, the initiation of cognitive control, and the coordination of behavioural responses (12). It consists of three main nodes: the dACC (thereby overlapping with the CCN), as well as the left and right anterior insula, and the inferior frontal gyri (12). In depression, the decoupling between the CCN and AN is thought to have repercussions for the functioning of the SN.

In a seminal fMRI study using an emotional go–no-go task, depressed patients showed elevated SN–CCN coactivation relative to healthy controls (14). This might indicate that, as the CCN struggles to activate to perform a cognitively demanding task, it co-opts the SN, perhaps in an effort to strengthen task performance. This SN–CCN coactivation is associated with heightened monitoring of emotional information, a failure to inhibit sadness-valenced distractors, and an exaggerated AMN response to sad information (14). Exaggerated AMN–SN connectivity is also linked to higher levels of depersonalization symptoms in depressed patients with a trauma history, perhaps stemming from poor ascription of salience to self-focused thoughts in vulnerable people (40). Conversely, outside of a cognitively demanding task, unmedicated people with depression show decreased activation of the SN bilaterally, which is linked to more severe somatic symptoms. Abnormal SN–AN connectivity correlates with overall symptom severity, and can be attenuated with training on cognitive-affective strategies leading to amelioration of anxiety and depression symptoms (see [6] for a review).

Summary: AN and SN in depression. Collectively, functional neuroimaging research to date indicates that: (i) poor activation of the CCN is linked to increased activity in the AN; (ii) there is increased connectivity between the AN and AMN; and (iii) there is decreased activation of the SN overall that occurs in the context of exaggerated coactivation of the SN with the CCN, AMN, and AN. It has been speculated that the diminished cognitive control of emotion highlighted by functional neuroimaging may lead to reduced 'top-down' regulation of negative emotional responses, biased information processing for sad or self-critical information, and aberrant reward processing (4, 14). The latter may well underpin the emotion symptom dimension pathognomonic of depression (6). Dysfunction of the mood-regulating circuitry is at least in part modifiable with successful pharmacological or psychological therapy (15), and may provide biomarkers of the illness with which to monitor the efficacy of treatment (21).

A Dynamic Neurocognitive Network Model Of Depression

The growing body of neuroimaging data outlined in this chapter suggests that many of the characteristic features of depression—anhedonia, dysphoria, rumination, intrusive negative thoughts, affectively biased cognitive processing, and reduced goal-directed behaviour—can be attributed to abnormal dynamics between two neurocognitive networks.

The general structure of this neurocognitive model broadly corresponds with previous ones based on neuroimaging and behaviour alike (see [6] for a review). Although speculative, the model is useful in that it suggests that the atypical dynamics between neurocognitive and affective networks accounts for the heterogeneous, pleomorphic co-occurrence of various depressive features, whereby in *Diagnostic and Statistical Manual of Mental Disorders*, 5th edition (DSM-5) criteria its two cardinal affective symptoms and nine associated somatic and cognitive features give rise to >1000 idiosyncratic configurations of presenting symptoms. Moreover, initial evidence suggests that these aberrant dynamics may be intrinsic to the organization of the brain, are evident at the first episode of illness, could represent a vulnerability factor for refractory or recurrent illness, and provide a potential biological marker of treatment response.

Conclusions

Better understanding of the underlying neurobiology of depressive symptoms has the potential to improve the precision of psychiatric medicine. Conceivable advances to stem from future neurocognitive studies include: (i) narrowing the search for in vivo biomarkers of depression that are evident on non-invasive investigations such as neuroimaging; (ii) broadening research parameters to include patients with a depressive biomarker but subclinical depressive symptom; and (iii) linking a patient's unique clinical presentation to proximal brain networks to define individually tailored anatomical, cognitive, or neurochemical targets for treatment, with follow-up scanning used to track functional network normalization as a marker of disease remission. Such an approach is in keeping with guidelines for gold-standard psychiatric research (3) and would bring the management of depression in line with what is routinely done in many other areas of medicine today.

References

1. American Psychiatric Association. *Diagnostic and Statistical Manual of Mental Disorders*, fifth edition. Arlington, VA: American Psychiatric Association; 2013.

2. World Health Organization. *ICD-10 Classifications of Mental and Behavioural Disorder: Clinical Descriptions and Diagnostic Guidelines.* Geneva: World Health Organization; 1992.

3. Insel T, Cuthbert B, Garvey M, et al. Research domain criteria (RDoC): toward a new classification framework for research on mental disorders. Am J Psychiatry 2010;167:748–51.

4. Mayberg HS. Modulating dysfunctional limbic-cortical circuits in depression: towards development of brain-based algorithms for diagnosis and optimised treatment. Br Med Bull 2003;65:193–207.

5. Sporns O. The human connectome: a complex network. Ann NY Acad Sci 2011; 1224:109–25.

6. Rayner G, Jackson G, Wilson S. Cognition-related brain networks underpin the symptoms of unipolar depression: evidence from a systematic review. Neurosci Biobehav Rev 2016;61:53–65.

7. Smith SM, Fox PT, Miller KL, et al. Correspondence of the brain's functional architecture during activation and rest. Proc Natl Acad Sci 2009;106:13040–5.

8. Andrews-Hanna JR. The brain's default network and its adaptive role in internal mentation. Neuroscientist 2012;18:251–70.

9. Buckner RL, Andrews-Hanna JR, Schacter DL. The brain's default network: anatomy, function, and relevance to disease. Ann N Y Acad Sci 2008;1124:1–38.

10. Tailby C, Rayner G, Wilson S, Jackson G. The spatiotemporal substrates of autobiographical recollection: using event-related ICA to study cognitive networks in action. NeuroImage 2017;152:237–48.

11. Sheline YL, Price JL, Yan Z, et al. Resting-state functional MRI in depression unmasks increased connectivity between networks via the dorsal nexus. Proc Natl Acad Sci U S A 2010;107:11020–5.

12. Seeley WW, Menon V, Schatzberg AF, et al. Dissociable intrinsic connectivity networks for salience processing and executive control. J Neurosci 2007;27:2349–56.

13. Grimm S, Boesiger P, Beck J, et al. Altered negative BOLD responses in the default-mode network during emotion processing in depressed subjects. Neuropsychopharmacol 2009;34:932–43.

14. Elliot R, Rubinsztein JS, Sahakian BJ, et al. The neural basis of mood-congruent processing biases in depression. Arch Gen Psychiatry 2002;59:597–604.

15. Delaveau P, Jabourian M, Lemogne C, et al. Brain effects of antidepressants in major depression: a meta-analysis of emotional processing studies. J Affect Disord 2001;130:66–74.

16. Posner J, Hellerstein JD, Gat I, et al. Antidepressants normalize the default mode network in patients with dysthymia. JAMA Psychiatry 2013;70:373–82.

17. Guo W, Cui X, Liu F, et al. Increased anterior default-mode network homogeneity in first-episode, drug-naive major depressive disorder: a replication study. J Affect Disord 2018;225:767–72.

18. Hamilton JP, Farmer M, Fogelman P, Gotlib IH. Depressive rumination, the default-mode network, and the dark matter of clinical neuroscience. Biol Psychiatry 2015;78:224–30.

19. Zhu X, Zhu Q, Shen H, Liao W, Yuan F. Rumination and default mode network subsystems connectivity in first-episode, drug-naive young patients with major depressive disorder. Sci Rep 2017;7:43105.

20. Grimm S, Ernst J, Boesiger P, et al. Reduced negative BOLD responses in the default-mode network and increased self-focus in depression. World J Biol Psychiatry 2011;12:627–37.

21. Hamilton JP, Chen G, Thomason ME, et al. Investigating neural primacy in major depressive disorder: multivariate Granger causality analysis of resting-state fMRI time-series data. Mol Psychiatry 2011;16:763–72.

22. Marchand WR, Lee JN, Johnson S, et al. Striatal and cortical midline circuits in major depression: implications for suicide and symptom expression. Prog Neuropsychopharmacol Biol Psychiatry 2012;36:290–9.

23. Gibbs BR, Rude SS. Overgeneral autobiographical memory as depression vulnerability. Cogn Ther Res 2004;28:511–26.

24. Beck AT. The evolution of the cognitive model of depression and its neurobiological correlates. Am J Psychiatry 2008;165:969–77.

25. Pizzagalli DA. Frontocingulate dysfunction in depression: toward biomarkers of treatment response. Neuropsychopharmacol 2011;36:183–206.

26. Fox MD, Snyder AZ, Vincent JL, et al. The human brain is intrinsically organized into dynamic, anticorrelated functional networks. Proc Natl Acad Sci U S A 2005;102:9673–8.

27. Vasic N, Walter H, Sambataro F, et al. Aberrant functional connectivity of dorsolateral prefrontal and cingulate networks in patients with major depression during working memory processing. Psychol Med 2009;39:977–87.

28. Buchanan A, Wang X, Gollan JK. Resting state functional connectivity in women with major depressive disorder. J Psychiatr Res 2014;59:38–44.

29. Foland-Ross LC, Hamilton JP, Joormann J, et al. The neural basis of difficulties disengaging from negative irrelevant material in major depression. Psychological Sci 2013;24:334–44.

30. Stange JP, Bessette KL, Jenkins LM, et al. Attenuated intrinsic connectivity within cognitive control network among individuals with remitted depression: temporal stability and association with negative cognitive styles. Hum Brain Mapp 2017;38:2939–54.

31. Korgaonkar M, Grieve SM, Etkin A, et al. Using standardized fMRI protocols to identify patterns of prefrontal circuit dysregulation that are common and specific to cognitive and emotional tasks in major depressive disorder: first wave results from the iSPOT-D study. Neuropsychopharmacol 2013;38:863–71.

32. Hamilton JP, Furman DJ, Chang C, et al. Default-mode and task-positive network activity in major depressive disorder: implications for adaptive and maladaptive rumination. Biol Psychiatry 2011;70:327–33.

33. Marchetti I, Koster EH, Sonuga-Barke EJ, et al. The default mode network and recurrent depression: a neurobiological model of cognitive risk factors. Neuropsychol Rev 2012;22:229–51.

34. Nemeroff CB, Vale WW. The neurobiology of depression: inroads to treatment and new drug discovery. J Clin Psychiatry 2005;66:5–13.

35. Buhle JT, Silvers JA, Wager TD, et al. Cognitive reappraisal of emotion: a meta-analysis of human neuroimaging studies. Cereb Cortex 2014;24:2981–90.

36. Tao H, Guo S, Ge T, et al. Depression uncouples brain hate circuit. Mol Psychiatry 2013;18:101–11.

37. Galynker II, Cai J, Ongseng F, et al. Hypofrontality and negative symptoms in major depressive disorder. J Nucl Med 1998;39:608–12.

38. Dichter GS, Felder JN, Smoski MJ. The effects of Brief Behavioral Activation Therapy for depression on cognitive control in affective contexts: an fMRI investigation. J Affect Disord 2010;126:236–44.

39. Mayberg HS, Brannan SK, Tekell JL, et al. Regional metabolic effects of fluoxetine in major depression: serial changes and relationship to clinical response. Biol Psychiatry 2000;48:830–43.

40. Parlar M, Densmore M, Hall GB, Frewen PA, Lanius RA, McKinnon MC. Relation between patterns of intrinsic network connectivity, cognitive functioning, and symptom presentation in trauma-exposed patients with major depressive disorder. Brain Behav 2017;7: e00664.

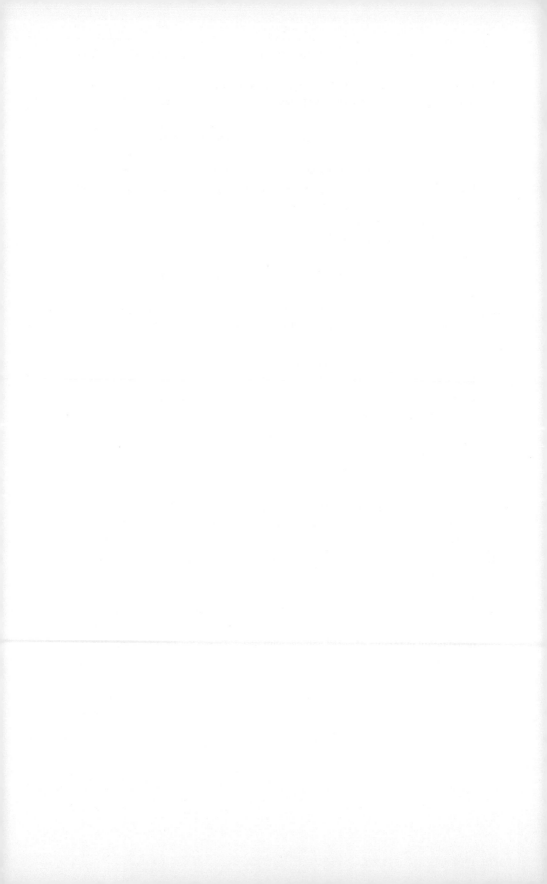

13

Networks of Cognitive Processes: Functional and Anatomical Correlates of Cognition, Emotions, and Social Cognition

John D. Medaglia

Introduction

How can the human mind occur in the physical universe? The cognitive psychologist John R. Anderson reviewed the critical foundations for *cognitive architectures* as models of the mind and their representation in human brains (1). With approximately 80 billion neurons and 100 trillion connections, the specific configuration of neural tissue enables human cognition via computations that occur within a complex network organization (2).

Human cognitive systems evolved from basic neural systems that processed basic sensory inputs and guided actions to approach or avoid stimuli. Over aeons, natural selection shaped systems that represented simple and complex relationships within and between objects in the environment and the ability to enact behaviours that modify the environment. Presumably, internal states such as perception and emotion became increasingly prominent and consciousness became richer. Gradually and inexorably, evolution shaped the neural systems that mediate modern human flourishing and suffering.

To describe neurocognitive organization at a high level, we can concisely consider major cognitive functions supported by the brain. Then, we can describe the coarse spatiotemporal organization of cognitive systems in brain networks, which allows us to celebrate progress to date and identify the intriguing paths before us.

Cognitive Organization in the Brain

Henceforth, we consider cognition to be processes organized into major networks (systems of interconnected regions that include millions or billions of neurons) in the human brain. These networks presumably involve many coordinated and competitive mechanisms that support the computational bases of cognition. Here, we group cognitive systems into a heuristic taxonomy that emphasizes distinct roles of systems with respect to our relationships with the world around us. Critically, these systems can be evaluated within an emerging interdisciplinary framework called *cognitive network neuroscience* (3).

A Converging High-Level Perspective on Cognitive Networks

Driven by research in anatomical and functional neuroimaging, a consistent picture of high-level cognitive network organization in the brain is emerging. Anatomical networks measured with white matter tractography demonstrably mediate and organize activity in observable functional systems (4). A number of major systems can be reliably observed that are consistent with data from multiple neural and behavioural modalities (5). *Henceforth are described systems predominantly identified in functional data analyses. For many of these systems, there are known anatomical networks that support the interactions within and between functional systems.* Evidence suggests that there are a number of relatively stable major networks that are organized as sets of highly interactive regions organized into *modules*. These modules are associated with distinct cognitive functions (6, 3, 5) and interact with varying patterns of within- and between-module associations thought to represent underlying fluctuations in communicative neural states (Figure 13.1).

Despite ongoing debates, some primary cognitive systems remain persistent objects of study, and we have gained substantial insight into how they are represented in the brain. Henceforth, we will focus on functional and anatomical systems commonly identified in network analysis that are putatively responsible for sensation, perception, action, control, learning, emotion, decision-making, and language. Given that various perspectives exist about the organization of major cognitive networks, it is useful to clarify the basis of the cognitive networks frequently discussed in network neuroscience. Specifically, these networks are often identified using data-driven techniques in conjunction with behavioural paradigms to identify distinct cognitive systems. The interactions within and between these systems provide the bases for human cognition. Notably, some sensory (e.g. olfactory and gustatory) and subcortical systems (e.g. the basal ganglia and cerebellum, which are known to functionally and anatomically communicate with the neocortically focused networks described herein [7]) tend to be underrepresented in large-scale network analyses in neuroimaging data, so they will be mentioned as contributors to major cognitive systems as relevant below.

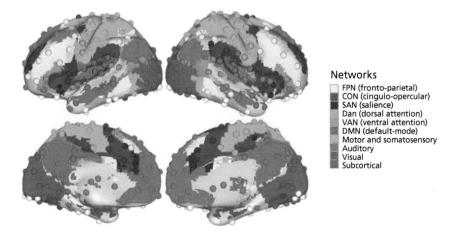

Networks
- FPN (fronto-parietal)
- CON (cingulo-opercular)
- SAN (salience)
- Dan (dorsal attention)
- VAN (ventral attention)
- DMN (default-mode)
- Motor and somatosensory
- Auditory
- Visual
- Subcortical

Figure 13.1 Major cognitive networks in the brain. Resting state functional connectivity analyses from functional magnetic resonance imaging (fMRI) frequently recover stable, internally communicating major networks. Each colour represents a different network defined by network community detection algorithms applied to measures of intrinsic fMRI associations. While specific maps vary by study, the systems illustrated here are frequently and reliably recovered. These networks can be associated with major cognitive functions as semiautonomous brain *modules*, and distributed interactions between these systems are thought to facilitate our rich repertoire of mental functions.

Adapted from *Neuron,* 72, 4, Power JD, Cohen AL, Nelson SM, Wig GS, Barnes KA, Church JA, et al. Functional network organization of the human brain, pp. 665–678. Copyright © 2011 Elsevier Inc. All rights reserved.

Sensation, perception, and action

Sensory, perceptual, and motor systems provide the boundaries of the input–output relationship between the environment's influence on us and our influence on the environment. Anatomically, *primary sensory systems* receive tactile, visual, gustatory, olfactory, and auditory input from the world. Our motor systems involve the primary motor cortex, which mediates outgoing signals to muscles to control behaviour. The primary motor cortex interacts with supplementary motor planning areas and mechanisms in the basal ganglia and cerebellum that coordinate fine motor movements (8).

These regions forward-process input to multisensory (or *multimodal*) regions that integrate information from distinct senses (9). Finally, high-level cortical *hubs* interact with multimodal regions. Hubs are features of networks that are highly 'central' to information processing, which makes them candidates for integrating and segregating processes in the brain (10). This hierarchy has been suggested by network analyses that examine connectivity organization seeded in primary sensory regions in a stepwise fashion, which recovers the hierarchical structure of sensation, multimodal, and high-level systems (Figure 13.2).

Control, Learning, Emotion, and Decision-Making

Intact and precise sensory, perceptual, and motor systems serve as the gatekeepers of complex integrating and multimodal functions such as cognitive control, learning, emotion, and decision-making. Increasingly, cognitive psychologists

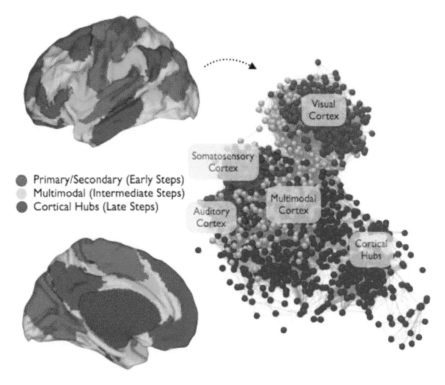

Figure 13.2 A hierarchy associating sensorimotor and hub regions. Resting-state functional magnetic resonance imaging data reveal an intrinsic hierarchy from sensorimotor to cognitive hub regions. Red represents primary and secondary sensorimotor regions identified in steps immediately following seeds placed in primary sensory regions. Green regions are the multimodal integration network, which receives input from multiple sensory regions and partially overlaps with the cingulo-opercular control system. Finally, blue represents cortical hubs, which are prominently observed in cognitive control and default mode-related regions.

Reproduced from *Journal of Neuroscience*, 32, 31, Sepulcre J, Sabuncu MR, Yeo TB, Liu H, Johnson KA, Stepwise connectivity of the modal cortex reveals the multimodal organization of the human brain, pp. 10649–10661. Copyright (2012) Society for Neuroscience.

and neuroscientists study the dynamic interplay between sensation, perception, and action systems with higher-ordered regions supporting other functions.

Generally considered to be 'up' the processing hierarchy, 'higher-ordered' processes in the brain coordinate diverse cognitive functions and behaviour. Among these processes are those that guide thought and action in the context of goals (cognitive control), store information about the world (learning and memory), add valence to experiences (emotion), and select among thoughts and actions (decision-making).

Cognitive Control

In network neuroscience, systems including the frontoparietal, dorsal and ventral attention networks, and cingulo-opercular network contribute to cognitive control. The frontoparietal network serves as a hub system among other major networks (11). This has been posited to explain the ubiquitous recruitment of the frontoparietal network in challenging and novel conditions to facilitate task adaptation, generally supporting set maintenance and task switching (11). The dorsal and ventral attention networks are thought to mediate top-down voluntary allocation of attention to location or features and shifting attention in response to unattended or unexpected stimuli, respectively (12). Cingulo-opercular regions administer control over within-set specific responses (e.g. selecting, inhibiting, or retrieving specific responses [13]) at an intermediate level of cognitive processing between dorsal attention and frontoparietal control systems.

Although beyond the scope of this chapter, it is critical to note that subcortical systems are heavily interactive in cognitive control processes. In general, it is thought that neocortical control systems interact with subcortical regions to guide behaviour optimally in the context of competing strong alternatives (14). Cortico–subthalamic–palladial pathways dynamically interact during response selection in circuits that mediate between cognitive control and action (15). In addition, the evolutionarily recent lateral aspects of the cerebellum heavily interact with cognitive control and multimodal networks (16). Deficits in inhibition, set shifting, and fluency have been observed following focal cerebellar lesions (17), and some theoretical accounts suggest that the cerebellum contributes the same coordinating and pattern learning mechanisms crucial to motor function to neocortical association and control systems (18). Thus, our models of cognition should eventually encapsulate the distinct contributions of these extended cortico–subcortical systems in generating controlled thought and action.

Learning and Memory

Learning is a process whereby skills, facts, and preferences about the world are encoded into the brain for later use. Notably absent from many large-scale descriptions of cognitive networks is a system for learning. We should expect this to be the case if learning is produced by changing representations via interactions within and between major networks. Indeed, there is reason to believe that cognitive control and learning are inversely proportional, and that evolutionary selection favoured delayed maturation of the cognitive control systems that are critical to learning early in life (19). Decreased overall demands for frontoparietal control mechanisms may be observed following learning (20). Thus, while individuals may rely on a set of robust relationships between the frontoparietal network and other systems in diverse tasks, changes in the degree of expression of common interactions between networks may represent task adaptation. Across neurodevelopment, evidence suggests that the expression of frontoparietal and memory system states is associated with better cognitive control and memory functioning, suggesting that these systems are interactive throughout early life into adulthood (21). Notably, the default mode network has also been referred to as an 'episodic memory network' (22) and is active when people remember past events (23).

While large-scale network interactions may be critical to learning and memory, some specific regions provide distinct contributions. In particular, the hippocampus, striatum, mammillary bodies, and the amygdala and the pathways involving these regions are crucial to different types of memory. The hippocampus is thought to be involved in spatial and declarative learning and memory, although debates remain as to whether its role is to map stimuli rather than encode them into memory per se (24). The dorsal striatum interacts competitively and cooperatively with the hippocampus. Specifically, the dorsal striatum competes with the hippocampus when facilitating memory for response learning at the expense of place learning (25). In contrast, it cooperates with the hippocampus to promote cue learning and contextual fear conditioning (25). The mammillary bodies contain a set of nuclei that may be involved in at least two contributions to episodic memory, specifically by encoding head orientation and mediating theta-rhythm neural activity that may elicit long-term potentiation (26). The amygdala is thought to contribute to emotional memory (27) and the *memory enhancement effect*, which describes the increased likelihood of remembering events when they are emotionally charged (28). Collectively, these regions interact with other subcortical and cortical systems to facilitate memory.

Emotion

In the context of major brain networks, large-scale interactions between major networks are associated with basic emotional functions in a *psychological constructionist* perspective, suggesting that emotions are encoded at a conceptual level involving coordinated interactions between complex systems (29).

In this view, the conventional language that we use to refer to notions such as 'anger' or 'sadness' is not respected by the brain, but instead emotions are caused by more basic psychological operations that are not specific to emotion (29). In the constructionist view, 'core affect' refers to mental representations of changes in the body that are experienced with some degree of pleasure or displeasure paired with some degree of arousal. Core affect is not psychologically meaningful without attachment to an object (29). The network thought to contribute to core affect includes the amygdala, insula, medial orbitofrontal cortex, inferior orbitofrontal cortex, anterior cingulate cortex, thalamus, hypothalamus, bed nucleus of the tria terminalis, basal forebrain, posterior angular gyrus, ventromedial prefrontal cortex, dorsomedial prefrontal cortex, medial temporal lobe, and posterior cortex/retrosplenial area (29). Thus, this complex distributed network involves integrated cortico–subcortical processes that intersect with multiple large-scale cognitive networks, suggesting that even a 'basic' process like core affect requires substantial coordination between executive, error monitoring, memory, metabolic, interoceptive, and multimodal perceptual processes.

Emotion occurs when core affect is categorized using similar mechanisms to those that categorize other features of experience. That is, core affect gains its emotional meaning by valencing different aspects of bodily and environmental perception. In addition to the default mode network's role in episodic memory, it is involved in context-sensitive predictions about others' feelings, making meaning out of sensations (30). In addition, language networks (see below) anchor emotional categories via emotion words that refer to socially constructed abstract categories (31). Executive attention (a form of cognitive control often referring to directed attention and suppression) is thought to mediate the selection of conceptual representations that are brought to bear on interpreting core affect, attention to specific sensory representations, and whether core affect is in conscious awareness. Executive attention can also operate well outside awareness (32). Thus, the executive components of emotion are thought to involve the frontoparietal executive network and dorsal and ventral attention networks (29). Whether these general cognitive control systems contributed common or unique features to emotion processes remains largely an open question.

Decision-Making

In many ways, our choices define us. A discipline known as *decision science* has emerged to understand and predict how we make choices at the intersection of economics, marketing, and cognitive science. Decision-making tasks are often used to examine choices under uncertainty about sensory input or outcomes, differentiating targets and distractors, or integrating information from multiple senses, or preference-based decision-making (33). At the heart of decision science is the nature of the predictability of the rewarding or punitive outcomes of our behaviour, the weight of evidence favouring a choice as correct relative to another, relative rationality of idealized versus natural choices, and native preferences of the decision-maker. While tasks may differ in terms of design and the number of choices, tasks with simple discriminative judgements (i.e. selecting 'yes/no' or otherwise option A versus option B) form the basis of *two-alternative forced choice* tasks, from which much of decision neuroscience has emerged.

Decision-making dynamics result from a complex interplay between mechanisms that process rewards, represent expected gains, and control attention and working memory capacity. The reward component relies on subcortical systems such as the ventral tegmental area, nucleus accumbens, and mesocortical pathway, which are recruited to process positive and negative stimuli in reinforcement learning (34). In turn, reward processing and response selection circuits are thought to require alertness maintained by the noradrenergic locus coeruleus (35), dorsal and ventral attention networks (36), and cognitive control mechanisms, including 'top-down control' to maintain goals and meet task demands with supplementary conflict monitoring to mediate conflict resolution (37). These neural systems support interactions between the focus of attention, discriminative judgements, and the anticipation and consumption of rewards during decisions. Collectively, systems that support these functions encompass a significant portion of the brain's neural architecture. This is testimony to the importance and complexity of choices in our daily lives.

Social Cognition and Language

In the animal kingdom, humans possess unparalleled social cognitive and language abilities. However, we should avoid anthropocentric hubris; indeed, the systems that afford us the ability to understand and react to others and communicate through symbolic representations in speech patterns are at one extreme on an evolutionary continuum (38). Social cognitive and language abilities rely deeply on the systems reviewed previously: indeed, it is unlikely that completely separate neural systems evolved to regulate social and communicative abilities. Rather, social cognition and language are likely adaptations and extensions of prior neural architecture and functions. Social and communicative processes involve domain-general contributions from sensory, perceptual, control, learning, emotion, and decision-making systems (39). In addition, they involve potentially unique functions that allow us to empathize with others, possess a theory of mind, and formulate symbolic representations that we can express with verbal utterances.

Empathy and Theory of Mind

Empathy and theory of mind are crucial to navigating our social world. Empathy recruits emotion-related networks when processing the anticipated emotional states of others (40). In addition, a quantitative meta-analysis revealed that the dorsal anterior and anterior mid-cingulate cortices plus the insula and supplementary motor area are active during a range of empathic tasks (41). A dissociation among these regions is observed whereby the dorsal anterior mid-cingulate cortex is recruited in cognitive–evaluative empathy, whereas the right anterior insula is involved in only affective–perceptual empathy (41). Importantly, this network is modulated by trait, state, and contextual factors. Specifically, the salience network and reward-processing circuitry are involved in processing reward in social cognition. Dissociable features of the salience network are associated with distinct functions: empathy-related anterior insula activity may be associated with costly helping of in-group members, whereas ventral striatal and nucleus accumbens activity may be associated with not helping out-group members (42). Together, these findings suggest that basic expectations about social affiliation and potential rewards are at play when we decide whether to help others.

Our theory of mind—the ability to attribute mental states to oneself and others—is essential to empathy and to social cognition more generally. Interestingly, much of what has been termed a 'theory of mind network' (43) largely coincides with the default mode network (44). As a result, it has been proposed that functions otherwise associated with the default mode network such as episodic and autobiographical memory, prospection, emotional processing of others, social evaluation, and social categorization contribute to theory of mind (30). Over development, the failure of youths to reason and empathize about the mental states of others may result from relatively underdeveloped frontoparietal networks. Specifically, it has been posited that mature executive systems are necessary to suppress dominant self-centred perspectives in children, perhaps represented in the interplay between executive systems and default mode systems throughout childhood and adolescence (45).

Language

The language network is essential to our function in a complex, social world. In a stringent case, we can consider only 'high-level' language regions involved in language comprehension to the exclusion of cognitive control systems in the domain-general frontoparietal system, sensory systems, and motor/articulatory regions (39). Crucially, the temporally stable functional core of brain regions during language processing involves predominantly the more exclusive set of regions plus regions in the lateral frontal cortex likely to be recruited in cognitive

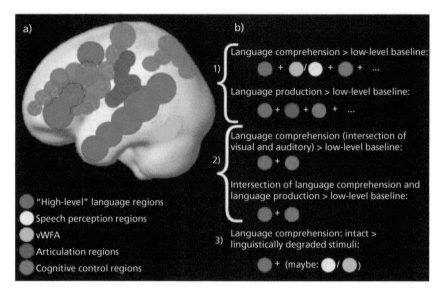

Figure 13.3 The language network under different definitions. a) A schematic depiction of five sets of brain regions that are sometimes included in the language network. Red, the classic high-level language processing regions; yellow, speech perception regions; green, visual word-form area; pink, speech articulation regions; and blue, cognitive control regions. b) A schematic illustration of possible definitions of the language network, ranging from very liberal (1) to more conservative (2 and 3). vWFA, Visual word form area.

control tasks (46). Thus, we can leverage a strict definition of a language network relevant to the symbolic representations necessary for semantics, and this network can be ascribed to regions in the left lateral temporal, inferior frontal, and dorsal frontal areas (Figure 13.3). Notable, this stringently defined core of symbolic language processing overlaps with parts of the default mode, cingulo-opercular control, and frontoparietal control networks defined in graph theoretical studies. Thus, we should continue to examine which aspects of language systems are truly language-specific versus domain-general control and symbolic representation mechanism.

What Does a Network Approach Add to Cognitive Science?

The emerging consensus about major cognitive systems in the brain has coincided with growing promise for a unifying framework in which to analyse and describe brain networks. Examining the human *connectome*—an explicit representation of the brain as a network—allows us to describe and understand complexity in the human brain with concise statistics and principles (47). This gives us the ability to understand the role of individual parts that comprise a system (e.g. neurons or entire brain regions) in the context of the greater whole (individual systems or the whole brain).

Some of the findings from cognitive network neuroscience resulted from mathematical concepts and tools based in *graph theory* to represent and analyse brain networks. *Graph theory is a branch of formal mathematics that studies the properties of 'graphs', which elegantly represent network components and connections.* Concisely, a brain graph can be represented by the graph *G=V,E*, where *V* contains a set of *vertices* (or often, 'nodes') and *E* is the set of edges associated with the nodes. Commonly, nodes represent individual elements of the system such as neurons or brain regions, and edges represent anatomical connections or functional interactions between nodes. Thus, a single *G* can be constructed to represent the nodes and edgewise relationships between many elements in a brain network. In addition, many *G* representations can be concatenated to encode a temporal graph that represents network organization that may vary in time. Further, networks can also be *multiplexed* to encode numerous features of organization across spatiotemporal scales (48).

Several key concepts are commonly applied in brain network analysis. First, we often examine the role of nodes in the network by describing their *centrality* in the network, which refers to statistics that represent the connectivity of nodes with their neighbours and their roles in pathways across the network. At the *mesoscale* level of organization, investigators examine the *community structure* of networks, which refers to how groups of regions are organized into communities or 'modules' of shared features or associations. These modules are analogous to the cognitive systems described throughout this chapter. At the *macroscale* level of organization, investigators examine the general organization of the graph, often including the inferred efficiency of information transformation via several distinct mathematical representations. Collectively, these notions provide mathematical approaches to study neurocognitive systems within a broader effort to study complex systems known as *network science*. Graph theoretic analysis in network neuroscience is a rapidly growing frontier and may one day help us to define a generalized framework within which to describe and understand cognitive systems (3, 5).

Conclusion

The networks discussed here are grounded in a rapidly growing literature that identifies large-scale network modules in the brain. Indeed, interactions within and between modules are a sensible focus for defining cognitive maps, and neuro-imaging modalities provide limited sensitivity to the 'ground truth' of neural function and cognitive correlates and causes. However, as the field rapidly develops, the promise of cognitive network neuroscience may be increasingly to unify diverse researchers from mathematics, computational science, engineering, psychology, and cognitive neuroscience. With a shared interest in representing the complexity of the human brain, we may one day understand how it produces the mind.

References

1. Anderson JR. *How can the Human Mind Occur in the Physical Universe?* Oxford: Oxford University Press; 2009.

2. Herculano-Houzel S. The remarkable, yet not extraordinary, human brain as a scaled-up primate brain and its associated cost. Proc Natl Acad Sci 2012;109(Suppl. 1):10661–8.

3. Medaglia JD, Lynall ME, Bassett DS. Cognitive network neuroscience. J Cogn Neurosci 2015;27(8):1471–91.

4. Hermundstad AM, Brown KS, Bassett DS, et al. Structurally-constrained relationships between cognitive states in the human brain. PLoS Comput Biol 2014;10(5):e1003591.

5. Bassett DS, Sporns O. Network neuroscience. Nature Neurosci 2017;20(3):353–364.

6. Power JD, Cohen AL, Nelson SM, et al. Functional network organization of the human brain. Neuron 2011;72(4):665–78.

7. Bostan AC, Dum RP, Strick PL. Cerebellar networks with the cerebral cortex and basal ganglia. Trends Cogn Sci 2013;17(5):241–54.

8. Gazzaniga M, Ivry RB, Mangun GR. *Cognitive Neuroscience.* New York: W.W. Norton & Company; 2013.

9. Sepulcre J, Sabuncu MR, Yeo TB, Liu H, Johnson KA. Stepwise connectivity of the modal cortex reveals the multimodal organization of the human brain. J Neurosci 2012;32(31):10649–61.

10. van den Heuvel MP, Sporns O. Network hubs in the human brain. Trends Cogn Sci 2013;17(12):683–96.

11. Cole MW, Reynolds JR, Power JD, Repovs G, Anticevic A, Braver TS. Multi-task connectivity reveals flexible hubs for adaptive task control. Nature Neurosci 2013;16(9):1348–55.

12. Corbetta M, Shulman GL. Control of goal-directed and stimulus-driven attention in the brain. Nature Rev Neurosci 2002;3(3):201–15.

13. Ridderinkhof KR, Van Den Wildenberg WP, Segalowitz SJ, Carter CS. Neurocognitive mechanisms of cognitive control: the role of prefrontal cortex in action selection, response inhibition, performance monitoring, and reward-based learning. Brain Cogn 2004;56(2):129–40.

14. Aron AR, Robbins TW, Poldrack RA. Inhibition and the right inferior frontal cortex. Trends Cogn Sci 2004;8(4):170–7.

15. Frank MJ. Hold your horses: a dynamic computational role for the subthalamic nucleus in decision making. Neural Networks 2006;19(8):1120–36.

16. Stoodley CJ, Schmahmann JD. Functional topography in the human cerebellum: a meta-analysis of neuroimaging studies. Neuroimage 2009;44(2):489–501.

17. Bellebaum C, Daum I. Cerebellar involvement in executive control. The Cerebellum 2007;6(3):184–92.

18. Koziol LF, Budding D, Andreasen N, et al. Consensus paper: the cerebellum's role in movement and cognition. The Cerebellum 2014;13(1):151–77.

19. Thompson-Schill SL, Ramscar M, Chrysikou EG. Cognition without control: when a little frontal lobe goes a long way. Curr Dir Psychol Sci 2009;18(5):259–63.

20. Bassett DS, Wymbs NF, Porter MA, Mucha PJ, Carlson JM, Grafton ST. Dynamic reconfiguration of human brain networks during learning. Proc Natl Acad Sci 2011;108(18):7641–6.

21. Medaglia JD, Satterthwaite TD, Kelkar A, et al. Brain state expression and transitions are related to complex executive cognition in normative neurodevelopment. NeuroImage 2018;166:293–306.

22. Vincent JL, Snyder AZ, Fox MD, et al. Coherent spontaneous activity identifies a hippocampal-parietal memory network. J Neurophysiol 2006;96(6):3517–31.

23. Schacter DL, Addis DR, Buckner RL. Remembering the past to imagine the future: the prospective brain. Nature Rev Neurosci 2007;8(9):657–61.

24. Eichenbaum H. Hippocampus: mapping or memory? Curr Biol 2000;10(21): R785–7.

25. Kathirvelu B, Colombo PJ. Effects of lentivirus-mediated CREB expression in the dorsolateral striatum: memory enhancement and evidence for competitive and cooperative interactions with the hippocampus. Hippocampus 2013;23(11):1066–74.

26. Vann SD, Aggleton JP. The mammillary bodies: two memory systems in one? Nature Rev Neurosci 2004;5(1):35–44.

27. LaBar KS, Cabeza R. Cognitive neuroscience of emotional memory. Nature Rev Neurosci 2006;7(1):54–64.

28. Adolphs R, Cahill L, Schul R, Babinsky R. Impaired declarative memory for emotional material following bilateral amygdala damage in humans. Learning Memory 1997;4(3):291–300.

29. Lindquist KA, Wager TD, Kober H, Bliss-Moreau E, Barrett LF. The brain basis of emotion: a meta-analytic review. Behav Brain Sci 2012;35(3):121–43.

30. Andrews-Hanna JR. The brain's default network and its adaptive role in internal mentation. Neuroscientist 2012;18(3):251–70.

31. Barrett LF. The future of psychology: connecting mind to brain. Perspectives Psychol Sci 2009;4(4):326–39.

32. Barrett LF, Tugade MM, Engle RW. Individual differences in working memory capacity and dual-process theories of the mind. Psychol Bull 2004;130(4):553.

33. Angela JY. Decision-Making Tasks. Encyclopedia of computational neuroscience 2015:761–66.

34. Cohen JY, Haesler S, Vong L, Lowell BB, Uchida N. Neuron-type specific signals for reward and punishment in the ventral tegmental area. Nature 2012;482(7383):85.

35. Aston-Jones G, Cohen JD. An integrative theory of locus coeruleus—norepinephrine function: adaptive gain and optimal performance. Annu Rev Neurosci 2005;28:403–50.

36. Vossel S, Geng JJ, Fink GR. Dorsal and ventral attention systems: distinct neural circuits but collaborative roles. Neuroscientist 2014;20(2):150–9.

37. Petersen SE, Posner MI. The attention system of the human brain: 20 years after. Annu Rev Neurosci 2012;35:73–89.

38. Adolphs R. The neurobiology of social cognition. Curr Opin Neurobiol 2001;11(2):231–9.

39. Fedorenko E, Thompson-Schill SL. Reworking the language network. Trends Cogn Sci 2014;18(3):120–6.

40. De Vignemont F, Singer T. The empathic brain: how, when and why? Trends Cogn Sci 2006;10(10):435–41.

41. Fan Y, Duncan NW, de Greck M, Northoff G. Is there a core neural network in empathy? An fMRI based quantitative meta-analysis. Neurosci Biobehav Rev 2011;35(3):903–11.

42. Hein G, Silani G, Preuschoff K, Batson CD, Singer T. Neural responses to ingroup and outgroup members' suffering predict individual differences in costly helping. Neuron 2010;68(1):149–60.

43. Siegal M, Varley R. Neural systems involved in'theory of mind'. Nature Rev Neurosci 2002;3(6):463–71.

44. Spreng RN, Mar RA, Kim AS. The common neural basis of autobiographical memory, prospection, navigation, theory of mind, and the default mode: a quantitative meta-analysis. J Cogn Neurosci 2009;21(3):489–510.

45. Sherman LE, Rudie JD, Pfeifer JH, Masten CL, McNealy K, Dapretto M. Development of the default mode and central executive networks across early adolescence: a longitudinal study. Dev Cogn Neurosci 2014;10:148–59.

46. Chai LR, Mattar MG, Blank IA, Fedorenko E, Bassett DS. Functional network dynamics of the language system. Cerebral Cortex 2016;26(11):4148–59.

47. Bassett DS, Gazzaniga MS. Understanding complexity in the human brain. Trends Cogn Sci 2011;15(5):200–9.

48. Betzel RF, Bassett DS. Multi-scale brain networks. Neuroimage 2017;160:73–83.

14

The Neurobiology
of Emotion–Cognition Interactions

Thalia Richter, Alexander J. Shackman, Tatjana Aue,
and Hadas Okon-Singer

Emotion and cognition have long been viewed as two separate mental faculties, largely based on subjective differences between emotional and cognitive experience. Yet, an increasing body of research highlights the bidirectional influences between cognitive and emotional systems (1). These recent developments have been made possible by the emergence of powerful new tools for objectively assessing emotion and brain function

This chapter reviews evidence for the mutual modulatory relationships between emotional and cognitive functions, as well as for the neural circuits supporting these relationships. We discuss the influence of emotional information on different aspects of attention. We further elaborate on the flexibility of cognitive biases toward emotional information, as well as the plasticity of the neural connections supporting these biases. We then discuss the influence of cognitive strategies on emotions. Finally, we point to limitations of existing research and suggest future scientific directions. A better understanding of the mutual influences between emotional and cognitive processes is of great theoretical and clinical importance. Such an understanding may also contribute to the development of specific interventions for individuals with prominent emotional and cognitive disturbances, including patients with schizophrenia, substance abuse, and internalizing disorders.

The Influence of Emotion on Cognition
Biased Attention to Threat

Ample evidence indicates that humans are particularly sensitive to threat-related stimuli (i.e. snakes, spiders, threatening faces [2]), probably owing to the evolutionary importance of selective responses to potentially dangerous aspects of the environment. Biased attention to emotional stimuli can be measured using a variety of methods that compare reaction time and accuracy rates between neutral and emotional items.

The focus of attention is determined by a delicate balance between *exogenous* (stimulus-driven) and *endogenous* (goal-directed) mechanisms (3). Sussman et al. (4) highlight the influence of goal-directed neurocognitive mechanisms—those related to internal goals, moods, and motivational states (e.g. looking for a friendly face in social gatherings)—on the prioritized perception of relevant stimuli. Such prestimulus factors lead to anticipatory search behaviours that allow fast detection of sources of potential reward or threat. An extended brain network is involved in endogenous processing of emotional stimuli, including frontoparietal (intraparietal sulcus, frontal eye field, and fusiform gyrus), sensory, and limbic regions. Neural circuits that involve limbic areas can facilitate enhanced attention via at least two mechanisms: directly, via projections from the basolateral nucleus of the amygdala to cortical sensory areas (e.g. fusiform face area); and indirectly, via projections to neuromodulatory systems in the basal forebrain and brainstem that, in turn, can modulate sensory cortical areas (i.e. increase the neuronal signal-to-noise ratio [5]). Accumulating evidence highlights the role of the amygdala in biased attention and demonstrates that manipulations that potentiate amygdala reactivity can also enhance attentional bias to threatening stimuli (for details see [5]). For example, Herry et al. (6) used a translational approach in mice and humans to show that unpredictability led to amygdala-dependent avoidance and anxiety behaviours. Amygdala damage in humans was shown to disrupt the prioritized processing of threat-related faces in crowded stimulus arrays (7). The amygdala was also found to play a key role in redirecting gaze (i.e. overt attention) to those features of the face, such as the eyes and the brows, that are most diagnostic of threat, trustworthiness, anger, and fear (8). Furthermore, there is evidence for increased connectivity between frontoparietal and sensory regions and the amygdala in response to informative cues for emotional stimuli (9). There is also evidence for increased connectivity between frontal regions and face-sensitive visual areas when participants must decide whether visual objects are faces or not (10).

Endogenous influences are of major importance when investigating depressed and anxious individuals, who tend to expect increased probability and cost for negative events (i.e. expectancy biases [11]). Indeed, threat sensitivity and maladaptive attention biases are more salient among depressed and anxious individuals (e.g. 12, 13). These biases can be manifested in both covert and overt attention by heightened vigilance to threat, difficulty in disengaging attention from threat, and/or avoidance of threatening stimuli (e.g. 11). Recent views highlight the role of dysfunctional expectancy biases in anxiety. Dysfunctional expectancy has been suggested to be associated with abnormal functioning of prefrontal–limbic–striatal–sensory pathways (14). Indeed, patients with social anxiety disorder showed increased amygdala activation and exaggerated behavioural interference when performing tasks that assess attentional bias to fear, such as the emotional Stroop or dot-probe tasks (15).

Dysfunctional biases already exist in populations *at risk* for developing psychopathology. For example, individuals with elevated levels of dispositional negativity—those who are prone to more intense, frequent, or persistent negative affect—are more likely to show elevated heightened reactivity to threat-related cues and to be characterized by significant attentional biases to threat (5). From a longitudinal perspective, attentional biases to threat-related cues have been shown to moderate the impact of dispositional negativity on the development of internalizing symptoms among youth. For example, White et al. (16) demonstrated that, among young people with an early childhood history of extreme dispositional negativity, those in the subset that also showed an attentional bias to threat-related cues on the dot-probe task were most likely to exhibit social withdrawal and elevated anxiety symptoms later in development.

The Influence of Threat on Executive Functions

Executive functioning is an umbrella term referring to a set of cognitive processes necessary for controlling behaviour. That is, these processes are essential in monitoring behaviours that facilitate the attainment of chosen goals. One of these functions is *working memory*, which holds important information regarding our current thoughts, feelings, and behaviour by directing attention towards internal representations (17). The capacity of working memory is determined by the ability to filter irrelevant information in the environment (18). However, evidence shows that task-irrelevant emotional information gains prioritized access to working memory (19), an effect that is more robust among individuals with, or dispositioned to, emotional disorders (20). The exaggerated representation of emotional information in working memory disrupts endogenous attention and other control mechanisms. This deficit may be a contributing factor to the heightened negative affect (i.e. anxiety, sadness) characterizing these populations (14). The tendency of anxious individuals to experience heightened distress and intrusive thoughts may be explained by allocation of excess storage capacity to threat, even when it is completely irrelevant to the task at hand and even when it is not present in the external world (21). Once lodged in working memory, threat-related information is poised to bias the stream of information processing (i.e. attention, memory retrieval, and action), thus promoting worry and other maladaptive cognitions (22).

Related to the evidence regarding enhanced distractibility in working memory, various studies have shown a reduced ability to disregard distracting emotional stimuli and to *focus attention* on a target among depressed and anxious individuals (23). The most common method of examining selectiveness of attention among these populations is the emotional Stroop task (24), in which participants are asked to attend to only one aspect of a written word (e.g. its colour) and ignore its distracting other characteristics (e.g. its emotional meaning). Findings demonstrate that the negative meanings of words interfere with attention among anxious and depressed patients, reflected by longer response latencies compared to healthy controls (25). Similar findings were demonstrated when participants were asked to determine the location of a picture target and to ignore emotional or neutral flankers that could appear in congruent and non-congruent locations (26). Anxious—but not depressed—participants showed attentional interference when faced with negative distractors (27). These findings demonstrate a specific deficiency in selective attention among anxious individuals during threat distraction.

Dysfunctional selective attention has been associated with abnormal activity in prefrontal, limbic, and sensory regions. For example, Mitterschiffthaler et al. (25) employed the emotional Stroop task and found significant engagement of the left rostral anterior cingulate cortex (ACC) and the right precuneus during the presentation of sad words, as well as a positive correlation between rostral ACC activation and response latencies for the sad words among depressed patients compared to controls. Fales et al. (28) reported a combination of enhanced amygdala reactivity and attenuated prefrontal reactivity among depressed patients in trials where they failed to ignore emotional distractors. Likewise, Kaiser et al. (29) showed that the level of depressive symptoms positively predicted the level of activation in the dorsal ACC and posterior cingulate cortex in response to negative distractors on the emotional Stroop, as well as correlating positively with higher connectivity between these areas. The researchers concluded that this connectivity between areas associated with cognitive control and internal attention systems suggests that, when depressed individuals are confronted with negative information, their elevated attention to internal thoughts and their difficulty in adaptively allocating resources in the environment interfere with goal-directed behaviour.

Deficiency in ignoring distractors may be related to a deficit in *cognitive control*, which refers to processes that enable regulating, coordinating, and sequencing thoughts and actions according to behavioural goals that are maintained internally. In situations when conflicting reactions must be modified based on contextual information, the control processes help make our behaviour as adaptive as possible (30). Accumulating evidence shows the disruptive influence of emotional distractors on cognitive control among healthy individuals (31) and even more significantly among depressed and anxious participants (32). In emotional-cued tasks in which individuals must strategically activate proactive control in a particular context (32), depressed as well as highly ruminative or worried individuals showed deficits manifested in longer response latencies or lower accuracy rates relative to healthy participants (e.g. 31, 33). In electrophysiological and neuroimaging studies of conflict and control, depressed individuals showed attenuated neural responses and anxious participants showed heightened responses compared to healthy controls (for a review see [32]).

Flexible Changes in the Relations Between Cognition and Emotion

Accumulating evidence suggests that attentional biases are plastic and can be altered by early and adult life experiences or interventions (34). Type of caregiving and type of parental communication were found to be associated with children's performance on inhibition, working memory, and cognitive flexibility tasks (35). Moreover, there is evidence that clinically effective cognitive behavioural and pharmacological treatments for anxiety also tend to reduce attentional biases to threat-related cues (36).

In light of the above, studies on adult interventions, such as cognitive training of adaptive allocation of attention or improvement of inhibitory functions, aim to reduce attentional biases presented in different mental disorders when reacting to emotional stimuli. In non-clinical samples, attention modification has been shown to reduce distress and behavioural signs of anxiety (e.g. 37). There is also evidence for neural plasticity following the training (e.g. 38). In adult clinical samples, medium-to-small treatment effects have been observed compared to placebo training (34, 39). However, recent reviews highlight some important limitations of existing protocols for attentional bias modification (see discussion in [40]).

The Influence of Cognition on Emotion

In daily life, we use a variety of cognitive strategies to regulate our emotions (e.g. 41). There is evidence that circuits involved in attention and working memory play a crucial role in emotion regulation (42). One frequently used and relatively effortless strategy aimed at reducing distress elicited from stimuli in the environment is attentional avoidance/deployment, manifested in shifting of attention away from the source of distress (41). Aue et al. (43) found that participants with arachnophobia who exhibited enhanced activation of the amygdala and dorsal striatum during exposure to spider images also executed more visual avoidance, suggesting that this strategy was aimed at regulating their extreme fear. This finding is in line with evidence highlighting the regulation of subcortical regions during attention avoidance (44). Another strategy considered to be an automatic attentional defence against unpleasant stimuli is repression of negative feelings aroused from emotional content away from awareness (45). Studies indicate that individuals who frequently exhibit this strategy tend not to recognize and label negative emotions (46) and report experiencing less negative emotion during mood induction. However, they also exhibit various deficiencies in cognitive and social skills, as well as enhanced physiological reactivity (47). Taken together, these findings show the complexity of repression as a strategy for emotion regulation.

Two strategies that require more effort and volition are distraction and reappraisal. Distraction is executed by generating a mental representation of something unrelated to the presented stimuli, while reappraisal involves generating an alternate meaning for the stimuli (48). Strauss et al. (49) pointed out that, while both distraction and reappraisal decrease amygdala response and increase activation in prefrontal and cingulate cortices, distraction leads to a larger decrease in the amygdala and a greater increase in prefrontal and parietal regions. This difference may be due to different demands on attention imposed by each strategy or their influence on different stages of emotion generation. Other strategies for regulating emotional states, such as cognitive reappraisal (50), require making efforts to maintain an explicit regulatory goal or model and depend on a working memory circuit encompassing the lateral prefrontal cortex (PFC) and posterior parietal cortex (PPC) (51). Consistent with this perspective, individual differences in working memory capacity are predictive of reappraisal success (42). Work using transcranial direct-current stimulation demonstrates that the lateral PFC is crucial for emotion regulation (52). In addition, recent evidence shows that the human ability to choose adaptive emotion regulation strategies is flexible, depending on the emotional context (e.g. reappraise when the stimulus is mildly aversive and distract when it is highly aversive [53]).

Ehring et al. (54) suggest that individuals who are vulnerable to depression fail to regulate their emotions successfully and sometimes regulate their emotions in situations when this is not necessary or functional. In addition, even when they do use adaptive strategies, they may extract less benefit from them, as they frequently fail to inhibit negative information (as in the case of repetitive rumination). Johnstone et al. (55) showed abnormal neural reactivity among depressed individuals during failure to regulate emotions. This abnormality was manifested in counterproductive enhanced activation of the right PFC and lack of engagement of left lateral–ventromedial prefrontal circuitry, crucial for the downregulation of amygdala responses to negative stimuli.

The Integration of Emotion and Cognition

Accumulating behavioural and neural-based evidence has led to the growing recognition that cognition and emotion are tightly interwoven. Neuroimaging studies demonstrate brain colocalization of key emotional and cognitive processes

(56); electrophysiological studies show that prototypical cognitive control signals (e.g. no-go N2, error-related negativity) systematically covary with emotional traits and states (57); and there is evidence for cognitive biases during negative or threatening states as well as among populations showing abnormal emotions. Indeed, a number of brain regions that are widely conceptualized as 'cognitive' are also involved in emotional processing. For example, the dorsolateral PFC, traditionally considered a key player in reasoning and higher cognition (58), also contributes to the top-down control of emotion and motivated behaviour (51) by gating working memory and focusing attention in the face of emotional distraction (e.g. 59).

Conversely, the amygdala, a canonical 'emotional' region, plays an important role in regulating higher cognitive functions by influencing the brainstem neurotransmitter systems orchestrating the quality of information processing (60). In situations that require rapid and immediate reactions to the environment, the amygdala guides attention and allocates resources from the PFC to adapt behaviour (61).

Conclusions and Future Directions

The findings reviewed here demonstrate that threat-related cues and emotional states influence a variety of attentional and executive functions. Cognitive biases have been demonstrated among healthy individuals, at-risk populations, and psychiatric patients. Other work indicates that executive attention plays a key role in the regulation of emotion. These mutual relationships between emotional and cognitive functions are subserved by a diffused neural network that includes the amygdala, insula, frontoparietal, midcingulate, sensory, and brainstem regions. This robust influence of emotional— mainly negative—information on attentional and executive function is nevertheless plastic and is modulated by experience.

The work we have reviewed suggests that emotion influences a number of specific cognitive processes. However, the vast majority of studies have only examined one cognitive process at a time, leaving the exact nature of the interrelationships unclear. This gap has motivated recent work aimed at understanding relationships between different kinds of emotional biases (11). For example, Everaert et al. (62) demonstrated that deficient inhibitory control over negative items is related to attention bias, which in turn predicts interpretation bias and depressive symptoms. A better understanding of the similarities and differences in processing biases between anxiety and depression may offer important insights for future diagnosis and treatment.

As demonstrated here and elsewhere (1), emotional cues, states, traits, and disorders can profoundly influence key elements of cognition, including orienting, selective attention, working memory, and cognitive control. There is also evidence that neural pathways involved in expectancy, executive functions, and working memory contribute to the regulation of emotional reactions. Evidence further shows that neural regions (e.g. dorsolateral PFC, middle cingulate cortex) and processes (e.g. attention, working memory, cognitive control) that are conventionally associated with cognition play a central role in emotional states, traits, and disorders. This evidence is in line with a recent model emerging from anatomical and neuroimaging findings. This model proposes that a non-hierarchical diffuse neural network, which includes cortical, thalamic, and midbrain areas, supports bidirectional and non-linear connections between emotion, cognition, motivation, and action (63).

Open questions remain regarding the dynamic mutual influences of the cognitive and neural systems modulating emotional processing. The development of advanced data acquisition and analysis methods may help to resolve these questions. Exciting developments in neuroimaging analysis offer opportunities for better characterizing the dynamics of valence processing and of interactions between neural networks. Developing a deeper understanding of the interplay between emotion and cognition is a matter of theoretical as well as practical importance. Many of the most common, costly, and challenging neuropsychiatric disorders involve prominent disturbances of both cognition and emotion, suggesting that these disorders can be conceptualized as disorders of the emotional–cognitive brain.

References

1. Okon-Singer H, Hendler T, Pessoa L, Shackman AJ. The neurobiology of emotion–cognition interactions: fundamental questions and strategies for future research. Front Hum Neurosci 2015;9:58.

2. Carretié L. Exogenous (automatic) attention to emotional stimuli: a review. Cogn Affect Behav Neurosci 2014;14:1228–58.

3. Egeth HE, Yantis S. Visual attention: control representation and time course. Annu Rev Psychol 1997;48:269–77.

4. Sussman TJ, Jin J, Mohanty A. Top-down and bottom-up factors in threat-related perception and attention in anxiety. Biol Psychol 2016;121:160–72.

5. Hur, J., Stockbridge, M. D., Fox, A. S. & Shackman, A. J. (in press). Dispositional negativity, cognition, and anxiety disorders: An integrative translational neuroscience framework. Progress in Brain Research.

6. Herry C, Bach DR, Esposito F, et al. Processing of temporal unpredictability in human and animal amygdala. J Neurosci 2007;27(22):5958–66.

7. Bach DR, Hurlemann R, Dolan RJ. Impaired threat prioritisation after selective bilateral amygdala lesions. Cortex 2015;63:206–13.

8. Oosterhof NN, Todorov A. Shared perceptual basis of emotional expressions and trustworthiness impressions from faces. Emotion 2009;9:128–33.

9. Mohanty A, Egner T, Monti JM, Mesulam MM. Search for a threatening target triggers limbic guidance of spatial attention. J Neurosci 2009;29(34):10563–72.

10. Summerfield C, Egner T, Greene M, Koechlin E, Mangels J, Hirsch J. Predictive codes for forthcoming perception in the frontal cortex. Science 2006;314(5803):1311–14.

11. Aue T, Okon-Singer H. Expectancy biases in fear and anxiety and their link to biases in attention. Clin Psychol Rev 2015;42:83–95.

12. Bar-Haim Y, Lamy D, Pergamin L, Bakermans-Kranenburg MJ, Van Ijzendoorn MH. Threat-related attentional bias in anxious and nonanxious individuals: a meta-analytic study. Psychol Bull 2007;133(1):1–24.

13. Crocker LD, Heller W, Warren SL, O'Hare AJ, Infantolino ZP, Miller GA. Relationships among cognition emotion and motivation: implications for intervention and neuroplasticity in psychopathology. Front Hum Neurosci 2013;7:261.

14. Grupe DW, Nitschke JB. Uncertainty and anticipation in anxiety: an integrated neurobiological and psychological perspective. Nat Rev Neurosci 2013;14:488–501.

15. Boehme S, Ritter V, Tefikow S, et al. Neural correlates of emotional interference in social anxiety disorder. PLoS ONE 2015;10:e0128608.

16. White LK, Degnan KA, Henderson HA, et al. Developmental relations between behavioral inhibition anxiety and attention biases to threat and positive information. Child Dev 2017;88:141–55.

17. Koshino H. Effects of working memory contents and perceptual load on distractor processing: when a response-related distractor is held in working memory. Acta Psychologica 2017;172:19–25.

18. Awh E, Vogel EK. The bouncer in the brain. Nature Neurosci 2008;11:5–6.

19. Moran TP. Anxiety and working memory capacity: a meta-analysis and narrative review. Psychol Bull 2016;142(8):831–64.

20. Stout DM, Shackman AJ, Larson CL. Failure to filter: anxious individuals show inefficient gating of threat from working memory. Front Hum Neurosci 2013;7:1–10.

21. Shackman AJ, Tromp DPM, Stockbridge MD, Kaplan CM, Tillman RM, Fox AS. Dispositional negativity: an integrative psychological and neurobiological perspective. Psychol Bull 2016;142:1275–314.

22. Thiruchselvam R, Hajcak G, Gross JJ. Looking inward: shifting attention within working memory representations alters emotional responses. Psychol Sci 2012;23(12):1461–6.

23. Snyder HR. Major depressive disorder is associated with broad impairments on neuropsychological measures of executive function: a meta-analysis and review. Psychol Bull 2013;139(1):81–132.

24. Gotlib IH, McCann CD. Construct accessibility and depression: an examination of cognitive and affective factors. J Personality Social Psychol 1984;47(2):427.

25. Mitterschiffthaler MT, Williams SCR, Walsh ND, et al. Neural basis of the emotional Stroop interference effect in major depression. Psychol Med 2008;38(2):247–56.

26. Lichtenstein-Vidne L, Henik A, Safadi Z. Task relevance modulates processing of distracting emotional stimuli. Cognition Emotion 2012;26(1):42–52.

27. Lichtenstein-Vidnea L, Okon-Singer H, Cohen N, et al. Attentional bias in clinical depression and anxiety: the impact of emotional and non-emotional distracting information. Biol Psychol 2017;122:4–12.

28. Fales CL, Barch DM, Rundle MM, et al. Altered emotional interference processing in affective and cognitive-control brain circuitry in major depression. Biol Psychiatry 2008;63(4):377–84.

29. Kaiser RH, Andrews-Hanna JR, Spielberg JM, et al. Distracted and down: neural mechanisms of affective interference in subclinical depression. Social Cogn Affective Neurosci 2014;10(5):654–63.

30. Braver TS. The variable nature of cognitive control: a dual mechanisms framework. Trends Cogn Sci 2012;16(2):106–13.

31. Kalanthroff E, Cohen N, Henik A. Stop feeling: inhibition of emotional interference following stop-signal trials. Front Hum Neurosci 2013;7:78.

32. Paulus MP. Cognitive control in depression and anxiety: out of control? Curr Opinion Behav Sci 2015;1:113–20.

33. Beckwé M, Deroost N, Koster EH, De Lissnyder E, De Raedt R. Worrying and rumination are both associated with reduced cognitive control. Psychol Res 2014;78(5):651–60.

34. MacLeod C, Clarke PJ. The attentional bias modification approach to anxiety intervention. Clin Psychol Sci 2015;3(1):58–78.

35. Spruijt AM, Dekker MC, Ziermans TB, Swaab H. Attentional control and executive functioning in school-aged children: linking self-regulation and parenting strategies. J Exp Child Psychol 2017;166:340.

36. Van Bockstaele B, Verschuere B, Tibboel H, De Houwer J, Crombez G, Koster EH. A review of current evidence for the causal impact of attentional bias on fear and anxiety. Psychol Bull 2014;140:682–721.

37. MacLeod C, Mathews A. Cognitive bias modification approaches to anxiety. Annu Rev Clin Psychol 2012;8:189–217.

38. Cohen N, Margulies DS, Ashkenazi S, et al. Using executive control training to suppress amygdala reactivity to aversive information. NeuroImage 2016;125:1022–31.

39. Price RB, Wallace M, Kuckertz JM, et al. Pooled patient-level meta-analysis of children and adults completing a computer-based anxiety intervention targeting attentional bias. Clin Psychol Rev 2016;50:37–49.

40. Okon-Singer H. The role of attention bias to threat in anxiety: mechanisms modulators and open questions. Curr Opinion Behav Sci 2018;19:26–30.

41. Gross JJ. Emotion regulation: current status and future prospects. Psychol Inquiry 2015;26:1–26.

42. Etkin A, Büchel C, Gross JJ. The neural bases of emotion regulation. Nature Rev Neurosci 2015;16(11):693–700.

43. Aue T, Hoeppli ME, Piguet C, Sterpenich V, Vuilleumier P. Visual avoidance in phobia: particularities in neural activity autonomic responding and cognitive risk evaluations. Front Hum Neurosci 2013;7:194.

44. Okon-Singer H, Mehnert J, Hoyer J, et al. Neural control of vascular reactions: impact of emotion and attention. J Neurosci 2014;34:4251–59.

45. Bonanno GA, Singer JL. Repressive personality style: theoretical and methodological implications for health and pathology. In: JL Singer (ed.). *Repression and Dissociation*. Chicago IL: University of Chicago Press, 1990: pp. 435–70.

46. Lane RD, Sechrest L, Riedel R, Shapiro DE, Kaszniak AW. Pervasive emotion recognition deficit common to alexithymia and the repressive coping style. Psychosomatic Med 2000;62(4):492–501.

47. Mauss IB, Bunge SA, Gross JJ. Automatic emotion regulation. Social Personality Psychology Compass 2007;1(1):146–67.

48. McRae K, Hughes B, Chopra S, Gabrieli JD, Gross JJ, Ochsner KN. The neural bases of distraction and reappraisal. J Cogn Neurosci 2010;22(2):248–62.

49. Strauss GP, Ossenfort KL, Whearty KM. Reappraisal and distraction emotion regulation strategies are associated with distinct patterns of visual attention and differing levels of cognitive demand. PloS One 2016;11(11):e0162290.

50. Heller AS, Johnstone T, Shackman AJ, et al. Reduced capacity to sustain positive emotion in major depression reflects diminished maintenance of fronto-striatal brain activation. Proc Natl Acad Sci U S A 2009;106:22445–50.

51. Buhle JT, Silvers JA, Wager TD, et al. Cognitive reappraisal of emotion: a meta-analysis of human neuroimaging studies. Cerebral Cortex 2014;24:2981–90.

52. Feeser M, Prehn K, Kazzer P, Mungee A, Bajbouj M. Transcranial direct current stimulation enhances cognitive control during emotion regulation. Brain Stimulation 2014;7(1):105–12.

53. Sheppes G, Scheibe S, Suri G, Radu P, Blechert J, Gross JJ. Emotion regulation choice: a conceptual framework and supporting evidence. J Exp Psychol: General 2014;143(1):163.

54. Ehring T, Tuschen-Caffier B, Schnülle J, Fischer S, Gross JJ. Emotion regulation and vulnerability to depression: spontaneous versus instructed use of emotion suppression and reappraisal. Emotion 2010;10(4):563.

55. Johnstone T, van Reekum CM, Urry HL, Kalin NH, Davidson RJ. Failure to regulate: counterproductive recruitment of top-down prefrontal-subcortical circuitry in major depression. J Neurosci 2007;27(33):8877–84.

56. de la Vega A, Chang LJ, Banich MT, Wager TD, Yarkoni T. Large-scale meta-analysis of human medial frontal cortex reveals tripartite functional organization. J Neurosci 2016;36:6553–62.

57. Cavanagh JF, Shackman AJ. Frontal midline theta reflects anxiety and cognitive control: meta-analytic evidence. J Physiol Paris 2014;109(1–3):3–15.

58. Miller EK, Cohen JD. An integrative theory of prefrontal cortex function. Annu Rev Neurosci 2001;24:167–202.

59. Peers PV, Simons JS, Lawrence AD. Prefrontal control of attention to threat. Front Hum Neurosci 2013;7:24.

60. Shansky RM, Lipps J. Stress-induced cognitive dysfunction: hormone neurotransmitter interactions in the prefrontal cortex. Front Hum Neurosci 2013;7:123.

61. Arnsten AF. Stress signalling pathways that impair prefrontal cortex structure and function. Nat Rev Neurosci 2009;10:410–22.

62. Everaert J, Grahek I, Koster EH. Individual differences in cognitive control over emotional material modulate cognitive biases linked to depressive symptoms. Cognition Emotion 2017;31(4):736–46.

63. Pessoa L. A network model of the emotional brain. Trends Cogn Sci 2017;21(5):357–71.

15

Clinical Characteristics of Social Cognitive Processes in Major Depressive Disorder

Katharina Foerster, Silke Joergens, and Bernhard T. Baune

Introduction

Social cognition—the ability to identify, perceive, and interpret socially relevant cues in relation to oneself and to others (1)—affects performance in interpersonal relationships as well as work performance; thus, it influences performance in everyday life. However, social cognition is a rarely investigated domain of cognitive impairment in major depressive disorder (MDD), although social cognitive dysfunction describes a core depressive symptom with broad influence on the functionality of a patient. A dysfunction in how a patient perceives and interprets emotional stimuli and mental states influences at least partly their social interaction and hence their treatment response to psychotherapy. Therefore, social cognitive function is an important contributor to the course of disease and is considered an indicator of treatment response (2).

The negative interpretation bias to sad facial expressions and oversensitivity to negative feedback are core clinical features of MDD and are associated with an unfavourable course of depression (3). This chapter focuses on how clinical characteristics (symptom severity, duration and intensity of illness, course of disease) influence social cognitive performance in MDD and how clinical research could achieve more consistent findings to elucidate the role of social cognitive function in the pathophysiology of MDD.

Affect Perception

The impairment of social functioning is an important feature of MDD (4). Patients with depression show decreased social interaction (5) and experience less reward value within social interaction (6). Previous investigations of social cognitive functions mostly focus on socially relevant cues like facial expressions. A recent meta-analysis found that patients with MDD show impaired facial affect recognition (7). A repeatedly reported effect in the psychological literature is *the negative interpretative bias*—the tendency of depressed patients to interpret a facial expression as more negative compared to interpretation by healthy controls. This interpretation bias has been backed up by evidence from a larger review (8). Interestingly, patients with MDD seem not to show perceptive deficits concerning the recognition accuracy across all facial expressions. Evidence suggests that the aberrations concerning facial affect recognition represent a pronounced phenomenon of *sensitivity* towards negative facial expressions. It has been repeatedly shown that patients with MDD perceive ambiguous faces as negative (9–15) and classify happy facial expressions more often as neutral when compared to healthy controls (3, 9). Additionally, studies have shown that patients with MDD perceive happy facial expressions with less intensity (16, 17).

Owing to an expansion in media transmitting techniques, social signals are often transmitted only via one channel; for instance, via the visual channel in text messages. Therefore, the communication of social signals through other modalities than facial expressions has become more important within relationships. Auditory emotional processing as another modality can be divided into the processing of verbal emotional information (via semantic content) and non-verbal emotional information (via prosody). Comparable to the results from research on facial affect perception, patients with MDD show a negative bias towards ambiguous prosodic information such as stimuli that represent surprise (18), an impairment towards the recognition of prosodic stimuli with a positive and negative valence (19, 20), and towards non-verbal vocalizations (e.g. screams [10]). Inpatients with MDD only show impaired affective prosody perception when there is a mismatch of emotional tone and semantic content (19), which has been referred to as executive dysfunction. While adults with MDD have not shown an impaired identification of prosodic content in semantically neutral sentences (18), depressed children were impaired in the categorization of emotional tone that matched the semantic content of the sentence (21).

Theory of Mind

Theory of mind (ToM) describes the ability to infer the mental states of others from socially relevant cues to understand and predict their behaviour (22). ToM consists of cognitive and affective compounds. Cognitive ToM or 'mentalizing' refers to the ability to infer the beliefs and intentions of others. Affective ToM refers to the ability to infer the emotional state of others.

The majority of evidence hints towards an impairment of patients with MDD in affective ToM (23–27). However, one study observed depressed patients to be selectively accurate in identifying negative emotional states while they did not differ in performance for neutral and positive emotional states compared to control subjects (28). This evidence fits well with previous results considering social cognitive dysfunction as a subtle and vulnerable phenomenon. In a recent review (29), it was argued that ToM deficits in MDD were focused around emotional, but not cognitive, processing. However, there has been evidence to suggest that patients with MDD have difficulties in cognitive ToM tasks compared to healthy controls (24, 25, 30). Patients with MDD were impaired in the interpretation of first- and second-order questions to social interactions (30) and the identification of faux pas in social situations (24, 31). MDD is also associated with less emotional awareness towards the thoughts (and feelings) of others compared to controls, but not towards their own emotional state (32). Compared to the compelling evidence found for affective ToM, only one study found that cognitive ToM deficits are limited to difficulties in integrating contextual information about other people or sequences of events (28) and three other studies found no difference in cognitive ToM between control and depressed subjects (33–35).

Clinical Characteristics

It has been suggested that patients in symptomatic remission might also be highly sensitive towards negative emotions: one study found that remitted patients identify anger more easily compared to controls (36), while another study found fear to be more easily identified by remitted patients (37). It has also been reported that a greater emotional intensity is required to identify happy expressions than in controls (38). Another important clinical subgroup is patients in a chronic state of depression. Some treatment strategies for chronically depressed patients address ToM dysfunction where patients are guided to falsify misinterpretations in social interactions; for example, the Cognitive Behavioural Analysis System of Psychotherapy (39, 40). This treatment approach seems to be well reasoned because patients with mentalizing dysfunction show an increased risk for relapse (41). Clinical features such as suicidal behaviours (42), excessive rumination (43), anxiety (27), and psychotic symptoms (24, 25) have also been associated with ToM dysfunction.

Prediction of Treatment Response

The prediction of treatment response becomes more important as healthcare and socioeconomic costs due to MDD have been rising. The association of social cognitive impairment with treatment response is particularly important because of its key role for the psychotherapeutic and psychiatric treatment process in depression. Of interest in this context is the finding that psychoanalytic group therapy was associated with an improved emotional awareness for others (32). On the pharmacological side, a randomized controlled trial found that acute administration of citalopram improves the recognition accuracy towards stimuli depicting fear compared to placebo (37). A longitudinal study found that only patients who recovered within the interval showed a reduced reaction towards negative emotions after a 6-week interval (2). Social cognitive dysfunction appears to be reversible by treatment with antidepressants as patients under pharmacological treatment show social cognitive dysfunction compared to the control subjects, while untreated depressed patients show social cognitive dysfunction (36). The reversibility might also be dependent on the antidepressant dose, with higher doses being associated with more accurate perception towards sad facial expressions (3). In a longitudinal study, patients' social cognitive performance was the same between baseline and at 6-month follow-up, while symptom severity had decreased during this time (44, 45). This might indicate that specific intervention targeting emotional processing via medication or psychotherapy induces change in social cognitive function. It has been suggested that social cognitive function should be targeted during therapy to prevent relapse (29). The effect of treatment on social cognitive function could also contribute to the partly inconsistent results observed in the field since treatment with antidepressants is quite common, but most often is not considered as a covariate in studies. To enhance the understanding on the relationship between treatment response and social cognitive function, large-scale longitudinal interventional studies with greater follow-up intervals would be required. Taken together, these studies suggest social cognitive impairment as a state feature of MDD and a predictor of treatment response that appears to be reversible through psychotherapeutic and pharmacological treatment.

Few studies investigated the effect of the severity of depression on social cognitive performance (27, 32, 46). Patients with severe depression performed worse on social cognitive tasks than those with mild depression (46). Studies that split the depressed group into 'mild-to-moderate' and 'severe' groups reported pronounced impaired social cognitive function in the severe group only (27). More severe depression was also associated with aberrant performance on specific emotional categories: while some studies found higher severity to be associated with an attenuated response towards happy stimuli (3, 47), others found severity to be associated with higher accuracy in recognizing sad stimuli (13, 14).

Increased symptom severity of depression may also be associated with reduced ToM function, as shown in a study that found a relationship between poor understanding towards the mental state of others and heightened depressive severity (28). Moreover, certain severe depressive symptoms, such as suicidal and psychotic features, have been related to impaired social cognitive function (24, 25, 42).

Tests for Social Cognitive Function

Although interesting patterns on social cognitive function in depression have emerged, results are still inconsistent. Various reasons could contribute to such inconsistency. Among others, methodological aspects, such as the use of varying social cognitive measures with sometimes unknown psychometric properties, contribute to the disparity within the field. Table 15.1 provides an overview of the more commonly used tests in social cognitive function research, including psychometric properties that could be used for guidance in future research. The Wechsler ACS Social Perception Subtest is especially relevant for clinical research because it is the only measurement that contains 15 comparative clinical groups. Future studies should use measurements that on the one hand meet certain psychometric properties (large normative samples, stability, reliability, and validity of the measure) and consider tasks that use multimodal stimuli and dynamic settings on the other hand.

Conclusions

Most of the evidence supports the observation that patients with MDD show a negative bias towards ambiguous emotional information in all domains of social perception (facial affect, prosody, verbal content, and ToM); patients with MDD appear to be more accurate in detecting negative information and they tend to misinterpret ambiguous or neutral information as negative compared to healthy controls. These aberrations of social cognition relate to overall symptom severity of depression and treatment response and tend to vary during the course of depression. An important topic for further research will be to investigate the possible consequences of digital social interaction for patients with MDD. Digital treatment tools (mental health apps) and digital communication with health professionals are becoming more common and there is a gap in social cognitive research concerning the processing of digital social cues. A recommendation for future research is the coherent use of standardized, normed, reliable, and valid tests for social cognitive function. This chapter provides an overview of commonly used tests of social cognitive function to assist with instrument choices for future research.

Table 15.1 Social cognitive tests and their psychometric properties

Social cognitive test, abbreviation (source): methodological description	Test–retest reliability	Internal consistency	Sample (size, clinical group)
Affect recognition			
Facial Expressions of Emotion Stimuli and Tests, *Ekman60* (48): faces of 10 actors displaying the six basic emotions (from the Ekman and Friesen photograph series) are displayed and the participants have to detect the emotions. The Ekman and Friesen photos (49) are a commonly used and validated series of photographs depicting facial emotion (50). The measure is considered as a discriminative instrument for FTD and depression (51).	0.77	n.r.	227 HC N=25 mild FTD, N=33 HC (51) Test–retest reliability (52)
Perception of Affect Task, *PAT* (53): 140-item measure of the ability to match emotions to stimuli, four subtasks that require the subject to match verbal or non-verbal emotion stimuli with verbal or non-verbal emotion responses; the PAT uses Ekman and Friesen's (1978) photograph series.	n.r.	0.72–0.88	N=176 (53)
Bell-Lysaker Emotional Recognition Test, *BLERT* (54): audiovisual affect recognition task designed to elicit a person's ability to discriminate seven affect states given facial, voice-tonal, and upper body movement cues; 21 vignettes (same actor in each 10-s vignette) in which an affect is portrayed.	0.77	0.87	Clinical sample available: schizophrenia N=54 HC: N=56 (55)
Florida Affect Battery (56): battery with 10 subtests in three domains: prosody, facial affect, cross-modal (happiness, sadness, anger, fear as emotional stimuli and a neutral condition).	0.89–0.97	n.r.	N=164 N=20 for retest reliability Norms from patients with brain injury and children
Wechsler Advanced Clinical Solutions—Social Perception Subtest (57): social cognitive battery with three tests for prosody and facial affect perception and multimodal affect perception.	0.60–0.70	0.69–0.81	N=800*; 15 clinical groups (1)

Social interaction

Levels of Emotional Awareness, *LEAS* (58): a projective instrument that describes in two to four sentences 20 scenes with two characters. The subjects describe their anticipated feelings and those of the other person. Interrater reliability ranges from 0.84 to 0.91 (59).	n.r.	LEAS A 0.81 LEAS B 0.76	N=40 Interrater reliability: N=364
Interpersonal Reactivity Index (60): a self-report instrument with four scales: perspective-taking, fantasy, empathic concern, personal distress. Few subscales correlate with other empathy measures (Hogan Empathy Scale, Mehrabian and Epstein Emotional Empathy (61).	0.62–0.71	0.71–0.77	N=1161*
MSCEIT-Managing-Emotions: Mayor–Salovey–Caruso Emotional Intelligence Test—Managing Emotion Branch (62): a measure that predicts consequences of self and other's thoughts, feelings and actions; International Scoring System for a consensus-based social cognition measure.	0.86	Split half reliability: 0.93	N=2112* emotions expert sample with N=21
Bar-On Emotional Quotient Inventory, *EQ-I* (63): 133-item inventory, 13 subscales that cluster into four factors: intrapersonal, interpersonal, adaptability, and stress management (factors are highly correlated), and two subscales for general mood.	0.72–0.80	0.97	N=3831*

Theory of mind

Social Cognition and Emotional Assessment, *SEA* (64): a test of identification of facial emotions, a reversal/extinction task, a behavioural control task, a ToM test, and an apathy scale.	n.r.	n.r.	N=22 FTD N=22 AD/MCI N=30 HC
EMOTICOM (65): a test battery that assesses four core domains of affective cognition: emotion processing, motivation, impulsivity, and social cognition. It contains 17 different tasks.	Emotion: 0.34–0.86 Social Cognition: 0.58–0.94	n.r.	N=200

(continued)

Table 15.1 Continued

Social cognitive test, abbreviation (source): methodological description	Test–retest reliability	Internal consistency	Sample (size, clinical group)
The Awareness of Social Interference Test, *TASIT/TASIT-S* (66): a test for higher label social cognition with film clips of everyday interactions. While Part 1 assesses emotion recognition, Parts 2 and 3 assess the ability to detect literal (sincerity and lies) and non-literal (sarcasm) conversational remarks, as well as the ability to make judgements about the thoughts, intentions, and feelings of speakers.	0.74–0.88	High level of item cohesiveness	N=116 with severe chronic brain injury N=32 retested N=283* (67)
The Frith–Happé animations, *FHA*—the social perception task, animated **triangles task** (68): silent animations where the participant has to infer the intentions of triangles and their relationship; the authors reported an interrater consistency of 86% for accuracy and 90% for description type (four raters).	n.r.	n.r.	N=27 ASD, N=23 children with general intellectual impairment, N=26 HC 8-year-olds N=28 HC adults
The Reading the Mind in the Eyes Task—Revised, *Eyes* (69): the subject has to classify the emotional state of a person via the photographic depiction of the person's eyes.	0.83	0.61	N=239 HC N=15 adults with Asperger syndrome

AD, Alzheimer's dementia; ASD, Autism spectrum disorder; FTD, frontotemporal dementia—a neurological disease associated with social cognitive dysfunction; HC, healthy controls; MCI, mild cognitive impairment; n. r., not reported; ToM, theory of mind. A range in reliability indicates the use of more than one scale/section in a test; psychometric properties were acquired through secondary literature if the primary study/manual was not accessible. *Indicates the availability of a large normative sample.

References

1. Kandalaft MR, Didehbani N, Cullum CM, et al. The Wechsler ACS Social Perception Subtest: a preliminary comparison with other measures of social cognition. J Psychoeduc Assess 2012;30(5):455–65.

2. Dannlowski U, Kersting A, Donges US, Lalee-Mentzel J, Arolt V, Suslow T. Masked facial affect priming is associated with therapy response in clinical depression. Eur Arch Psychiatry Clin Neurosci 2006;256(4):215–21.

3. Surguladze SA, Young AW, Senior C, Brébion G, Travis MJ, Phillips ML. Recognition accuracy and response bias to happy and sad facial expressions in patients with major depression. Neuropsychology 2004;18(2):212–18.

4. Levendosky AA, Okun A, Parker JG. Depression and maltreatment as predictors of social competence and social problem-solving skills in school-age children. Child Abuse Negl 1995;19(10):1183–95.

5. Gotlib IH, Lee CM. The social functioning of depressed patients: a longitudinal assessment. J Soc Clin Psychol 1989;8(3):223–37.

6. Nezlek JB, Hampton CP, Shean GD. Clinical depression and day-to-day social interaction in a community sample. J Abnorm Psychol 2000;IOQ(i):11–19.

7. Dalili MN, Penton-Voak IS, Harmer CJ, Munafò MR. Meta-analysis of emotion recognition deficits in major depressive disorder. Psychol Med 2015;45:1135–44.

8. Bourke C, Douglas K, Porter R. Processing of facial emotion expression in major depression: a review. Aust N Z J Psychiatry 2010;44(8):681–96.

9. Gur RC, Erwin RJ, Gur RE, Zwil AS, Heimberg C, Kraemer HC. Facial emotion discrimination: II. Behavioral findings in depression. Psychiatry Res 1992;42(3):241–51.

10. Naranjo C, Kornreich C, Campanella S, et al. Major depression is associated with impaired processing of emotion in music as well as in facial and vocal stimuli. J Affect Disord 2011;128(3):243–51.

11. Gur RE, McGrath C, Chan RM, et al. An fMRI study of facial emotion processing in patients with schizophrenia. Am J Psychiatry 2002;159(12):1992–9.

12. Hale WWI. Judgment of facial expressions and depression persistence. Psychiatry Res 1998;80:265–74.

13. Leppänen JM, Milders M, Bell JS, Terriere E, Hietanen JK. Depression biases the recognition of emotionally neutral faces. Psychiatry Res 2004;128(2):123–33.

14. Gollan JK, McCloskey M, Hoxha D, Coccaro EF. How do depressed and healthy adults interpret nuanced facial expressions? J Abnorm Psychol 2010;119(4):804–10.

15. Douglas KM, Porter RJ. Recognition of disgusted facial expressions in severe depression. Br J Psychiatry 2010;197(2):156–7.

16. Joormann J, Gotlib IH. Is this happiness I see? Biases in the identification of emotional facial expressions in depression and social phobia. J Abnorm Psychol 2006;115(4):705–14.

17. Yoon KL, Joormann J, Gotlib IH. Judging the intensity of facial expressions of emotion: depression-related biases in the processing of positive affect. J Abnorm Psychol 2009;118(1):223–8.

18. Kan Y, Mimura M, Kamijima K, Kawamura M. Recognition of emotion from moving facial and prosodic stimuli in depressed patients. J Neurol Neurosurg Psychiatry 2004;75(12):1667–71.

19. Uekermann J, Abdel-Hamid M, Lehmkämper C, Vollmoeller W, Daum I. Perception of affective prosody in major depression: a link to executive functions? J Int Neuropsychol Soc 2008;14(4):552–61.

20. Péron J, El Tamer S, Grandjean D, et al. Major depressive disorder skews the recognition of emotional prosody. Prog Neuro-Psychopharmacology Biol Psychiatry 2011;35(4):987–96.

21. Emerson CS, Harrison DW, Everhart DE. Investigation of receptive affective prosodic ability in school-aged boys with and without depression. Neuropsychiatry Neuropsychol Behav Neurol 1999;12(2):102–9.

22. Premack D, Woodruff G. Does the chimpanzee have a theory of mind? Behav Brain Sci 1978;1(4):515.

23. Szily E, Kéri S. Anomalous subjective experience and psychosis risk in young depressed patients. Psychopathology 2009;42:229–35.

24. Wang Y-G, Wang Y-Q, Chen S-L, Zhu C-Y, Wang K. Theory of mind disability in major depression with or without psychotic symptoms: a componential view. Psychiatry Res 2008;161:153–61.

25. Cao Y, Zhao Q-D, Hu L-J, et al. Theory of mind deficits in patients with esophageal cancer combined with depression. World J Gastroenterol 2013;19(19):2969–73.

26. Harkness KL, Washburn D, Theriault JE, Lee L, Sabbagh MA. Maternal history of depression is associated with enhanced theory of mind in depressed and nondepressed adult women. Psychiatry Res 2011;189(1):91–6.

27. Lee L, Harkness KL, Sabbagh MA, Jacobson JA. Mental state decoding abilities in clinical depression. J Affect Disord 2005;86(2–3):247–58.

28. Wolkenstein L, Schoenenberg M, Schirm E, Hautzinger M. I can see what you feel, but I can't deal with it: impaired theory of mind in depression. J Affect Disord 2011;132(1–2):104–11.

29. Weightman MJ, Air TM, Baune BT. A review of the role of social cognition in major depressive disorder. Front Psychiatry 2014;5:179.

30. Zobel I, Werden D, Linster H, et al. Theory of mind deficits in chronically depressed patients. Depress Anxiety 2010;27(9):821–8.

31. Cao B, Passos IC, Mwangi B, et al. Hippocampal volume and verbal memory performance in late-stage bipolar disorder. J Psychiatr Res 2016;73:102–7.

32. Donges U-S, Kersting A, Dannlowski U, Lalee-Mentzel J, Arolt V, Suslow T. Reduced awareness of others' emotions in unipolar depressed patients. J Nerv Ment Dis 2005;193(5):331–7.

33. Wilbertz G, Brakemeier E-L, Zobel I, Härter M, Schramm E. Exploring preoperational features in chronic depression. J Affect Disord 2010;124:262-9.

34. Bertoux M, Delavest M, de Souza LC, et al. Social cognition and emotional assessment differentiates frontotemporal dementia from depression. J Neurol Neurosurg Psychiatry 2012;83(4):411-16.

35. Bazin N, Brunet-Gouet E, Bourdet C, et al. Quantitative assessment of attribution of intentions to others in schizophrenia using an ecological video-based task: a comparison with manic and depressed patients. Psychiatry Res 2009;167(1-2):28-35.

36. Anderson IM, Shippen C, Juhasz G, et al. State-dependent alteration in face emotion recognition in depression. Br J Psychiatry 2011;198(4):302-8.

37. Bhagwagar Z, Cowen PJ, Goodwin GM, Harmer CJ. Normalization of enhanced fear recognition by acute SSRI treatment in subjects with a previous history of depression. Am J Psychiatry 2004;161(1):166-8.

38. LeMoult J, Joormann J, Sherdell L, Wright Y, Gotlib IH. Identification of emotional facial expressions following recovery from depression. J Abnorm Psychol 2009;118(4):828-33.

39. McCullough JP. Treatment for chronic depression: cognitive behavioral analysis system of psychotherapy (CBASP). J Psychother Integr 2003;13(3-4):241-63.

40. Klein DN, Leon AC, Li C, et al. Social problem solving and depressive symptoms over time: a randomized clinical trial of cognitive-behavioral analysis system of psychotherapy, brief supportive psychotherapy, and pharmacotherapy. J Consult Clin Psychol 2011;79(3):342-52.

41. Inoue Y, Yamada K, Kanba S. Deficit in theory of mind is a risk for relapse of major depression. J Affect Disord 2006;95(1-3):125-7.

42. Szanto K, Dombrovski AY, Sahakian BJ, et al. Social emotion recognition, social functioning, and attempted suicide in late-life depression. Am J Geriatr Psychiatry 2012;20(3):257-65.

43. Raes F, Hermans D, Williams JMG. Negative bias in the perception of others' facial emotional expressions in major depression. J Nerv Ment Dis 2006;194(10):796-9.

44. Suslow T, Dannlowski U, Lalee-Mentzel J, Donges U-S, Arolt V, Kersting A. Spatial processing of facial emotion in patients with unipolar depression: a longitudinal study. J Affect Disord 2004;83(1):59-63.

45. Milders M, Bell S, Platt J, Serrano R, Runcie O. Stable expression recognition abnormalities in unipolar depression. Psychiatry Res 2010;179(1):38-42.

46. Air T, Weightman MJ, Baune BT. Symptom severity of depressive symptoms impacts on social cognition performance in current but not remitted major depressive disorder. Front Psychol 2015;6:1-9.

47. Csukly G, Czobor P, Szily E, Takács B, Simon L. Facial expression recognition in depressed subjects. J Nerv Ment Dis 2009;197(2):98-103.

48. Young A, Perret D, Cabler A, Sprengelmeyer R, Ekman P. *Facial Expressions of Emotion: Stimuli and Tests (FEEST)*. St. Edmunds, UK: Thames Valley Test Company; 2002.

49. Ekman P, Friesen WV. *Pictures of Facial Affect.* Palo Alto: Consulting Psychologists Press; 1978.

50. Edwards J, Jackson HJ, Pattison PE. Emotion recognition via facial expression and affective prosody in schizophrenia: a methodological review. Clin Psychol Rev 2002;22(6):789–832.

51. Diehl-Schmid J, Pohl C, Ruprecht C, Wagenpfeil S, Foerstl H, Kurz A. The Ekman 60 Faces Test as a diagnostic instrument in frontotemporal dementia. Arch Clin Neuropsychol 2007;22(4):459–64.

52. Williams C, Daley D, Burnside E, Hammond-Rowley S. Measuring emotional intelligence in preadolescence. Pers Individ Diff 2009;47:316–20.

53. Rau J. A normative study of the perception of affect task. The University of Arizona. 1988;

54. Bryson G, Bell M, Lysaker P. Affect recognition in schizophrenia: a function of global impairment or a specific cognitive deficit. Psychiatry Res 1997;71(2):105–13.

55. Fiszdon JM, Johannesen JK. Functional significance of preserved affect recognition in schizophrenia. Psychiatry Res 2010;176(2–3):120–5.

56. Bowers B, Blonder LX, Heilman KM. Florida affect battery. 1992. https://neurology.ufl.edu/files/2011/12/Florida-Affect-Battery-Manual.pdf

57. Pearson. *Advanced Clinical Solutions for WAIS-IV and WMS-IV.* San Antonio, TX: Pearson; 2009.

58. Lane RD, Quinlan DM, Schwartz GE, Walker PA, Zeitlin SB. The levels of emotional awareness scale: a cognitive-developmental measure of emotion. J Pers Assess 1990;55(1&2):124–34.

59. Subic-Wrana C, Thomas W, Huber M, Köhle K. Levels of Emotional Awareness Scale (LEAS). Psychotherapeut 2001;46(3):176–81.

60. Davis MH. A multidimensional approach to individual differences in empathy. JSAS Cat Sel Doc Psychol 1980;10:85.

61. Davis MH. Measuring individual differences in empathy: evidence for a multidimensional approach. J Pers Soc Psychol 1983;44(1):113–26.

62. Mayer JD, Salovey P, Caruso DR, Sitarenios G. Measuring emotional intelligence With the MSCEIT V2.0. Emotion 2003;3(1):97–105.

63. Bar-On R. *The Bar-On Emotional Quotient Inventory (EQ-i): A test of emotional intelligence.* Toronto, Canada: Multi-Health Systems; 1997.

64. Funkiewiez A, Bertoux M, de Souza LC, Lévy R, Dubois B. The SEA (Social Cognition and Emotional Assessment): a clinical neuropsychological tool for early diagnosis of frontal variant of frontotemporal lobar degeneration. Neuropsychology 2012;26(1):81–90.

65. Bland AR, Chan RCK, Lau J, et al. EMOTICOM: a neuropsychological test battery to evaluate emotion, motivation, impulsivity, and social cognition. Front Behav Neurosci 2016;10(10):253389–25.

66. Honan CA, McDonald S, Sufani C, Hine DW, Kumfor F. The awareness of social inference test: development of a shortened version for use in adults with acquired brain injury. Clin Neuropsychol 2016;30(2):243–64.

67. McDonald S, Flanagan S, Rollins J, Kinch J. TASIT: A new clinical tool for assessing social perception after traumatic brain injury. J Head Trauma Rehabil 2003;18(3):219–38.

68. Abell F, Happé F, Frith U. Do triangles play tricks? Attribution of mental states to animated shapes in normal and abnormal development. Cogn Dev. 2000;15(1):1–16.

69. Baron-Cohen S, Wheelwright S, Hill J, Raste Y, Plumb I. The "Reading the Mind in the Eyes" Test Revised Version: a study with normal adults, and adults with Asperger syndrome or high-functioning autism. J Child Psychol Psychiatry 2001;42(2):241–51.

16

Understanding of Self and Others: Neurobiological Underpinnings of Social Cognition

Franziska K. Goer and Rebecca Elliott

Introduction

Major depressive disorder (MDD) has consistently been linked to disturbances in affective or 'hot' (emotionally salient) cognition, including the robust finding of negative affective biases and deficits in reward and punishment learning, which are thought to play a key role in the development and maintenance of the disorder (1–3). Neuroimaging studies suggest roles for limbic, subcortical, and prefrontal regions, including both dorsolateral and dorsomedial prefrontal cortices and anterior cingulate cortex (ACC; 4–6). This network of brain regions also underpins emotion regulation (7), which allows individuals, consciously or automatically, to alter aspects of emotion response. Maladaptive emotion regulation has been consistently implicated in depression (8).

These findings have been critical for deepening our understanding of the underlying mechanisms of depression and providing targets for established treatments; however, currently available treatments do not offer benefits to all depressed patients. Evidence suggests that many patients remain treatment-resistant even after two (50%; 9) or three (33%; 10) courses of antidepressant treatment. Furthermore, even when promoting successful remission of depressive symptoms, current treatments may provide only limited improvements in social functioning (11), despite this being of critical importance to patients' long-term outcomes.

Social cognition, the processes underlying interpersonal interactions (12), constitutes a higher-order integration and real-life application of many components of affective cognition, and may be a critical factor in functional outcomes, as has already been demonstrated in schizophrenia (13).

Cognitive processes underlying effective social interactions are complex and manifold, reflecting the intricate and dynamic nature of human social functioning. Research on social cognition has focused on self-referential processing, other-processing (including knowledge about internal states, motivations, and agency of others, known as 'theory of mind'), moral emotions, and social decision-making. The chapter will review these subcomponents of social cognition in depression and discuss the neural correlates in both patients with MDD and healthy controls (HC).

Social Cognition in Depression
Self-processing in Depression

Depression is associated with a cognitive bias toward negative self-focus. Classic studies on memory have demonstrated a significant 'self-reference effect' (14), in which self-related words are better recalled than words related to others (15). In line with observed negative processing biases, studies report that depressed individuals show increased recall accuracy for negatively valenced compared to positively valenced words that have been self-referentially encoded (16). The opposite pattern is observed in HC (17).

Heightened memory for negative self-referential stimuli is consistent with prominent cognitive theories of depression, including Beck's triad of depression consisting of negative views about oneself, the world, and the future (18). Furthermore, rumination, a maladaptive emotion regulation strategy involving fixated self-focused attention on past events, has been consistently linked to depression (19).

Neural Basis of Self-processing in Healthy Controls
Functional magnetic resonance imaging (fMRI) studies of HC have highlighted the importance of the medial prefrontal cortex (MPFC) in self-referential processing (20), including the self-reference effect (21). The MPFC is also a main functional hub of the default mode network (DMN; 22), which, along with other social cognitive roles, has been consistently linked to self-referential thought (23).

Neural Basis of Self-processing in Major Depressive Disorder
Aberrant MPFC activity appears to underlie negative self-referential processing biases observed in depression (24). Depression, along with other psychiatric disorders, has also been associated with hyperactivity and hyperconnectivity of the DMN (which incorporates the MPFC) during emotion-processing tasks (25, 26), as well as in the resting state (27). Hyperconnectivity and hyperactivity of the DMN in MDD may provide the neural basis of difficulty disengaging from self-referential thought during tasks, which may in turn contribute to maladaptive rumination. Supporting this hypothesis, a study found significant positive correlation between DMN dominance and depressive rumination in individuals with MDD (28).

Other-processing (Theory of Mind) in Depression

Theory of mind (ToM), the capacity to attribute mental states and intentions to other people, is essential for successful social interactions (29). ToM is a complex cognitive process that requires mentalizing (the ability to interpret others' mental states [30]), computations of social agency (who is responsible for a particular outcome in a social exchange), and an understanding of social norms (31).

A widely used first-order ToM task is the 'Reading the Mind in the Eyes' test (RMET), which requires participants to assign an emotional state to a picture of a set of eyes (32). Significant deficits in performance on this task have been observed in MDD (33, 34). A more recent study, however, reported unimpaired RMET performance (35). Findings should be cautiously interpreted, as researchers have argued that the RMET may more accurately be interpreted as a measure of emotion recognition than ToM (36).

Second-order ToM tasks require inference of other people's beliefs about another's mental state (37). This may be measured using second-order false belief tasks ('Person A thinks that person B thinks that ...' [38]) or faux pas tasks (involving a deviation from a social norm [39]). Significant deficits have been reported in depressed patients' ability to pass second-order ToM tasks in spite of unimpaired performance on the first-order RMET (35, 40). Importantly, these deficits have been found to be linked to poor clinical and social functioning outcomes (41, 42).

Neural Basis of Theory of Mind in Healthy Controls

Neural substrates of ToM in HC have been extensively studied using fMRI, which consistently implicates the bilateral temporoparietal junctions, MPFC, and the adjacent paracingulate cortex (43). The temporoparietal junction is thought to mediate lower-level perceptual processing, whereas the MPFC and paracingulate cortex mediate higher-order integration of complex social information about self, others, and their intentions (44).

Neural Basis of Theory of Mind in Major Depressive Disorder

There is a dearth of studies of the neural basis of possible ToM deficits in MDD. The limited research to date has focused on patients with bipolar disorder and has revealed decreased response of temporal regions and the insula associated with ToM (42). More studies are needed to investigate whether similar brain regions may underlie aberrant ToM in MDD.

Moral Emotions in Depression

Moral emotions are critical to social functioning in humans as they may promote adherence to social norms and motivate behaviour that is other-serving (aiming to satisfy certain moral standards) as oppose to maximizing self-interest (45). While traditionally research on moral emotions has focused on negative self-conscious emotions (particularly shame and guilt), the past decade has seen an extension of the concept to negative other-focused emotions (e.g. righteous anger, contempt) and positive moral emotions (e.g. gratitude, empathy [46]).

A recent systematic review revealed exaggerated levels of empathic stress but not empathic concern in depression (47). The authors defined empathic stress as the negative emotion resulting from observing another person's pain or negative experience that may promote behavioural withdrawal. Empathic concern, by contrast, was operationalized as other-orientated compassion that motivates prosocial approach behaviours (47). The selectively heightened empathic stress in depression is in line with the previously discussed findings of increased negative self-focus. A third type of empathy that encompasses perspective-taking (known as 'cognitive empathy') has also been found to be diminished in MDD and is associated with poorer psychosocial outcomes (47, 48).

The most studied moral emotions in the context of depression are the self-conscious and self-blaming emotions shame and guilt. MDD has been consistently associated with heightened levels of shame (49) and guilt (50). In fact, guilt constitutes one of the core diagnostic symptoms of MDD (51), and studies suggest that this symptom may be a strong predictor of suicide attempts (52). While shame does not constitute a discrete diagnostic criterion for MDD, various studies highlight its clinical relevance. Both shame and guilt have been independently associated with suicidal ideation (53). Shame may even constitute a risk factor for developing MDD; a longitudinal study that found shame levels at age 3 years predicted development of MDD in later life (50).

Neural Basis of Moral Emotions in Healthy Controls

Prior to the advent of neuroimaging, neuropsychological case studies provided insight into the neurobiological underpinnings of moral emotions. The widely cited case of Phineas Gage, and subsequent single case studies, indicated that damage to the ventral frontal cortex impacts social behaviour while sparing general cognitive abilities (54, 55).

Neuropsychological studies have been able to investigate more discriminate effects of such lesions on various forms of social cognition. For example, a study of 33 patients with PFC lesions found profound deficits in interpersonal judgements on a social perception task, particularly in those patients with orbitofrontal cortex (OFC) lesions (56). Another study found that cognitive empathy was impaired in patients with bilateral ventromedial prefrontal cortex (VMPFC) damage while affective empathy was impaired in those with inferior frontal gyrus damage (57). VMPFC damage has also been associated with abnormal moral judgements in hypothetical moral dilemmas (58).

More recently, neuroimaging studies have provided additional evidence for the neurobiological underpinnings of moral emotions. These studies have revealed a neural network underlying moral emotion that includes the MPFC, superior temporal sulcus (STS), and anterior temporal cortex (59). For example, an fMRI study in which participants passively watched pictures of emotionally charged scenes revealed response of the OFC, MPFC, and STS specifically during scenes with moral content (60). fMRI studies investigating ethical decision-making (61) and hypothetical moral judgements (62) revealed responses in comparable brain regions.

Neuroimaging studies of specific moral emotions, such as guilt, have highlighted the role of the ACC. Recent fMRI studies have found selective subgenual (sg)ACC response to guilt compared to various control emotions, including indignation (63, 64) and anger and sadness (65). These responses may be especially pronounced in guilt scenarios accompanied by social consequences (66).

Neural Basis of Moral Emotions in Major Depressive Disorder
There has been a dearth of studies directly investigating the neural underpinnings of moral emotions in depression. A recent fMRI study using a task designed to elicit social/moral emotions found decreased MPFC activation to images depicting social interactions in individuals with remitted MDD (rMDD) compared to HC (67). Another fMRI study of participants with rMDD found decreased coupling between the right superior anterior temporal lobe (ATL) and the subgenual cingulate cortex/septal region (SCSR) for guilt versus indignation (63). Furthermore, ATL–SCSR connectivity was negatively correlated with self-blame. A recent study in rMDD found heightened activation of the right amygdala and posterior insula during shame relative to guilt, providing initial evidence for an at least partially distinct neural basis of shame versus guilt in depression (68).

Regions that have been implicated in the experience of guilt and shame, especially the sgACC, have also been implicated more generally in MDD (69). Moreover, studies have proposed that sgACC metabolism may be a biomarker for successful psychotherapy (70) and antidepressant treatment response (71). However, more studies are needed to investigate the neural substrates of moral emotions in depression directly.

Social Decision-making in Depression

Decision-making in the context of social interactions (social decision-making) allows for successful interpersonal cooperation, including altruistic behaviour and economic exchange (72). The extent of our willingness to cooperate and exchange with others is a highly intricate and dynamic process that is influenced by social emotions and feelings of trust (73, 74).

Choose Cooperate (C) or Defect (D)		Your Partner	
		C	D
You	C	You get 5 Partner gets 5	You get 0 Partner gets 8
	D	You get 8 Partner gets 0	You get 1 Partner gets 1

Figure 16.1 Numbers indicate points or monetary gain (i.e. higher numbers relate to a more desirable outcome).

Adapted from *Frontiers in Psychology*, 4, Pulcu E, Zahn R, Elliott R, The role of self-blaming moral emotions in major depression and their impact on social-economical decision making. © 2013 Pulcu, Zahn and Elliott. Reproduced under the terms of the Creative Commons Attribution 3.0 Unported (CC BY 3.0) license. (https://creativecommons.org/licenses/by/3.0/)

Two frequently applied paradigms to study social exchange are the Ultimatum Game (UG) and the Prisoner's Dilemma (PD). In the UG, the participant (proposer) is asked to split an amount of money with another participant (respondent). The proposer decides how to split this money. The respondent then decides whether to accept this offer or reject the offer (in which case neither player receives any money). Classic economic theory, which assumes that all players act rationally, suggests that the proposer should offer the smallest amount of money, which the respondent should in turn accept (75). This, however, does not reflect actual human behaviour. Proposers tend to offer 40–50% (76), while 'unfair' offers below 25% are rejected up to 80% of the time (77). This behaviour has been observed cross-culturally and appears to be independent of the monetary amount (78).

In the PD, a participant is given the choice to either cooperate or defect with a partner. They are informed of the predetermined payoff matrix, which depends on the choice (defect/cooperate) made by *both* participants (Figure 16.1). Importantly, participants are not informed of the other player's decision prior to making their own, leading to an uncertain environment. The PD may involve a single round or, more commonly, several rounds in succession (known as the iterated PD). While economic game theory postulates that the dominant strategy of a rational agent should be to select defection, this does not generally reflect observed human behaviour, which is highly dynamic and strongly influenced by the previous choices made by the other player (79).

Neural Basis of Social Decision-making in Healthy Controls
fMRI studies of HC playing the UG and PD have highlighted the involvement of the dorsal striatum (specifically the caudate nucleus), insula, dorsolateral PFC (DLPFC), and OFC. Insula activation is positively correlated with degree of unfairness (80, 81), consistent with the theory that negative affective states drive

rejection decisions as the insula mediates experience of and regulation of nega-tive emotion (82). fMRI studies of the UG have also highlighted the role of the DLPFC, thought to be involved in the cognitive task of maximizing rewards (81). Another study found that response of the OFC, frequently implicated in emotion regulation (7), was correlated with acceptance of unfair offers (80).

Neural Basis of Social Decision-making in Major Depressive Disorder
Relatively few studies to date have used economic exchange games to probe social decision-making in the context of depression. A recent study found that symp-tomatic patients were more likely to defect in the PD (83). Another study reported a negative correlation between depressive symptoms and reciprocal cooperation in the PD and UG (84). By contrast, a study of depressed/anxious adolescents reported higher levels of reciprocal cooperation in the PD (85). Clearly further studies using economic exchange games are needed to elucidate the behavioural pattern of cooperation and social decision-making in depression.

A handful of fMRI studies have sought to investigate possible neural under-pinnings of aberrant social decision-making in depression. A recent fMRI study of the UG revealed that, in the absence of behavioural differences, only HC, and not MDD, participants demonstrated a positive correlation between fairness of offers and activation in two striatal brain regions, the nucleus accumbens and the dorsal caudate (86). A different study investigating altruistic decision-making in individuals with rMDD found that patients had significantly higher sgACC acti-vation in response to charitable donations. Additional studies are clearly needed, as behavioural results to date have been inconsistent and the neural underpin-nings of possible increased cooperative and altruistic behaviour in MDD need to be further investigated.

Conclusion

The studies reviewed in this chapter point to several social cognitive abnormalities in MDD and emerging evidence for a neural network underlying these observed differences. Key brain areas identified include prefrontal cortex (particularly the OFC, MPFC, and DLPFC), temporal–parietal regions, and sgACC. Increased negative self-focus appears to be associated with aberrant MPFC activity and both hyperactivity and hyperconnectivity of the DMN. While ToM deficits have been observed in depressed patients, no imaging studies to date have been conducted to investigate possible biological substrates. Evidence from bipolar disorder points to hypoactivation of the MPFC, associated with difficulty passing ToM tasks. The review of moral emotions highlighted several unique characteristics in depressed individuals, including increased experiences of shame and guilt (as-sociated with sgACC activation) and decreased MPFC activation while watching moral content. Studies using social economic exchange games to investigate social decision-making in MDD have been inconclusive at both behavioural and neural levels. Some have suggested heightened reciprocal cooperation and altruistic behaviours, but other studies have not reported these abnormalities.

Since social cognition depends on more basic components of affective cognition, it is no surprise that the key brain areas identified in this chapter show distinct overlap with areas previously identified in 'hot' cognition. Furthermore, many of these areas have been implicated in depression and maladaptive emotion regulation (particularly rumination). As discussed, however, evidence on the neural underpinnings of social cognition in depression is limited to date, and more research is needed to elucidate possible biological mechanisms that give rise to social cognitive deficits. This is especially pertinent given the limitations of existing psychotherapies and pharmacological treatments of depression, and the potential for enhanced social cognition to be associated with better social functioning outcomes. Functional outcomes, closely linked to patient wellbeing and quality of life, represent an important target for novel therapies that extend traditional therapeutic targets of symptom reduction.

References

1. Elliott R, Zahn R, Deakin JF, Anderson IM. Affective cognition and its disruption in mood disorders. Neuropsychopharmacology 2011;36(1):153–82.

2. Gotlib IH, Joormann J. Cognition and depression: current status and future directions. Annu Rev Clin Psychol 2010;6:285–312.

3. Roiser JP, Sahakian BJ. Hot and cold cognition in depression. CNS Spectr 2013;18(3):139–49.

4. Clark L, Chamberlain SR, Sahakian BJ. Neurocognitive mechanisms in depression: implications for treatment. Annu Rev Neurosci 2009;32:57–74.

5. Davidson RJ, Pizzagalli D, Nitschke JB, Putnam K. Depression: perspectives from affective neuroscience. Annu Rev Psychol 2002;53:545–74.

6. Drevets WC. Neuroimaging and neuropathological studies of depression: implications for the cognitive-emotional features of mood disorders. Curr Opin Neurobiol 2001;11(2):240–9.

7. Ochsner KN, Gross JJ. Cognitive emotion regulation: insights from social cognitive and affective neuroscience. Curr Dir Psychol Sci 2008;17(2):153–8.

8. Joormann J, Vanderlind WM. Emotion regulation in depression: the role of biased cognition and reduced cognitive control. Clin Psychol Sci 2014;2(4):402–21.

9. Souery D, Oswald P, Massat I, et al. Clinical factors associated with treatment resistance in major depressive disorder: results from a European multicenter study. J Clin Psychiatry 2007;68(7):1062–70.

10. Rush AJ, Trivedi MH, Wisniewski SR, et al. Acute and longer-term outcomes in depressed outpatients requiring one or several treatment steps: a STAR* D report. Am J Psychiatry 2006;163(11):1905–17.

11. Renner F, Cuijpers P, Huibers M. The effect of psychotherapy for depression on improvements in social functioning: a meta-analysis. Psychol Med 2014;44(14): 2913–26.

12. Frith CD, Frith U. Social cognition in humans. Curr Biol 2007;17(16):R724–32.

13. Fett A-KJ, Viechtbauer W, Penn DL, van Os J, Krabbendam L. The relationship between neurocognition and social cognition with functional outcomes in schizophrenia: a meta-analysis. Neurosci Biobehav Rev 2011;35(3):573–88.

14. Rogers TB, Kuiper NA, Kirker WS. Self-reference and the encoding of personal information. J Pers Soc Psychol 1977;35(9):677–88.

15. Symons CS, Johnson BT. The self-reference effect in memory: a meta-analysis. Psychol Bull 1997;121(3):371–94.

16. Wisco BE. Depressive cognition: self-reference and depth of processing. Clin Psychol Rev 2009;29(4):382–92.

17. D'Argembeau A, Comblain C, Van der Linden M. Affective valence and the self-reference effect: influence of retrieval conditions. Br J Psychol 2005;96(Pt 4):457–66.

18. Beck A. *Cognitive Therapy and the Emotional Disorders*. New York: New American Library; 1976.

19. Nolen-Hoeksema S, Wisco BE, Lyubomirsky S. Rethinking rumination. Perspect Psychol Sci 2008;3(5):400–24.

20. Mitchell JP, Macrae CN, Banaji MR. Encoding-specific effects of social cognition on the neural correlates of subsequent memory. J Neurosci 2004;24(21):4912–17.

21. Macrae CN, Moran JM, Heatherton TF, Banfield JF, Kelley WM. Medial prefrontal activity predicts memory for self. Cereb Cortex 2004;14(6):647–54.

22. Buckner RL, Andrews-Hanna JR, Schacter DL. The brain's default network: anatomy, function, and relevance to disease. Ann N Y Acad Sci 2008;1124:1–38.

23. Andrews-Hanna JR, Smallwood J, Spreng RN. The default network and self-generated thought: component processes, dynamic control, and clinical relevance. Ann N Y Acad Sci 2014;1316:29–52.

24. Lemogne C, Delaveau P, Freton M, Guionnet S, Fossati P. Medial prefrontal cortex and the self in major depression. J Affect Disord 2012;136(1–2):e1–e11.

25. Grimm S, Ernst J, Boesiger P, et al. Reduced negative BOLD responses in the default-mode network and increased self-focus in depression. World J Biol Psychiatry 2011;12(8):627–37.

26. Sheline YI, Barch DM, Price JL, et al. The default mode network and self-referential processes in depression. Proc Natl Acad Sci U S A 2009;106(6):1942–7.

27. Kaiser RH, Andrews-Hanna JR, Wager TD, Pizzagalli DA. Large-scale network dysfunction in major depressive disorder: a meta-analysis of resting-state functional connectivity. JAMA Psychiatry 2015;72(6):603–11.

28. Hamilton JP, Furman DJ, Chang C, et al. Default-mode and task-positive network activity in major depressive disorder: implications for adaptive and maladaptive rumination. Biol Psychiatry 2011;70(4):327–33.

29. Frith C, Frith U. Theory of mind. Curr Biol 2005;15(17):R644–6.

30. Frith CD, Frith U. The neural basis of mentalizing. Neuron 2006;50(4):531–4.

31. Kishida KT, King-Casas B, Montague PR. Neuroeconomic approaches to mental disorders. Neuron 2010;67(4):543–54.

32. Baron-Cohen S, Wheelwright S, Hill J, Raste Y, Plumb I. The 'Reading the Mind in the Eyes' Test revised version: a study with normal adults, and adults with Asperger syndrome or high-functioning autism. J Child Psychol Psychiatry Allied Disciplines 2001;42(2):241–51.

33. Lee L, Harkness KL, Sabbagh MA, Jacobson JA. Mental state decoding abilities in clinical depression. J Affect Disord 2005;86(2–3):247–58.

34. Wang Y-g, Wang Y-q, Chen S-l, Zhu C-y, Wang K. Theory of mind disability in major depression with or without psychotic symptoms: a componential view. Psychiatry Res 2008;161(2):153–61.

35. Wolkenstein L, Schönenberg M, Schirm E, Hautzinger M. I can see what you feel, but I can't deal with it: impaired theory of mind in depression. J Affective Disord 2011;132(1):104–11.

36. Oakley BF, Brewer R, Bird G, Catmur C. Theory of mind is not theory of emotion: a cautionary note on the Reading the Mind in the Eyes Test. J Abnorm Psychol 2016;125(6):818–23.

37. Baron-Cohen S, Jolliffe T, Mortimore C, Robertson M. Another advanced test of theory of mind: evidence from very high functioning adults with autism or Asperger syndrome. J Child Psychol Psychiatry 1997;38(7):813–22.

38. Miller SA. Children's understanding of second-order mental states. Psychol Bull 2009;135(5):749–73.

39. Baron-Cohen S, O'Riordan M, Jones R, Stone V, Plaisted K. A new test of social sensitivity: detection of faux pas in normal children and children with Asperger syndrome. J Autism Dev Disord 1999;29(5):407–18.

40. Zobel I, Werden D, Linster H, et al. Theory of mind deficits in chronically depressed patients. Depress Anxiety 2010;27(9):821–8.

41. Fischer-Kern M, Fonagy P, Kapusta ND, et al. Mentalizing in female inpatients with major depressive disorder. J Nerv Ment Dis 2013;201(3):202–7.

42. Cusi AM, Nazarov A, Holshausen K, Macqueen GM, McKinnon MC. Systematic review of the neural basis of social cognition in patients with mood disorders. J Psychiatry Neurosci 2012;37(3):154–69.

43. Siegal M, Varley R. Neural systems involved in 'theory of mind'. Nat Rev Neurosci 2002;3(6):463–71.

44. Van Overwalle F. Social cognition and the brain: a meta-analysis. Hum Brain Mapp 2009;30(3):829–58.

45. Haidt J. The moral emotions. Handbook Affective Sci 2003;11:852–70.

46. Tangney JP, Stuewig J, Mashek DJ. Moral emotions and moral behavior. Annu Rev Psychol 2007;58:345–72.

47. Schreiter S, Pijnenborg GH, Aan Het Rot M. Empathy in adults with clinical or subclinical depressive symptoms. J Affect Disord 2013;150(1):1–16.

48. Cusi AM, Macqueen GM, Spreng RN, McKinnon MC. Altered empathic responding in major depressive disorder: relation to symptom severity, illness burden, and psychosocial outcome. Psychiatry Res 2011;188(2):231–6.

49. Tangney JP, Wagner P, Gramzow R. Proneness to shame, proneness to guilt, and psychopathology. J Abnorm Psychol 1992;101(3):469–78.

50. Luby J, Belden A, Sullivan J, et al. Shame and guilt in preschool depression: evidence for elevations in self-conscious emotions in depression as early as age 3. J Child Psychol Psychiatry 2009;50(9):1156–66.

51. Association AP. Diagnostic and Statistical Manual of Mental Disorders, 5th edition. Arlington, VA: American Psychiatric Publishing; 2013.

52. Bi B, Xiao X, Zhang H, et al. A comparison of the clinical characteristics of women with recurrent major depression with and without suicidal symptomatology. Psychol Med 2012;42(12):2591–8.

53. Bryan CJ, Morrow CE, Etienne N, Ray-Sannerud B. Guilt, shame, and suicidal ideation in a military outpatient clinical sample. Depress Anxiety 2013;30(1):55–60.

54. Damasio H, Grabowski T, Frank R, Galaburda AM, Damasio AR. The return of Phineas Gage: clues about the brain from the skull of a famous patient. Science 1994;264(5162):1102–5.

55. Eslinger PJ, Damasio AR. Severe disturbance of higher cognition after bilateral frontal lobe ablation: patient EVR. Neurology 1985;35(12):1731–41.

56. Mah L, Arnold MC, Grafman J. Impairment of social perception associated with lesions of the prefrontal cortex. Am J Psychiatry 2004;161(7):1247–55.

57. Shamay-Tsoory SG, Aharon-Peretz J, Perry D. Two systems for empathy: a double dissociation between emotional and cognitive empathy in inferior frontal gyrus versus ventromedial prefrontal lesions. Brain 2009;132(3):617–27.

58. Koenigs M, Young L, Adolphs R, et al. Damage to the prefrontal cortex increases utilitarian moral judgements. Nature 2007;446(7138):908–11.

59. Takahashi H, Yahata N, Koeda M, et al. Brain activation associated with evaluative processes of guilt and embarrassment: an fMRI study. Neuroimage 2004;23(3):967–74.

60. Moll J, de Oliveira-Souza R, Eslinger PJ, et al. The neural correlates of moral sensitivity: a functional magnetic resonance imaging investigation of basic and moral emotions. J Neurosci 2002;22(7):2730–6.

61. Heekeren HR, Wartenburger I, Schmidt H, Schwintowski H-P, Villringer A. An fMRI study of simple ethical decision-making. Neuroreport 2003;14(9):1215–19.

62. Greene JD, Sommerville RB, Nystrom LE, Darley JM, Cohen JD. An fMRI investigation of emotional engagement in moral judgment. Science 2001;293(5537):2105–8.

63. Green S, Lambon Ralph MA, Moll J, Deakin JF, Zahn R. Guilt-selective functional disconnection of anterior temporal and subgenual cortices in major depressive disorder. Arch Gen Psychiatry 2012;69(10):1014–21.

64. Zahn R, Moll J, Paiva M, et al. The neural basis of human social values: evidence from functional MRI. Cereb Cortex 2009;19(2):276–83.

65. Basile B, Mancini F, Macaluso E, et al. Deontological and altruistic guilt: evidence for distinct neurobiological substrates. Hum Brain Mapp 2011;32(2):229–39.

66. Morey RA, McCarthy G, Selgrade ES, et al. Neural systems for guilt from actions affecting self versus others. Neuroimage 2012;60(1):683–92.

67. Elliott R, Lythe K, Lee R, et al. Reduced medial prefrontal responses to social interaction images in remitted depression. Arch Gen Psychiatry 2012;69(1):37–45.

68. Pulcu E, Lythe K, Elliott R, et al. Increased amygdala response to shame in remitted major depressive disorder. PLoS One 2014;9(1):e86900.

69. Drevets WC, Savitz J, Trimble M. The subgenual anterior cingulate cortex in mood disorders. CNS Spectr 2008;13(8):663–81.

70. Siegle GJ, Carter CS, Thase ME. Use of FMRI to predict recovery from unipolar depression with cognitive behavior therapy. Am J Psychiatry 2006;163(4):735–8.

71. Mayberg HS, Brannan SK, Mahurin RK, et al. Cingulate function in depression: a potential predictor of treatment response. Neuroreport 1997;8(4):1057–61.

72. Rilling JK, Sanfey AG, Aronson JA, Nystrom LE, Cohen JD. The neural correlates of theory of mind within interpersonal interactions. Neuroimage 2004;22(4):1694–703.

73. King-Casas B, Tomlin D, Anen C, et al. Getting to know you: reputation and trust in a two-person economic exchange. Science 2005;308(5718):78–83.

74. Pulcu E, Zahn R, Elliott R. The role of self-blaming moral emotions in major depression and their impact on social-economical decision making. Front Psychol 2013;4:310.

75. Kagel JH, Roth AE. *The Handbook of Experimental Economics, Volume 2: The Handbook of Experimental Economics*. Princeton: Princeton University Press; 2016.

76. Nowak MA, Page KM, Sigmund K. Fairness versus reason in the ultimatum game. Science 2000;289(5485):1773–5.

77. Camerer CF. *Behavioral Game Theory: Experiments in strategic interaction*. Princeton: Princeton University Press; 2011.

78. Crockett MJ. The neurochemistry of fairness: clarifying the link between serotonin and prosocial behavior. Ann N Y Acad Sci 2009;1167:76–86.

79. Hilbe C, Traulsen A, Sigmund K. Partners or rivals? Strategies for the iterated prisoner's dilemma. Games Econ Behav 2015;92:41–52.

80. Tabibnia G, Satpute AB, Lieberman MD. The sunny side of fairness: preference for fairness activates reward circuitry (and disregarding unfairness activates self-control circuitry). Psychol Sci 2008;19(4):339–47.

81. Sanfey AG, Rilling JK, Aronson JA, Nystrom LE, Cohen JD. The neural basis of eco-nomic decision-making in the Ultimatum Game. Science 2003;300(5626):1755–8.

82. Calder AJ, Lawrence AD, Young AW. Neuropsychology of fear and loathing. Nat Rev Neurosci 2001;2(5):352–63.

83. Pulcu E, Thomas EJ, Trotter PD, et al. Social-economical decision making in current and remitted major depression. Psychol Med 2015;45(6):1301–13.

84. Clark CB, Thorne CB, Hardy S, Cropsey KL. Cooperation and depressive symptoms. J Affective Disord 2013;150(3):1184–7.

85. McClure EB, Parrish JM, Nelson EE, et al. Responses to conflict and cooper-ation in adolescents with anxiety and mood disorders. J Abnorm Child Psychol 2007;35(4):567–77.

86. Gradin V, Pérez A, MacFarlane J, et al. Abnormal brain responses to social fair-ness in depression: an fMRI study using the Ultimatum Game. Psychol Med 2015;45(6):1241–51.

17

Emotional and Cognitive Consequences of Social Rejection: An Entry Door to Major Depression

Philippe Fossati, Sophie Hinfray, Anna Fall, Cédric Lemogne, and Jean-Yves Rotge

Introduction

Major depressive disorder (MDD) is a frequent and disabling mental disorder with great risk of recurrence and chronicity (1). Depressed individuals display an increased risk of natural mortality, especially from cardiovascular diseases, and poor social outcomes. These poor health and social outcomes may add to the burden of the symptoms and contribute themselves to worsen the course of the disease.

Interpersonal factors are among the strongest predictors of the onset and course of a major depressive episode. Even though interpersonal models of depression have recently emerged in the literature to explain the onset and maintenance of depressive symptoms (2), little attention has been paid to the biological mechanisms of social difficulties of depressed patients.

Depression is tightly linked to social exclusion. Social exclusion and threat to social acceptance (TSA; Box 17.1) are common life experiences and the most frequently studied environmental risk factors of MDD in large epidemiological studies (3).

We propose here to summarize the literature about the relationships between social exclusion, rejection sensitivity, and major depression, with a special emphasis on emotional and cognitive consequences of social rejection.

We will describe how social acceptance can be viewed as a homeostatic state that calls for monitoring and regulation in healthy subjects. According to this proposal, we will then suggest that MDD could result from a global impairment within the set of biological, cognitive, emotional, and behavioural responses that regulate and maintain homeostasis of social acceptance.

Box 17.1 Definitions

Social acceptance: signals from other people meaning that they wish to include someone in their groups and relationships. Here we consider social acceptance and social inclusion as equivalent terms.

Social rejection: signals from other people meaning explicitly that someone is not wanted in their groups and relationships. People can be exposed to acute or chronic social rejection.

Social exclusion: being kept apart from others.

Ostracism: being deliberately left out of a group by exclusion and rejection.

Threat to social acceptance: threat resulting from social rejection, exclusion, or ostracism.

Rejection sensitivity: a dispositional trait characterized by anxious expectation of being rejected, ready perception of signals of social rejection and overreaction (emotionally or behaviourally) to rejection. Rejection sensitivity may be determined by genetic and learning (i.e. interpersonal trauma during childhood) factors.

Self-esteem: subjective evaluation of one's worth as a person, feeling that one is 'good enough'.

State self-esteem: momentary fluctuations in a person's feeling about himself/herself.

Trait self-esteem: person's general appraisal of his/her value.

Overview of SENSO (SENsitivity to SOcial Signals): A Model of Social Acceptance Homeostasis

Belonging to a social group is a fundamental human need (4). Baumeister and Leary defined belonging as a need to form and maintain social bonds and at least a minimum quantity of interpersonal relationships. This need is thought to be innate among human beings. In gregarious animal species, including humans, being alone means a higher risk of death, and the drive to form and maintain interpersonal bonds is an adaptive way to secure resources, gain access to reproduction, and promote survival.

We postulate here that social acceptance is a byproduct of a homeostatic system in healthy subjects. This system monitors and regulates the TSA by reestablishing or disrupting inclusion to the social group.

People may be socially excluded because of personal features that others may consider undesirable, including incompetence, immorality, or unattractiveness. Social exclusion may also result from several situations, including, for instance, forced separation by a loved one or being ostracized. We consider here that social exclusion (being kept apart from others) and social rejection (an explicit declaration that an individual or a group is not wanted) are equivalent signals regarding our homeostatic response.

TSA induces transient or persistent changes in the perceived level of social acceptance and activates an integrated and coordinated set of specific biological, cognitive, and emotional responses (Figure 17.1). This set of responses to TSA signals allows selecting behaviours that engage one in seeking or in avoiding social relationships while probing social acceptance status.

Some authors proposed different pathways to understand how social signals are integrated to estimate the likelihood of further exclusion or inclusion. Allen and Badcock (5) proposed that the ratio between our social value to others and our social burden on others could monitor our integration status. We propose, based on Leary's Sociometer theory (6), that self-esteem monitors social acceptance and contributes to trigger a set of emotional and biological adaptive changes.

Many psychologists have assumed that high self-esteem is essential to psychological health. Consistent with this view, high self-esteem has been associated with psychological wellbeing, whereas low self-esteem has been associated

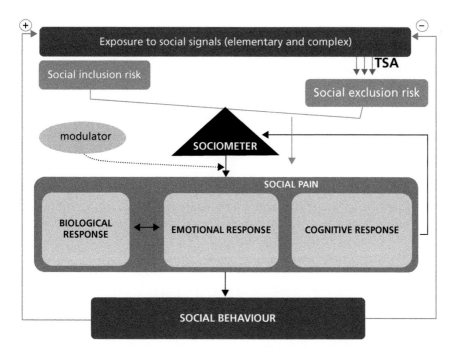

Figure 17.1 The SENSO Framework. TSA, Threat to social acceptance; + indicates a prosocial behaviour that decreases the TSA and increases social reconnection; – indicates an 'antisocial' or avoidant behaviour that decreases the probability of social reconnection.

with greater levels of depression, anxiety, and other psychological problems (7). According to the sociometer theory, self-esteem is a gauge that measures the quality of people's relationships with others and makes the individual aware of the possibility of social exclusion. From this perspective, self-esteem is a marker of how people believe they are perceived by their social environment, whereas behaviours driven by motivational effects of self-esteem are not intended to keep self-esteem stable per se, but to avoid social exclusion or social devaluation.

By emphasizing the social component of self-esteem, Leary and Baumeister suggest that we integrate and translate social cues into state self-esteem. State self-esteem is the fluctuant part of self-esteem, whereas trait self-esteem is the more stable part and reflects the general sense of how persons feel about themselves (6).

State self-esteem is lowered by events that may trigger a negative judgement from familiar others (for instance, failure) or from direct negative evaluation from others (criticism, rejection). On the contrary, state self-esteem is increased with success, signs of love, or congratulations. Participants report lower state self-esteem after social rejection. Moreover, participants who experiment with social acceptance report a boost in their level of state self-esteem (8). Finally, chronic exposure to social rejection may also dampen trait self-esteem (9).

Following the translation of social cues of inclusion or exclusion, our framework proposes that state self-esteem is a major trigger of the coordinated set of adaptive responses to TSA. Our proposal includes a direct pathway from perception of social exclusion or TSA to adaptive responses bypassing a change in state self-esteem (Figure 17.1).

Genetics, childhood experiences, attachment style, personality traits, and social support act as 'trait' modulators, explaining interindividual differences in the sensitivity to TSA and the regulation of social acceptance (10).

We hypothesize that this integrated and coordinated set of responses following TSA signals is impaired in MDD and results in an abnormal homeostatic state of social acceptance and an increased sensitivity to social rejection signals in depressed patients and in subjects prone to depression.

We describe in more detail some components of the SENSO model and their putative impairment in MDD.

Perception of Social Signals

Social signals may be differentiated into basic (i.e. facial or body expression, for example) or complex (verbal) signals. It is beyond the scope of this chapter to describe in detail the biological signature of perception and integration of these social signals. In healthy subjects, the processing of social signals involves a complex network of brain regions encompassing the social brain, including the amygdala, the temporal pole, the superior temporal sulcus, the anterior cingulate, the insula, and medial prefrontal cortices. Most of these regions are associated with the emotional brain, suggesting strong relationships between social processing and emotion processing (11). Likewise, as we value primary rewards such as food or sexual stimuli, we value social outcomes. The human ventral striatum, known to play a key role in reward processing, displays activation related to a broad spectrum of social signals (12). Thus verbal and non-verbal social signals are used to inform us of both our social environment and our level of social acceptance in this environment.

Usually depressed patients and subjects at risk for depression (e.g. subjects with personal history of childhood abuse or neglect and/or genetic risk factors for depression) are prone to seek and thus perceive negative social signals and to interpret those signals as a threat to their social acceptance. Moreover, altered empathy has been described in depressed individuals with impaired ability to perceive and identify pain and related emotions in others. This impairment in emotional and empathetic processes may reinforce the interpersonal difficulties of depressed patients and increase their sensitivity to social stressors (13).

Social Exclusion and Fundamental Needs

The past decade has witnessed a proliferation of research on consequences of perceiving a TSA. Through analyses of diaries, Williams and Jarvis (14) showed that most people experience a TSA once a day. This can result, for example, from perceiving an angry face, an insult, or an act of ignorance. TSA may jeopardize at least four fundamental human needs: maintenance of a reasonably high self-esteem; sense of belonging; sense of personal control over one's social environment; and sense of meaning of life. Feeling psychologically distressed when detecting a TSA is adaptive and most likely has strong evolutionary roots for maintaining the success of the individual and the group.

To explore emotional, cognitive, behavioural, and biological reactions to social rejection, the Cyberball game has become a gold-standard over the past few years (14). The Cyberball is a minimally socially interactive ball game in which participants are ignored and excluded by two other players. During the game, the participant is led to believe that he or she plays a ball-tossing game with two other real players over the internet. In fact, the reactions of these two other players are computer-generated to induce feelings of exclusion in the participant. The participant is usually told that the task is designed to study his or her mental imagery ability. In the exclusion condition, the participant will generally get the ball for no more than two or three tosses, whereas in the inclusion condition, the participant gets 30% of the tosses. After exclusion, subjects report substantial changes in meeting their fundamental needs. Self-reports of belonging, sense of control, meaningful experience, and self-esteem are lower for people excluded compared to those included in the Cyberball task (10). These measures are usually well intercorrelated and the effects of exclusion during the Cyberball game on fundamental needs are robust and reproducible.

Many studies have used the Cyberball paradigm to determine the brain regions implicated in social exclusion. They showed that social rejection triggers a brain response that shares some similarities with brain responses to physical pain, activating regions that usually process the negative affect and the distress associated with physical pain (10, 15). Indeed, social rejection activates the ventrolateral prefrontal cortex, anterior cingulate cortex (ACC), and anterior insula. A meta-analysis by our group showed that the ventral part of the ACC—the subgenual cingulate (sgACC)—is particularly associated with self-reported distress triggered by social rejection (16). The sgACC is a key region in the pathophysiology of MDD (17). Interestingly, a study showed that the activation of the sgACC in adolescents submitted to a Cyberball exclusion predicted the incidence of depressive symptoms in the following year (18). One study with healthy subjects demonstrated that a strong experience of social rejection can even activate somatosensory areas that support sensory elements of physical pain (19). Hsu et al. (20) explored medication-free depressed patients with the Cyberball game and positron emission tomography scan with a radioligand binding to the opioid system. Compared to healthy controls, patients with MDD showed reduced endogenous opioid release in brain regions regulating stress and mood after social exclusion. According to the authors, altered endogenous opioid activity in MDD may hinder emotional recovery and increased sensitivity of depressed patients to negative social feedback. Overall these results support experience that social rejection literally hurts.

Social Exclusion and Emotional Responses

In healthy subjects, social exclusion can induce different types of emotional responses, including social anxiety, jealousy, shame, social pain, emotional numbness, embarrassment, anger, and sadness (21). According to Leary we distinguish two different types of emotion induced by social rejection: 1) the primary emotions related to the direct emotional response to the social threat (social anxiety, jealousy, shame, social pain); 2) the secondary emotions related to other features of the situation (e.g. loss) associated with social rejection (anger and sadness).

We hypothesize that subjects at risk for depression or depressed subjects will more likely and intensively react to TSA and will show increased levels of secondary emotions (sadness or anger) to healthy subjects.

Bauriel-Schmidt et al. (22) evaluated the emotional reaction of acutely and chronically depressed patients to the Cyberball exclusion condition and the moderating effects of attachment style. Both depressive groups reported significantly higher scores in negative mood during exclusion. This condition significantly lowered self-esteem only in the chronically depressed patients. These results were moderated by the attachment style: the 'organized' (more secure, connected to others) depressed patients showed less impact on self-esteem and planned to engage in pleasant activities following social exclusion, whereas 'disorganized' depressed patients adopted a passive behaviour (i.e. sleeping) after exclusion, reflecting social withdrawal.

Recently, in a set of experiments, we assessed the temporal dynamic of emotional response in healthy subjects and subjects with depressive symptoms following negative social feedback on personality trait (23, 24). Only 23% of healthy subjects reported sadness after negative feedback on their personality. Depression severity moderated the temporal dynamics of emotion after negative social feedback. Usually emotional reactions unfold across two phases in healthy subjects: emotion explosiveness, primarily reflecting whether the emotional episode has a steep versus a gentle start, and emotion accumulation, reflecting whether emotion intensity increases over time versus going back to baseline. In our experiments, the higher the depressive symptoms, the higher the accumulation score when subjects were self-immersed in their emotional experience. Adopting a self-distanced perspective before the feedback decreased the accumulation score only in subjects with depressive symptoms, suggesting strong relationships between emotional dynamics, self-regulatory processes, and depressive symptoms after exposure to negative social feedback (24). These results are consistent with Hsu et al.'s (20) findings showing difficulties in emotional recovery from social exclusion in a clinical population of depressed patients.

Cognitive Consequences of Social Exclusion

To avoid the negative emotional consequences of social exclusion, individuals must cope with these social stressors using cognitive resources and self-regulatory strategies. Cognitive control involves several processes engaged in conflict detection and response implementation. Studies on the effects of social exclusion on cognitive control produced contradictory results, with some studies showing impaired, normal, or increased cognitive control following exclusion. Conflicting results may reflect the use of different tasks to induce social exclusion and the tasks at hand for assessing cognitive control. For instance, in one recent study, Xu et al. (25) excluded subjects with the Cyberball game and assessed cognitive control with the go–no-go task. After exclusion, healthy subjects invested more attention in conscious conflict detection but less in conscious inhibition of impulsive responses. On the other hand, during unconscious cognitive control, excluded subjects devoted more attention to the unconscious inhibition of impulsive responses. Overall, this suggests that social exclusion calls for rebalancing attentional resources according to the cognitive demands of the task.

After social exclusion, subjects may prioritize the allocation of attentional resources toward the 'external world' and toward the processing of social cues that signal opportunity for social connection or social withdrawal. Thus, following social exclusion, subjects failed to recruit the dorsomedial prefrontal cortex (DMPFC) during the exposure to negative social scenes (26). The DMPFC is engaged in self-evaluation tasks as well as tasks that require theory of mind (27). Interestingly, in the same study (26), the level of DMPFC activity increased to a greater extent for positive social scenes than negative ones. Thus, two different regulatory strategies are at play to cope with social exclusion: avoidance of negative social stimuli (defensive behaviours) and increased attention to positive social signals that may reveal opportunities to reconnect socially (affiliative behaviours).

After social exclusion, subjects may also allocate attentional resources toward the internal world and increase self-focus attention. There is robust evidence that people emphasize their self-evaluation when facing TSA, a self-protection strategy in which people may downplay their negative personality traits and exaggerate their positive traits. In a study combining both social exclusion and self-evaluation, Hughes and Beer (28) described the neural bases of this self-protection strategy and found a specific role in self-enhancement for the medial orbital frontal cortex. The activity of this region was modulated by the degree of the perceived desirability of the self. Remarkably, regions involved in this protection strategy were not the classical regions engaged in emotion regulation, emphasizing the specificity of the interplay between social negative threat and self-related processes.

The increased self-focused attention triggered by social exclusion may also be maladaptive by reinforcing and maintaining the negative affect resulting from this social stress. Subjects sometimes activate rumination after exclusion, a repetitive thinking on the causes and consequences of emotion associated with increased self-focus.

There are complex bidirectional relationships between sensitivity to social rejection and rumination. Rejection sensitivity is a dispositional trait characterized by anxious expectations of being rejected, readlily perception of signals of rejection, and overreaction to rejection (29).

Both rejection sensitivity and rumination are risk factors for depression. In his interpersonal model of major depression, Joiner (30) suggested that rumination is the cognitive process that fuels the interpersonal mechanisms of depression. Subjects frequently ruminate on interpersonal problems.

In a prospective study, Pearson et al. (29) examined the longitudinal relationships between rumination and rejection sensitivity in currently depressed, previously depressed, and never depressed subjects. Baseline rejection sensitivity prospectively predicted increased rumination 6 months later after controlling for baseline rumination and depression. Rumination may represent a consequence rather than a cause for rejection sensitivity.

Hamilton et al. (31) proposed that depressive rumination is characterized by increased functional connectivity between the default mode network (DMN) and the sgACC. We have demonstrated the major role of the DMN in self-referential processing in healthy subjects and in depressed patients (32). It is noteworthy that brain regions related to rumination (DMN, sgACC) are also implicated in the processing of signals of social rejection (16). In the next section we reconciliate these two sets of findings.

SENSO Model, Rejection Sensitivity, and Major Depression

We have described a general homeostatic system that monitors the social acceptance of individuals. This system is activated in response to actual or putative threats to social acceptance. Our SENSO model describes a cascade of cognitive, emotional, and behavioural consequences of social exclusion. This model also emphasizes the role of specific regions—the sgACC, insula and DMN—in the detection and regulation of negative social signals. We have also evoked the role of rumination, cognitive control, and processes engaged in emotional regulation for monitoring social acceptance.

Such cognitive processes and brain regions are known to be key players in the pathophysiology of depression. Hence we propose that MDD is tightly linked to the processing of social exclusion and may represent a specific impairment in the homeostatic system that monitors social acceptance. We now summarize the impairment of SENSO in major depression and suggest new avenues for research in the field.

One major component of the SENSO dysfunction in MDD is 'rejection sensitivity'. People high in rejection sensitivity are at risk for depression and depressed patients are high in rejection sensitivity. Two specific features characterize people with high rejection sensitivity: 1) subjects expect to be rejected; and 2) subjects put high value in preventing social rejection. According to this formulation, the 'high expectancy–high value' susceptibility determines specific situations precipitating a depressive episode, situations where subjects cannot control the rejection. It is well known from epidemiological studies that the breakdown of an important relationship increases the risk for depression significantly, especially if the subject does not initiate this break. Consistent with this, a 6-month longitudinal study of college women revealed that women high in rejection sensitivity compared to those who are low became more depressed when they experienced a partner-initiated breakup but not when they experienced a self-initiated or mutually initiated breakup (33).

Following unique or repeated exposures to TSA, subjects high in rejection sensitivity will produce several emotional responses, mainly including sadness and anger. At the cognitive level, subjects high in rejection sensitivity will more likely activate ruminative processes and increase their self-focused attention. Rumination in this context reflects both the failed goal of preventing the social rejection perceived as a personal failure and the response to the secondary emotion (sadness and/or anger) associated with the loss induced by social rejection. Rumination will then dampen the executive resources and reinforce the negative emotional response. This will result in difficulties with adequate allocation of attentional resources toward the external world to cope with the social stress.

At the neural level we speculate that the TSA will activate the sgACC as a detector of social rejection. The sgACC transfers the signal information to the anterior dorsal part of the insula that calls for regulation. According to the triple network model (34), the anterior insula is a node that regulates the coordination between the DMN and the control executive network (CEN). Several studies (35) view major depression as a disorder of the functional connectivity and dynamics of neural networks involved in allocation of attentional resources to the internal and external worlds. Among these networks, the CEN, including the lateral prefrontal cortex and the parietal cortex, supports attention directed to the external world, whereas the DMN supports attention directed toward the internal world. The DMN includes the posterior cingulate cortex and the medial prefrontal cortex. It has been suggested that CEN–DMN cooperation may be altered in acute depressed patients as well as in remitted depression (36). Here we propose a specific situation that triggers and reveals this abnormal CEN–DMN cooperation, a situation where the subject is socially excluded and interprets this exclusion as a personal failure. Instead of synchronizing the CEN–DMN dynamics following social exclusion, subjects at risk for depression show increased connectivity between the DMN and the sgACC, and increased rumination and self-focused attention.

Some parts of this model need to be validated and further explored. It has to be demonstrated that social exclusion abnormally involves the CEN–DMN cooperation in subjects with high rejection sensitivity. However, preliminary results in healthy volunteers confirm the adaptive changes of large-scale brain networks after exposure to the Cyberball exclusion (37). Likewise, the specific roles of the sgACC and anterior insula in detection and regulation, respectively, during processing of social exclusion signals need to be tested.

Conclusion

In our social world, individuals are highly sensitive to how they are perceived and valued by others, and this sensitivity triggers adaptive mechanisms that monitor and regulate the human drive for social belonging. The homeostatic system that monitors the level of social acceptance is linked with fundamental cognitive and brain mechanisms that regulate emotion and behaviour. This system is impaired in acutely depressed patients and subjects at risk for depression, emphasizing the importance of social cognition in depression. Considering the ability of patients with major depression to navigate their social world would allow the development of specific treatments and tools for cognitive and social remediation. Overall, this may contribute to the development of personalized medicine tailored to the specific needs of patients.

References

1. Whiteford HA, Degenhardt L, Rehm J, et al. Global burden of disease attributable to mental and substance use disorders: findings from the Global Burden of Disease Study 2010. Lancet 2013;382(9904):1575–86.

2. Hames JL, Hagan CR, Joiner TE. Interpersonal processes in depression. Annu Rev Clin Psychol 2013;9:355–77.

3. Kendler KS, Hettema JM, Butera F, Gardner CO, Prescott CA. Life event dimensions of loss, humiliation, entrapment, and danger in the prediction of onsets of major depression and generalized anxiety. Arch Gen Psychiatry 2003;60(8):789–96.

4. Baumeister RF, Leary MR. The need to belong: desire for interpersonal attachments as a fundamental human motivation. Psychol Bull 1995;117(3):497–529.

5. Allen NB, Badcock PBT. The social risk hypothesis of depressed mood: evolutionary, psychosocial, and neurobiological perspectives. Psychol Bull 2003;129(6):887–913.

6. Leary MR, Baumeister RF. The nature and function of self-esteem: sociometer theory. Adv Exp Social Psychol 2000;32:1–62.

7. Creemers DHM, Scholte RHJ, Engels RCME, Prinstein MJ, Wiers RW. Damaged self-esteem is associated with internalizing problems. Front Psychol 2013;4:152.

8. Blackhart GC, Nelson BC, Knowles ML, Baumeister RF. Rejection elicits emotional reactions but neither causes immediate distress nor lowers self-esteem: a meta-analytic review of 192 studies on social exclusion. Personality Social Psychol Rev 2009;13(4):269–309.

9. Srivastava S, Beer JS. How self-evaluations relate to being liked by others: integrating sociometer and attachment perspectives. J Pers Soc Psychol 2005;89(6):966–77.

10. Eisenberger NI. Social pain and the brain: controversies, questions, and where to go from here. Annu Rev Psychol 2015;66(1):601–29.

11. Phillips ML, Drevets WC, Rauch SL, Lane R. Neurobiology of emotion perception I: the neural basis of normal emotion perception. Biol Psychiatry 2003;54(5):504–14.

12. Bhanji JP, Delgado MR. The social brain and reward: social information processing in the human striatum. WIREs Cogn Sci 2013;5(1):61–73.

13. Ratcliffe M. The phenomenology of depression and the nature of empathy. Med Health Care Philos 2014;17(2):269–80.

14. Williams KD, Jarvis B. Cyberball: a program for use in research on interpersonal ostracism and acceptance. Behav Res Methods 2006;38(1):174–80.

15. Eisenberger NI, Lieberman MD, Williams KD. Does rejection hurt? An FMRI study of social exclusion. Science 2003;302(5643):290–2.

16. Rotge JY, Lemogne C, Hinfray S, et al. A meta-analysis of the anterior cingulate contribution to social pain. Soc Cogn Affect Neurosci 2015;10(1):19–27.

17. Johansen-Berg H, Gutman DA, Behrens TEJ, et al. Anatomical connectivity of the subgenual cingulate region targeted with deep brain stimulation for treatment-resistant depression. Cereb Cortex 2008;18(6):1374–83.

18. Masten CL, Eisenberger NI, Borofsky LA, McNealy K, Pfeifer JH, Dapretto M. Subgenual anterior cingulate responses to peer rejection: a marker of adolescents' risk for depression. Dev Psychopathol 2011;23(01):283–92.

19. Kross E, Berman MG, Mischel W, Smith EE, Wager TD. Social rejection shares somatosensory representations with physical pain. Proc Natl Acad Sci U S A 2011;108(15):6270–5.

20. Hsu DT, Sanford BJ, Meyers KK, et al. It still hurts: altered endogenous opioid activity in the brain during social rejection and acceptance in major depressive disorder. Mol Psychiatry 2015;20(2):193–200.

21. Leary MR. Emotional responses to interpersonal rejection. Dialogues Clin Neurosci 2015;17(4):435–41.

22. Bauriel-Schmidt C, Jobst A, Gander M, et al. Attachment representations, patterns of emotion regulation, and social exclusion in patients with chronic and episodic depression and healthy controls. J Affect Disord 2017;210:130–8.

23. Résibois M, Verduyn P, Delaveau P, et al. The neural basis of emotions varies over time: different regions go with onset- and offset-bound processes underlying emotion intensity. Soc Cogn Affect Neurosci 2017;12(8):1261–71.

24. Résibois M, Kuppens P, Van Mechelen I, Fossati P, Verduyn P. Depression severity moderates the relation between self-distancing and features of emotion unfolding. Pers Individ Dif 2018;123:119–24.

25. Xu M, Li Z, Diao L, et al. Social exclusion modulates priorities of attention allocation in cognitive control. Sci Rep 2016;6:31282.

26. Powers KE, Wagner DD, Norris CJ, Heatherton TF. Socially excluded individuals fail to recruit medial prefrontal cortex for negative social scenes. Soc Cogn Affect Neurosci 2013;8(2):151–7.

27. Fossati P, Hevenor SJ, Graham SJ, et al. In search of the emotional self: an fMRI study using positive and negative emotional words. Am J Psychiatry 2003;160(11):1938–45.

28. Hughes BL, Beer JS. Protecting the self: the effect of social-evaluative threat on neural representations of self. J Cogn Neurosci 2013;25(4):613–22.

29. Pearson KA, Watkins ER, Mullan EG. Rejection sensitivity prospectively predicts increased rumination. Behav Res Ther 2011;49(10):597–605.

30. Joiner TE. Jr. Depression's vicious scree: self-propagating and erosive processes in depression chronicity. Clin Psychology: Science and Practice 2000;7:203–18.

31. Hamilton JP, Farmer M, Fogelman P, Gotlib IH. Depressive rumination, the default-mode network, and the dark matter of clinical neuroscience. Biol Psychiatry 2015;78(4):224–30.

32. Nejad AB, Fossati P, Lemogne C. Self-referential processing, rumination, and cortical midline structures in major depression. Front Hum Neurosci 2013;7:666.

33. Ayduk O, Downey G, Kim M. Rejection sensitivity and depressive symptoms in women. Pers Soc Psy Bulletin 2001;27(7):868–77.

34. Menon V. Large-scale brain networks and psychopathology: a unifying triple network model. Trends Cogn Sci (Regul Ed) 2011;15(10):483–506.

35. Kaiser RH, Andrews-Hanna JR, Wager TD, Pizzagalli DA. Large-scale network dysfunction in major depressive disorder. JAMA Psychiatry 2015;72(6):603–11.

36. Delaveau P, Arruda Sanchez T, Steffen R, et al. Default mode and task-positive networks connectivity during the N-Back task in remitted depressed patients with or without emotional residual symptoms. Hum Brain Mapp 2017;64:9–11.

37. Clemens B, Wagels L, Bauchmüller M, Bergs R, Habel U, Kohn N. Alerted default mode: functional connectivity changes in the aftermath of social stress. Sci Rep 2017;7:40180

18

Pharmacological Interventions for Cognitive Dysfunction in Major Depressive Disorder

Marco Solmi, Beatrice Bortolato, Nicola Veronese, Brendon Stubbs,
Nathan Herrmann, and Andre F. Carvalho

Introduction

Major depressive disorder (MDD) is a chronic mental illness with a lifetime prevalence of 14.6% and 11.1% in high-income and low-to-middle income countries, respectively (1). The treatment of MDD may include evidence-based pharmacological, psychotherapeutic, or neuromodulatory approaches (2). Evidence indicates that approximately 40% of patients with MDD achieve symptomatic remission with a first-line antidepressant agent (3). However, burdensome residual symptoms persist even among patients who meet the traditional criteria for remission (4), the effects of available treatments on psychosocial functioning appear to be modest (5), and psychosocial dysfunction may remain even during symptomatic remission (6, 7).

Growing evidence shows that MDD is associated with deficits across several cognitive domains (8, 9), and preliminary data suggest that deficits in certain cognitive domains may predict response to antidepressant drug treatment (10, 11).

Cognitive dysfunction may persist in a subset of patients with MDD even during symptomatic remission (8, 9), and explains a substantial proportion of psychosocial dysfunction that may affect a subgroup of patients even during remission (12–15). There is also replicated evidence that cognitive dysfunction may predict the onset of depressive symptoms (16, 17). Considering the framework proposed by Davis and colleagues (18), cognitive dysfunction appears to be a risk biomarker, a trait marker that is present during remission, a marker of progression in at least a subset of patients showing more severe impairment as a function of recurring affective episodes, and also a state or acuity marker of MDD with more marked deficits during depressive episodes.

The achievement of cognitive remission has been proposed as a novel treatment aim for MDD (19), and the effects of standard antidepressants, as well as of novel therapeutic targets, on MDD-related cognitive dysfunction have been a focus of increasing research attention (19, 20).

In this chapter, we initially discuss methodological challenges for the study of potential neurotherapeutic interventions for cognitive dysfunction in MDD. Furthermore, an appraisal of the current state of knowledge on pharmacological treatments (including potential novel neurotherapeutic targets for cognitive dysfunction in MDD) is provided. Lastly, suggestions to improve the design of future randomized clinical trials (RCTs) are provided.

Methodological Challenges

A recent systematic review and meta-analysis found that the treatment of MDD with monoaminergic antidepressants promotes modest beneficial effects on psychomotor speed and delayed recall (21). However, another systematic review indicated that antidepressant monotherapy could also improve verbal memory, while augmentation therapies appear to mitigate cognitive dysfunction in broader domains (22). Methodological challenges, as well as differences in design across trials, may limit the robustness of available evidence and may also explain the heterogeneity of findings (19, 21, 23).

Pseudospecificity

'Pseudospecificity' (23) means that observed procognitive effects of antidepressants and other treatments may be at least partly due to non-specific improvements in mood. Although some RCTs have attempted to assess putative direct and mood-independent effects of antidepressants upon cognitive performance by employing relatively novel statistical tools (e.g. path analysis) (24, 25), it may not be possible to quantify possible mood-dependent effects precisely (e.g. owing to residual confounding). In addition, few trials so far have specifically enrolled euthymic participants with MDD (i.e. participants in symptomatic remission) (23).

Screening and Assessment of Cognitive Dysfunction

Evidence points to a relatively weak correlation of self-perceived cognitive impairment and objectively assessed neuropsychological impairment among individuals with affective disorders (26–28), which may be a challenge to comparison of results across trials that used only one type of measurement (i.e. subjective tools versus objective neuropsychological tests). In addition, a recent systematic review observed that most RCTs that investigated putative cognitive enhancers for MDD did not screen for the presence of cognitive deficits at baseline (23). Therefore, the inclusion of participants with relatively intact cognitive performance at baseline and hence with little scope for improvement may limit the proper assessment of putative procognitive agents even if patients present with subjective cognitive complaints. In addition, the methods used to assess both subjective cognitive complaints and objective neuropsychological tests have varied across trials (15).

The Confounding Effects of Age

There is an acknowledged overrepresentation of older participants (i.e. aged >65 years) in trials that have evaluated possible cognitive effects of antidepressants (19), possibly introducing higher frequency of baseline non-MDD-related cognitive and higher prevalence of co-occurring medical and neurodegenerative conditions.

Other Methodological Limitations

Cognitive dysfunction was not the primary outcome in a substantial proportion of trials conducted to date, and the post hoc assessment of this symptomatic domain limits the strength of available evidence (19). Furthermore, as pointed out by Miskowiak and colleagues (23), several RCTs that assessed possible treatments for cognitive dysfunction in samples with MDD did not provide adequate information regarding allocation sequence and concealment.

The Effects of Antidepressants on Cognitive Dysfunction in Major Depressive Disorder

Some evidence indicates that treatment with antidepressant agents may improve certain cognitive domains among patients with MDD (21, 23), while other sources of data suggest that some antidepressants may make cognitive abilities deteriorate in patients with MDD (29–33). Anticholinergic effects may contribute to adverse cognitive effects associated with some antidepressants, most notably tricyclic antidepressants.

Previous studies conducted in healthy volunteers started to identify the prominence of cognition on the mechanism of action of antidepressants. For example, medial prefrontal cortex and core areas of the emotion network (including the anterior cingulate, amygdala, and thalamus) function increased in response to positive emotions, while it decreased in response to negative emotions (33). Together with previous cognitive experiments, a neuropsychological hypothesis for antidepressant drug action has been proposed (34). According to this framework, antidepressants may not work as direct mood enhancers.

In an 8-week multicentre placebo randomized trial citalopram did not improve cognition (35), while duloxetine (25) (N=207), compared to placebo (N=90), showed beneficial effects on global cognition, which appeared to be predominantly driven by effects on verbal learning and memory. In addition, post hoc path analysis suggested that 91% of the observed procognitive effects of duloxetine appeared to be mood-independent (25).

Two RCTs have assessed putative effects of tricyclic antidepressants on cognitive performance in samples with MDD. In a small (N=32), 12-week RCT comparing imipramine and placebo, imipramine improved short-term memory relative to placebo (36). The primary outcome of this trial was not specified, and the possibility of cognitive effects secondary to improvements in mood could not be ruled out (36). In a previous trial randomizing 90 symptomatic elderly participants with MDD to treatment with nortriptyline, phenelzine, or placebo for 7 weeks (37), no significant result emerged on cognition.

A sample of symptomatic participants with MDD was randomized to receive either nomifensine (100 mg/day; N=25), a noradrenaline–dopamine inhibitor, which was subsequently withdrawn from the market owing to the risk of haemolytic anaemia, or placebo (N=25) for 4 weeks (38). The nomifensine group exhibited significant improvements in memory, psychomotor speed, and visuospatial function relative to placebo.

In another RCT, no difference emerged among reboxetine, paroxetine, and placebo on cognition (39), although cognitive dysfunction was not the primary outcome.

Uncontrolled trials have investigated potential cognitive effects of other antidepressants on cognitive dysfunction in participants with MDD. For example, Tian and colleagues found significant improvement in executive control of attention in a sample of patients with MDD after 6 weeks of treatment with venlafaxine (40), while bupropion was found to improve verbal memory and mental processing in a small open-label study that enrolled 20 patients with MDD (41). Clearly these data deserve replication in well-designed RCTs and have been covered in previous reviews on this topic (15, 19, 22).

Vortioxetine is a multimodal antidepressant that is thought to act as an antagonist of the 5-HT$_3$ and 5-HT$_7$ serotonin receptors, a partial agonist of the 5-HT$_{1B}$ serotonin receptor, an agonist of the 5-HT$_{1A}$ receptor, and inhibits the serotonin transporter (42). In addition, owing to indirect 5-HT-mediated effects on glutamatergic neurotransmission as well as histaminergic effects, this compound was hypothesized as a candidate treatment for cognitive dysfunction in MDD (42, 43). Three RCTs have investigated vortioxetine's effects on cognition in samples with MDD (44–46). An initial RCT compared vortioxetine (5 mg/day; N=156) to duloxetine (active reference group; N=151) and placebo (N=145) in a sample of symptomatic participants with MDD (44). Cognitive improvement was the tertiary outcome. Vortioxetine improved processing speed and verbal memory compared to placebo. A second trial assessed cognitive dysfunction as the primary outcome in a large sample of symptomatic participants with MDD (45). Vortioxetine at both tested doses (i.e. 10 and 20 mg/day) improved the composite cognitive score and processing speed relative to placebo. Those findings were subsequently replicated in a large multicentre RCT (46), in which psychomotor speed was the primary outcome. Vortioxetine (but not duloxetine) significantly improved psychomotor speed relative to placebo. Results from these three RCTs underwent meta-analysis, and evidence indicated that vortioxetine led to small but significant improvements in scores of the Digit Symbol Substitution Test (DSST) and, to a substantial extent, those effects were independent of mood improvement. However, 'pseudospecific' cognitive effects cannot be ruled out because included RCTs did not enrol MDD participants who were euthymic.

Novel Therapeutic Targets

Some novel therapeutic targets have been tested as cognitive enhancers across RCTs (Table 18.1). Putative mechanisms of action, available evidence, as well as possible novel neurotherapeutic targets that still await proper testing, are discussed.

Apomorphine

The effects of a single-dose administration of apomorphine, a dopaminergic agent employed as a treatment of Parkinson's disease, were tested in a small, proof-of-concept, crossover trial of seven participants with melancholic MDD (47). No significant procognitive effects relative to placebo were observed.

Lisdexamfetamine Dimesylate

Lisdexamfetamine dimesylate (LDX) enhances noradrenaline and dopamine neurotransmission and is currently used as a treatment for attention deficit hyperactivity disorder and binge-eating disorder. A sample of patients with MDD in full or partial remission was randomized to LDX (20–70 mg/day; N=71) or placebo (N=72) for 9 weeks (48). An improvement in subjectively reported executive dysfunction in the LDX group relative to placebo was observed (primary

Table 18.1 Potential therapeutic targets for the treatment of cognitive dysfunction in major depressive disorder (MDD)

Agent	Putative mechanisms of action	Clinical evidence
Vortioxetine	5-HT$_3$/5HT$_7$ receptor antagonist; partial agonist at the 5-HT$_{1B}$ receptor; agonist at 5-HT$_{1A}$ receptor; inhibitor of the 5-HT transporter	Two multicentre RCTs having cognitive performance as the primary outcome measure were conducted in participants with MDD. Overall, vortioxetine displayed a significant procognitive effect over several domains, which was largely independent of the amelioration of affective symptoms. However, a recent meta-analysis found that the overall effect size was small (0.34).
Lisdexamfetamine dimesylate (LDX)	D-amphetamine prodrug; enhances the efflux of dopamine and noradrenaline in the CNS	An RCT found LDX augmentation to be efficacious in reducing self-reported executive dysfunction among participants with MDD (N=143) with residual depressive symptoms.
Erythropoietin (EPO)	Readily crosses the BBB and increases the production of BDNF	EPO improved verbal learning and memory in a preliminary RCT involving participants with treatment-resistant MDD (N=40). This effect was largely mood-independent. However, cognitive performance was not the primary outcome measure in this trial.
S-adenosyl methionine (SAMe)	Major methyl-donor; essential for the synthesis of several neurotransmitters; involved in the synthesis of glutathione	A post-hoc analysis of a preliminary RCT involving 40 SSRI-resistant participants with MDD found SAMe to improve in self-rated recall and word-finding difficulties compared to placebo.
Omega-3 PUFAs	Anti-inflammatory and antioxidant activities; increases the production of BDNF; diminishes microglia-related neuroinflammation	No published clinical trials to date have investigated the effects of omega-3 PUFAs on cognitive performance in samples with MDD.
Modafinil	Pleiotropic agent that targets several neurotransmitter systems (e.g. 5-HT, GABA, glutamate, orexin, and histamine).	A randomized single-dose proof-of-concept RCT that enrolled participants with MDD in remission found that modafinil improved verbal and working memory relative to placebo.

Galantamine	Rapidly reversible acetylcholinesterase inhibitor and a potent modulator of the nicotinic receptor; affects monoamines, GABA, and glutamate neurotransmitter systems.	Two preliminary RCTs have found no evidence for a procognitive effect of galantamine augmentation in participants with MDD.
Donepezil	An acetylcholinesterase inhibitor that also has possible antioxidant, neuroprotector, anti-inflammatory, and may also decrease glutamate excitotoxicity.	Two RCTs found no evidence of clear procognitive effects of donepezil augmentation in elderly patients with MDD.

BBB, Blood–brain barrier; BDNF, brain-derived neurotrophic factor; CNS, central nervous system; GABA, gamma-aminobutyric acid; MDD, major depressive disorder; PUFA, polyunsaturated fatty acids; RCT, randomized clinical trial; SSRI, selective serotonin reuptake inhibitor.

Source data from *Journal of Clinical Psychiatry*, 75, Keefe RS, McClintock SM, Roth RM, Doraiswamy PM, Tiger S, Madhoo M. Cognitive effects of pharmacotherapy for major depressive disorder: a systematic review, 2014.

outcome), while no improvements in objective neuropsychological scores were observed (secondary outcome). These results deserve replication.

Erythropoietin

A large body of data suggests that brain-derived erythropoietin (EPO) may have neuroprotective effects and may also stimulate neuroplasticity and have cognitive effects (49). A preliminary RCT assessed weekly EPO infusions (N=19; 40,000 UI) relative to saline (N=21) for 8 weeks among participants with treatment-resistant depression (50). Erythropoietin produced substantial effects on verbal memory compared to the control group. These effects were maintained in a 6-week follow-up after study completion. However, these results should be interpreted with caution and deserve replication because cognition was a tertiary outcome.

Metformin

Metformin is a first-line agent for the treatment of type 2 diabetes mellitus. Available preclinical evidence suggests that it may enhance hippocampal plasticity (51). However, preclinical and clinical evidence for putative neurocognitive effects across a number of conditions has been mixed (51). Symptomatic participants with MDD were randomized to metformin (1–2 g/day; N=29) or placebo (N=29) for 24 weeks. Notwithstanding, metformin significantly improved all assessed cognitive dimensions relative to placebo, those effects correlated with mood improvements, and hence pseudospecific effects cannot be ruled out.

Omega-3 polyunsaturated fatty acids

A recent meta-analysis suggests that adjunctive omega-3 polyunsaturated fatty acids (n-3 PUFAs) may improve depressive symptoms in patients with MDD (52), while preclinical data point to possible procognitive effects (53). Participants who were previously depressed were randomized to n-3 PUFAs (N=36) or placebo (N=35) for 4 weeks. No significant effects were observed on memory, attention, and cognitive reactivity (54).

Acetylcholinesterase inhibitors

Acetylcholinesterase inhibitors are cognitive enhancers used for the treatment of Alzheimer's disease, which appear to have pleiotropic mechanisms of action that may have a role upon cognition. Two RCTs have assessed potential procognitive effects of donepezil in MDD. In a small pilot study with 23 elderly patients with MDD who had been treated with open-label antidepressants, patients were randomized to donepezil or placebo for 12 weeks (55). Donepezil-treated patients appeared to have improvement in one measure of immediate recall. However, in a well-designed trial of participants with MDD, with or without mild cognitive impairment who had responded to initial antidepressant treatment, randomization to 24-month treatment with donepezil (N=67; 5–10 mg/day) or placebo (N=63) resulted in no significant differences (56).

In a pilot study, symptomatic participants with MDD were randomized to galantamine (8–16 mg/day; N=19) or placebo (N=19) in addition to antidepressant treatment for 24 weeks; there were no significant drug–placebo differences noted (55). In another RCT that enrolled participants with MDD who were in full or partial remission, 9-week augmentation treatment with galantamine or placebo (56) revealed no significant differences (57).

S-adenosyl methionine

S-adenosyl methionine (SAMe) works as a major methyl donor, facilitating the biosynthesis of several neurotransmitters and glutathione synthesis (58). A recent systematic review and meta-analysis suggests that adjunctive SAMe is efficacious for the treatment of MDD (57). In a trial that randomized 46 participants who had failed to respond to SSRI treatment to 6-week augmentation with either SAMe or placebo (59), SAMe improved the ability to recall information relative to placebo. However, these findings deserve replication because it was not specified whether cognitive function was a primary outcome, no objective neuropsychological assessment was conducted, and pseudospecific effects due to improvements in mood were possible.

Modafinil

Modafinil is a stimulant-like agent with a pleiotropic mechanism of action targeting serotonin, gamma-aminobutyric acid, glutamate, orexin, and histaminergic systems, among others (60). In a recent placebo RCT (61), participants who were treated with modafinil exhibited significant improvements in working and verbal memory relative to the placebo group, while no significant improvements in planning or sustained attention were observed. These promising findings, however, deserve replication in future RCTs of longer duration.

Melatonin/Agomelatine

Melatonin and agomelatine maintain circadian rhythms and regulate energy metabolism. They may exert neuroprotective and procognitive effects via anti-inflammatory and antioxidant properties, as well as enhance neuroplasticity and neurogenesis (62). A previous trial randomized symptomatic participants with MDD to treatment with melatonin (3 mg/day) plus buspirone (15 mg/day) or buspirone (15 mg/day) or placebo for 6 weeks (63). Participants who received melatonin plus buspirone exhibited significant improvements in subjectively reported global cognition relative to placebo. However, the possibility of mood-dependent pseudospecific effects cannot be ruled out. Both melatonin and agomelatine, an MT1/MT2 agonist and 5-HT$_{2C}$ antagonist, may modulate circadian rhythms and sleep disruption, which in turn may positively affect mood and cognition (62). Nevertheless, no published RCT has assessed putative effects of agomelatine on cognition in patients with MDD thus far.

Anti-inflammatory Agents

Peripheral immune activation and (neuro)-inflammation may contribute to the development of MDD (64, 65), and a recent study found inflammation to be associated with impairment in psychomotor speed in depression (66). Although evidence suggests that anti-inflammatory agents may mitigate depressive symptoms (67), no RCT to date has been performed.

Conclusion

Several steps may increase the methodological quality of RCTs aiming to assess effects of antidepressants or novel therapeutic targets for cognitive improvement in patients with MDD (Table 18.2). Evidence to date suggests that some antidepressants, most notably imipramine, duloxetine, and vortioxetine, may improve certain cognitive dimensions, namely psychomotor speed and delayed recall. In addition, several novel agents hold promise as cognitive enhancers for MDD, including LDX, EPO, SAMe, and modafinil. Yet replication in well-designed RCTs with cognitive performance as the primary outcome is warranted prior to the establishment of more definitive conclusions. Although the achievement of cognitive remission is a novel and unmet target in the treatment of MDD, the field awaits the approval of cognitive enhancers by regulatory bodies. The experience gained from more than three decades of research provides guidance for the conduct of methodologically robust RCTs that may enhance the robustness of the

Table 18.2 Suggestions to improve the methodological quality of future randomized clinical trial testing of neurotherapeutic agents for cognitive dysfunction related to major depressive disorder

Methodological aspect	Steps to improve methodological quality
'Pseudospecific' mood-dependent effects	Enrol participants with major depressive disorder in remission
'Ceiling effects'	Screen for cognitive dysfunction at inception and a priori define a threshold for enrolment in the trial
Inconsistency and differences in measures across studies	Always include an objective neuropsychological measure; further standardization of tests is required
Post-hoc assessment of cognition	Consider cognitive dysfunction as primary outcome; provide an a priori hierarchy of cognitive measures; publication and/or public availability of trial protocol in advance
Multiple cognitive measures	Provide statistical control for multiple comparisons; specify a hierarchy of measures
Randomization/allocation concealment	Provide an accurate a priori reporting of steps taken to ensure proper allocation concealment/randomization

evidence. To date the specific treatment of cognitive dysfunction in MDD should be weighed against possible safety and tolerability concerns associated with long-term treatment with antidepressant agents, including a possible higher risk of dementia and Alzheimer's disease (68, 69).

References

1. Bromet E, Andrade LH, Hwang I, et al. Cross-national epidemiology of DSM-IV major depressive episode. BMC Med 2011;9:90.

2. Kennedy SH, Lam RW, McIntyre RS, et al. Canadian Network for Mood and Anxiety Treatments (CANMAT) 2016 Clinical Guidelines for the Management of Adults with Major Depressive Disorder: Section 3. Pharmacological treatments. Can J Psychiatry 2016;61(9):540–60.

3. Trivedi MH, Rush AJ, Wisniewski SR, et al. Evaluation of outcomes with citalopram for depression using measurement-based care in STAR*D: implications for clinical practice. Am J Psychiatry 2006;163(1):28–40.

4. Nierenberg AA, Husain MM, Trivedi MH, et al. Residual symptoms after remission of major depressive disorder with citalopram and risk of relapse: a STAR*D report. Psychol Med 2010;40(1):41–50.

5. Kamenov K, Twomey C, Cabello M, Prina AM, Ayuso-Mateos JL. The efficacy of psychotherapy, pharmacotherapy and their combination on functioning and quality of life in depression: a meta-analysis. Psychol Med 2017;47(3):414–25.

6. Saris IMJ, Aghajani M, van der Werff SJA, van der Wee NJA, Penninx B. Social functioning in patients with depressive and anxiety disorders. Acta Psychiatr Scand 2017;136(4):352–61.

7. Sacchetti E, Frank E, Siracusano A, Racagni G, Vita A, Turrina C. Functional impairment in patients with major depression in clinical remission: results from the VIVAL-D-Rem, a nationwide, naturalistic, cross-sectional survey. Int Clin Psychopharmacol 2015;30(3):129–41.

8. Rock PL, Roiser JP, Riedel WJ, Blackwell AD. Cognitive impairment in depression: a systematic review and meta-analysis. Psychol Med 2014;44:2029–40.

9. Ahern E, Semkovska M. Cognitive functioning in the first-episode of major depressive disorder: a systematic review and meta-analysis. Neuropsychology 2017;31(1):52–72.

10. Gorlyn M, Keilp JG, Grunebaum MF, et al. Neuropsychological characteristics as predictors of SSRI treatment response in depressed subjects. J Neural Trans 2008;115(8):1213–19.

11. Pimontel MA, Rindskopf D, Rutherford BR, Brown PJ, Roose SP, Sneed JR. A meta-analysis of executive dysfunction and antidepressant treatment response in late-life depression. Am J Ger Psychiatry 2016;24(1):31–41.

12. Evans VC, Iverson GL, Yatham LN, Lam RW. The relationship between neurocognitive and psychosocial functioning in major depressive disorder: a systematic review. J Clin Psychiatry 2014;75(12):1359–70.

13. McIntyre RS, Lee Y. Cognition in major depressive disorder: a 'Systemically Important Functional Index' (SIFI). Curr Opin Psychiatry 2016;29(1):48–55.

14. Woo YS, Rosenblat JD, Kakar R, Bahk WM, McIntyre RS. Cognitive deficits as a mediator of poor occupational function in remitted major depressive disorder patients. Clin Psychopharmacol Neurosci 2016;14(1):1–16.

15. Baune BT, Miller R, McAfoose J, Johnson M, Quirk F, Mitchell D. The role of cognitive impairment in general functioning in major depression. Psychiatry Res 2010;176(2–3):183–9.

16. Simons CJ, Jacobs N, Derom C, et al. Cognition as predictor of current and follow-up depressive symptoms in the general population. Acta Psychiatr Scand 2009;120(1):45–52.

17. Franz CE, Lyons MJ, O'Brien R, et al. A 35-year longitudinal assessment of cognition and midlife depression symptoms: the Vietnam Era Twin Study of Aging. Am J Ger Psychiatry 2011;19(6):559–70.

18. Davis J, Maes M, Andreazza A, McGrath JJ, Tye SJ, Berk M. Towards a classification of biomarkers of neuropsychiatric disease: from encompass to compass. Mol Psychiatry 2015;20(2):152–3.

19. Bortolato B, Miskowiak KW, Kohler CA, et al. Cognitive remission: a novel objective for the treatment of major depression? BMC Med 2016;14:9.

20. Carvalho AF, Miskowiak KK, Hyphantis TN, Kohler CA, Alves GS, Bortolato B. Cognitive dysfunction in depression—pathophysiology and novel targets. CNS Neurol Disord Drug Targets 2014;13:1819–35.

21. Rosenblat JD, Kakar R, McIntyre RS. The cognitive effects of antidepressants in major depressive disorder: a systematic review and meta-analysis of randomized clinical trials. Int J Neuropsychopharmacol 2015;19(2):pii: pyv082.

22. Keefe RS, McClintock SM, Roth RM, Doraiswamy PM, Tiger S, Madhoo M. Cognitive effects of pharmacotherapy for major depressive disorder: a systematic review. J Clin Psychiatry. 2014;75:864–76.

23. Miskowiak KW, Ott CV, Petersen JZ, Kessing LV. Systematic review of randomized controlled trials of candidate treatments for cognitive impairment in depression and methodological challenges in the field. Eur Neuropsychopharmacol 2016;26(12):1845–67.

24. Mahableshwarkar AR, Zajecka J, Jacobson W, Chen Y, Keefe RS. A randomized, placebo-controlled, active-reference, double-blind, flexible-dose study of the efficacy of vortioxetine on cognitive function in major depressive disorder. Neuropsychopharmacol 2015;40:2025–37.

25. Raskin J, Wiltse CG, Siegal A, Sheikh J, Xu J, Dinkel JJ. Efficacy of duloxetine on cognition, depression, and pain in elderly patients with major depressive disorder: an 8-week, double-blind, placebo-controlled trial. Am J Psychiatry 2007;164:900–9.

26. Burdick KE, Endick CJ, Goldberg JF. Assessing cognitive deficits in bipolar disorder: are self-reports valid? Psychiatry Res 2005;136(1):43–50.

27. Srisurapanont M, Suttajit S, Eurviriyanukul K, Varnado P. Discrepancy between objective and subjective cognition in adults with major depressive disorder. Sci Rep 2017;7(1):3901.

28. Ott CV, Bjertrup AJ, Jensen JH, et al. Screening for cognitive dysfunction in unipolar depression: validation and evaluation of objective and subjective tools. J Affect Disord 2016;190:607–15.

29. Fava M, Graves LM, Benazzi F, et al. A cross-sectional study of the prevalence of cognitive and physical symptoms during long-term antidepressant treatment. J Clin Psychiatry 2006;67(11):1754–9.

30. Snyder HR. Major depressive disorder is associated with broad impairments on neuropsychological measures of executive function: a meta-analysis and review. Psychol Bull 2013;139(1):81–132.

31. Wroolie TE, Williams KE, Keller J, et al. Mood and neuropsychological changes in women with midlife depression treated with escitalopram. J Clin Psychopharmacol 2006;26(4):361–6.

32. Peretti S, Judge R, Hindmarch I. Safety and tolerability considerations: tricyclic antidepressants vs. selective serotonin reuptake inhibitors. Acta Psych Scand Suppl 2000;403:17–25.

33. Ma Y. Neuropsychological mechanism underlying antidepressant effect: a systematic meta-analysis. Mol Psychiatry 2015;20(3):311–19.

34. Harmer CJ, Goodwin GM, Cowen PJ. Why do antidepressants take so long to work? A cognitive neuropsychological model of antidepressant drug action. Br J Psychiatry 2009;195(2):102–8.

35. Culang ME, Sneed JR, Keilp JG, et al. Change in cognitive functioning following acute antidepressant treatment in late-life depression. Am J Ger Psychiatry 2009;17(10):881–8.

36. Glass RM, Uhlenhuth EH, Hartel FW, Matuzas W, Fischman MW. Cognitive dysfunction and imipramine in outpatient depressive. Arch Gen Psychiatry 1981;38(9):1048–51.

37. Georgotas A, McCue RE, Reisberg B, et al. The effects of mood changes and antidepressants on the cognitive capacity of elderly depressed patients. Int Psychoger 1989;1(2):135–43.

38. Jansen W, Siegfried K. Nomifensine in geriatric inpatients: a placebo-controlled study. J Clin Psychiatry 1984;45(4 Pt 2):63–7.

39. Ferguson JM, Wesnes KA, Schwartz GE. Reboxetine versus paroxetine versus placebo: effects on cognitive functioning in depressed patients. Int Clin Psychopharmacol 2003;18(1):9–14.

40. Tian Y, Du J, Spagna A, et al. Venlafaxine treatment reduces the deficit of executive control of attention in patients with major depressive disorder. Sci Rep 2016;6:28028.

41. Herrera-Guzman I, Gudayol-Ferre E, Lira-Mandujano J, et al. Cognitive predictors of treatment response to bupropion and cognitive effects of bupropion in patients with major depressive disorder. Psychiatry Res 2008;160(1):72–82.

42. Pehrson AL, Sanchez C. Serotonergic modulation of glutamate neurotransmission as a strategy for treating depression and cognitive dysfunction. CNS Spectr 2014;19(2):121–33.

43. Smagin GN, Song D, Budac DP, et al. Histamine may contribute to vortioxetine's procognitive effects; possibly through an orexigenic mechanism. Prog Neuropsychopharmacol Biol Psychiatry 2016;68:25–30.

44. Katona C, Hansen T, Olsen CK. A randomized, double-blind, placebo-controlled, duloxetine-referenced, fixed-dose study comparing the efficacy and safety of Lu AA21004 in elderly patients with major depressive disorder. Int Clin Psychopharmacol 2012;27(4):215–23.

45. McIntyre RS, Lophaven S, Olsen CK. A randomized, double-blind, placebo-controlled study of vortioxetine on cognitive function in depressed adults. Int J Neuropsychopharmacol 2014;17(10):1557–67.

46. Mahableshwarkar AR, Zajecka J, Jacobson W, Chen Y, Keefe RS. A randomized, placebo-controlled, active-reference, double-blind, flexible-dose study of the efficacy of vortioxetine on cognitive function in major depressive disorder. Neuropsychopharmacology 2015;40(8):2025–37.

47. Austin MP, Mitchell P, Hadzi-Pavlovic D, et al. Effect of apomorphine on motor and cognitive function in melancholic patients: a preliminary report. Psychiatry Res 2000;97(2–3):207–15.

48. Madhoo M, Keefe RS, Roth RM, et al. Lisdexamfetamine dimesylate augmentation in adults with persistent executive dysfunction after partial or full remission of major depressive disorder. Neuropsychopharmacology 2014;39(6):1388–98.

49. Miskowiak KW, Vinberg M, Harmer CJ, Ehrenreich H, Kessing LV. Erythropoietin: a candidate treatment for mood symptoms and memory dysfunction in depression. Psychopharmacology 2012;219(3):687–98.

50. Miskowiak KW, Vinberg M, Christensen EM, et al. Recombinant human erythropoietin for treating treatment-resistant depression: a double-blind, randomized, placebo-controlled phase 2 trial. Neuropsychopharmacology 2014;39(6):1399–408.

51. Ying MA, Maruschak N, Mansur R, Carvalho AF, Cha DS, McIntyre RS. Metformin: repurposing opportunities for cognitive and mood dysfunction. CNS Neurol Disord Drug Targets 2014;13(10):1836–45.

52. Schefft C, Kilarski LL, Bschor T, Kohler S. Efficacy of adding nutritional supplements in unipolar depression: a systematic review and meta-analysis. Eur Neuropsychopharmacol 2017;27(11):1090–109.

53. Knochel C, Voss M, Gruter F, et al. Omega 3 fatty acids: novel neurotherapeutic targets for cognitive dysfunction in mood disorders and schizophrenia? Current Neuropharmacol 2015;13(5):663–80.

54. Antypa N, Smelt AH, Strengholt A, Van der Does AJ. Effects of omega-3 fatty acid supplementation on mood and emotional information processing in recovered depressed individuals. J Psychopharmacol 2012;26(5):738–43.

55. Holtzheimer PE, 3rd, Meeks TW, Kelley ME, et al. A double blind, placebo-controlled pilot study of galantamine augmentation of antidepressant treatment in older adults with major depression. Int J Ger Psychiatry 2008;23(6):625–31.

56. Elgamal S, MacQueen G. Galantamine as an adjunctive treatment in major depression. J Clin Psychopharmacol 2008;28(3):357–9.

57. Sarris J, Murphy J, Mischoulon D, et al. Adjunctive nutraceuticals for depression: a systematic review and meta-analyses. Am J Psychiatry 2016;173(6):575–87.

58. Bottiglieri T. Folate, vitamin B(1)(2), and S-adenosylmethionine. Psychiatr Clin North Am 2013;36(1):1–13.

59. Levkovitz Y, Alpert JE, Brintz CE, Mischoulon D, Papakostas GI. Effects of S-adenosylmethionine augmentation of serotonin-reuptake inhibitor antidepressants on cognitive symptoms of major depressive disorder. J Affect Disord 2012;136(3):1174–8.

60. Gerrard P, Malcolm R. Mechanisms of modafinil: a review of current research. Neuropsychiatr Dis Treat 2007;3:349–64.

61. Kaser M, Deakin JB, Michael A, et al. Modafinil improves episodic memory and working memory cognition in patients with remitted depression: a double-blind, randomized, placebo-controlled study. Biol Psychiatry Cogn Neurosci Neuroimaging 2017;2(2):115–22.

62. Zaki NFW, Spence DW, BaHammam AS, Pandi-Perumal SR, Cardinali DP, Brown GM. Chronobiological theories of mood disorder. Eur Arch Psychiatry Clin Neurosci 2017;268:107–18.

63. Targum SD, Wedel PC, Fava M. Changes in cognitive symptoms after a buspirone-melatonin combination treatment for major depressive disorder. J Psychiatr Res 2015;68:392–6.

64. Kohler CA, Freitas TH, Maes M, et al. Peripheral cytokine and chemokine alterations in depression: a meta-analysis of 82 studies. Acta Psychiatr Scand 2017;135(5):373–87.

65. Miller AH, Raison CL. The role of inflammation in depression: from evolutionary imperative to modern treatment target. Nature Rev Immunol 2016;16(1):22–34.

66. Goldsmith DR, Haroon E, Woolwine BJ, et al. Inflammatory markers are associated with decreased psychomotor speed in patients with major depressive disorder. Brain Behav Immun 2016;56:281–8.

67. Kohler O, Benros ME, Nordentoft M, et al. Effect of anti-inflammatory treatment on depression, depressive symptoms, and adverse effects: a systematic review and meta-analysis of randomized clinical trials. JAMA Psychiatry 2014;71(12):1381–91.

68. Moraros J, Nwankwo C, Patten SB, Mousseau DD. The association of antidepressant drug usage with cognitive impairment or dementia, including Alzheimer disease: a systematic review and meta-analysis. Depress Anxiety 2017;34(3):217–26.

69. Carvalho AF, Sharma MS, Brunoni AR, Vieta E, Fava GA. The safety, tolerability and risks associated with the use of newer generation antidepressant drugs: a critical review of the literature. Psychother Psychosom 2016;85(5):270–88.

19

Psychological Interventions for Cognitive Dysfunction in Major Depressive Disorder

Claudia Woolf, Loren Mowszowski, and Sharon Naismith

Introduction

Major depressive disorder (MDD) is a chronic, disabling, and recurring psychiatric condition that currently affects 322 million people worldwide (1) or one in seven individuals across their lifetime (2). Depression is now recognized as the leading cause of disability worldwide (1) and is associated with increased functional impairment (3) and higher rates of mortality (4).

While pharmacological and psychological treatments for MDD are moderately effective, as many as 50% of patients across all age groups will not achieve remission with their first treatment (5). Ultimately, 20–30% will not achieve full recovery despite access to multiple interventions (6), and those individuals who do achieve full recovery remain at high risk for further episodes (7). In this context, the mechanisms that underpin the persistence and recurrence of depressive symptoms need to be elucidated to better inform treatment and outcomes.

It is well recognized that MDD is associated with cognitive dysfunction (8), of which two primary types have been delineated: (a) cognitive biases, which include distorted information appraisal or attentional allocation toward negative stimuli and away from positive stimuli; and (b) cognitive deficits, which include impairments in neuropsychological functioning in specific cognitive domains. For many individuals, while cognitive biases in MDD improve with treatment, cognitive or neuropsychological deficits persist despite resolution of depressive symptoms (9). This is particularly troubling as cognitive impairment in MDD is reportedly associated with disability (3), burden, and duration of illness (10, 11), and, at least in elderly patients, response to antidepressant treatment (12). It is therefore not surprising that one of the most prominent and persistent predictors of functional deficits (13) and reduced quality of life (14) in MDD is neuropsychological impairment. Hence, symptomatic remission of low mood is insufficient as the predominant goal of treatment for MDD. Rather, treatment goals should equally address factors affecting the persistence and recurrence of symptoms, including neuropsychological deficits.

In this chapter, we will briefly review the underlying neurobiological mechanisms of neuropsychological dysfunction in MDD, followed by a discussion of treatment approaches targeting cognitive deficits in MDD.

Cognitive Dysfunction in Major Depressive Disorder

Neuropsychological dysfunction is now well established as a core feature of depression (15), with a diminished ability to think or concentrate and (or) indecisiveness listed as key diagnostic criteria in the *Diagnostic and Statistical Manual of Mental Disorders*, 5th edition (DSM-5) classification of MDD (16). The profile is typically thought to resemble a 'fronto-subcortical' pattern, with deficits in executive functioning and processing speed being most pronounced, followed by changes in learning/memory (15, 17–19). While there is considerable heterogeneity in presentation, figures suggest that impaired neuropsychological function (of a moderate effect size) may be evident in around two-thirds of all depressed patients (20, 21). In fact, a recent meta-analysis of cognitive symptoms in first episode MDD of 644 young adult patients with a mean age of 39.36 years (standard deviation [SD] 10.21) and 570 healthy controls across 13 different studies demonstrated that patients with first-episode MDD had significant impairment in psychomotor speed (effect size 0.48), attention (effect size 0.36), and visual learning and memory (effect size 0.53) compared with healthy controls (8). Within the domain of executive function, attentional switching (effect size 0.22), verbal fluency (effect size 0.59), and cognitive flexibility (effect size 0.53) were worse in patients with MDD. In terms of the evidence for cognitive dysfunction in patients remitted from depression, Hasselbalch et al. (22) included 500 remitted patients (of younger, middle, and older age) and 472 controls, and revealed impaired neuropsychological performance (on at least one test) in nine of the 11 included studies.

Mechanisms Underpinning Neuropsychological Dysfunction in Depression

Studying the neurobiological basis of neuropsychological dysfunction in depression may help to elucidate potential treatment targets. While many studies focus on the underlying mechanisms of emotional disturbance or cognitive biases (for example, negative bias, response to failure, etc.) in the acute phase of a depressive episode, fewer studies have investigated the neural correlates of neuropsychological impairment in MDD.

Of the studies that have investigated the neural correlates of neuropsychological impairment in MDD, most have focused on executive tasks that depend on functional integrity of the prefrontal cortices, with somewhat heterogeneous findings. That is, a number of studies report reduced cortical activity on different measures of executive function in depressed patients (23), while other studies report increased cortical activity (24). Considerably fewer studies have focused on the neurobiological underpinnings of other neuropsychological domains in MDD. For example, while memory complaints are the most common of the neuropsychological symptoms reported by depressed patients, there are few studies that explore the neuronal basis for memory impairment in depression and, again, these studies report mixed findings (25, 26). Discrepancies may reflect variability in patient demographics and task differences.

Other evidence demonstrates neurochemical abnormalities in the anterior cingulate and prefrontal cortices in depression and in remitted states (27–29). Interestingly, there is also evidence that suggests that hippocampal spectroscopic markers have differential relationships with neuropsychological functioning depending on depression history (30).

Structural neuroanatomical changes have also been widely reported in MDD, particularly in regions known to be important for memory and other relevant neuropsychological functions. For example, hippocampal volume changes are consistently observed and such changes persist after the resolution of depressive symptoms (17, 30, 31). An empiric study of clinical patients showed that years of untreated illness was significantly associated with hippocampal volume loss (32), a finding that is consistent with a body of work suggesting that antidepressant medication may be neuroprotective (33). In addition, other studies demonstrate that MDD is associated with volumetric reductions in several other discrete brain regions, including the frontal cortex, orbitofrontal cortex, cingulate cortex, and striatum (34).

In terms of understanding the impact of these structural and functional neurobiological changes, studies to date suggest that a progressive process takes place in recurring MDD (35), and that this may be a primary driver for ensuing neuropsychological impairment. Specifically, it is thought that neurotoxic effects of depression occur via downregulation of the hypothalamic–pituitary–adrenocortical axis, neurotoxic effects of glucocorticoids, and reduced expression of neurotrophins (36). Other factors, such as cerebrovascular disease, reactive oxygen and nitrogen species, immunological and inflammatory changes, as well as amyloid deposition, are also thought to contribute (37).

Importantly, however, depression alone does not appear to fully mediate the extent of neuropsychological deficits in MDD. Rather, comorbid medical burden and concomitant brain changes are also likely to contribute to neuropsychological deficits. In fact, the presence of cardiovascular disease appears to be particularly pertinent, especially for older people (38). The strong interplay between white matter disease and depression has led to the 'vascular depression' hypothesis (39, 40), which is characterized by structural changes on magnetic resonance imaging and 'depression dysexecutive syndrome'. Indeed, the neuropsychological implications of this syndrome were recently emphasized in a large study of 217 older subjects with MDD (41) and have also been replicated in smaller cohorts of patients with MDD (11, 42).

In light of the evidence linking depression with underlying structural, functional, and neurochemical brain changes, it is unsurprising that MDD has emerged as a 'risk factor' for substantial long-term functional impairment (3), which is likely secondary, at least in part, to neuropsychological impairment (13).

Current Treatment Options for Cognitive Impairment in Depression

Given that there is a growing realization that neurocognitive deficits in MDD may: a) worsen the burden and duration of illness (10); b) contribute to ongoing functional impairment (14); and c) represent a risk factor for cognitive decline and dementia (43), treatment of neurocognitive impairment in MDD needs to be considered a priority. Below, we outline the available evidence for a variety of interventions in relation to addressing cognitive deficits in MDD.

First, a number of studies have examined the clinical impact of pharmacological agents for targeting cognitive impairments in a number of psychiatric disorders (44). However, data supporting the efficacy of such pharmacological strategies in MDD is at best preliminary. In any case, the strongest evidence to date supports the use of serotonin and noradrenaline reuptake inhibitors (SNRIs; e.g. duloxetine), which target multiple neurochemical systems simultaneously and are associated with improvement in a global cognitive composite indexed by increases in measures of verbal learning and recall (45). There is also evidence for some selective serotonin reuptake inhibitors (SSRIs; e.g. sertraline) showing improvements in memory (45), psychomotor speed, and executive function (46, 47). However, epidemiological and longitudinal data suggest that global cognitive decline does not differ based on antidepressant use (48). Overall, the effect of antidepressants on cognitive functioning still remains an emerging area of investigation and, despite some promising findings, there is a paucity of large randomized controlled trials (RCTs) with objective cognitive measures as primary endpoints, which limits the strength and reliability of any conclusions.

Second, psychotherapeutic strategies have proven efficacy for treatment of cognitive biases and subjective cognitive complaints in MDD and, while psychotherapy programmes that utilize cognitive rehabilitation techniques have been investigated in schizophrenia (49) and bipolar depression (50) and may also be effective for neurocognitive symptoms in MDD (51), there are very few studies that investigate the efficacy of psychotherapy in neuropsychological impairment in MDD.

Third, behavioural strategies, such as physical exercise, have proven beneficial effects not only for depressive symptoms but also for objective cognition, even in those with mild cognitive impairment (52). Given this, it is not surprising that physical exercise has also been associated with neuroplastic changes in the hippocampus, demonstrating the potential capacity of exercise to induce longer-lasting cognitive benefits (52). However, a recent meta-analysis did not find an effect of exercise on cognition in a depressed cohort. In saying that, interventions combining physical and cognitive activity significantly improved global cognition (53). Overall, physical exercise represents a promising area of investigation, yet further research is certainly required.

Fourth, stimulation-based therapies, including electroconvulsive therapy, transcranial magnetic stimulation, and transcranial direct current stimulation (tDCS), are posited to induce neuroplastic properties. For example, there is some evidence to suggest that electroconvulsive therapy increases the expression of brain-derived neurotrophic factor and therefore induces neuroplasticity (see review [54]). In addition, a recent meta-analysis demonstrated promising support for the utility of transcranial magnetic stimulation in improving cognitive functioning in adults with treatment-resistant MDD (55). Recently, similar interest has grown regarding the beneficial effects of repeated tDCS for improving cognition, irrespective of concurrent improvements in mood, in those with depression (56). Therefore, stimulation-based therapies may represent a promising approach to targeting cognitive deficits in MDD, although further research is needed.

Finally, cognitive remediation is a novel intervention that is proposed not only to only improve neuropsychological impairment but also general functioning. Cognitive remediation encompasses cognitive stimulation, cognitive training (CT), and cognitive rehabilitation (Figure 19.1) (see [57] for an overview). Of these, CT is gaining increasing prominence owing to its potential to maintain and potentially enhance cognitive function. An operational definition has been delineated to differentiate CT from other cognitive remediation approaches: CT is defined as repetitive practice directly training specific neuropsychological skills on exercises (58, 59). The underlying premise is that intensive cognitive exercises build or restore brain and cognitive integrity, promoting neuroplasticity and providing greater resilience against neuropathology, thereby maintaining function (60).

As shown in Figure 19.1, CT programmes enhance cognition by providing theoretically driven strategies and skills, usually involving 'guided practice' in compensatory as well as restorative techniques to improve neuropsychological weaknesses and strengthen intact skills. Compensatory methods aim to bypass neuropsychological deficits and teach alternative approaches to achieve goals. Restorative methods typically incorporate repetitive drill-and-practice exercises (on computer), targeting specific cognitive domains to improve neuropsychological functioning in those areas (57, 58).

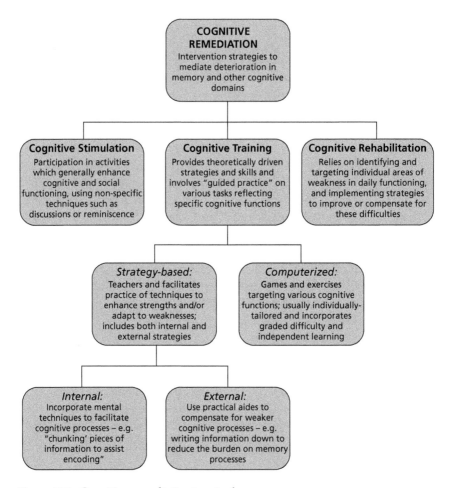

Figure 19.1 Cognitive remediation terminology.

Reproduced from *International Psychogeriatrics*, 22, 4, Mowszowski L, Batchelor J, Naismith SL, Early intervention for cognitive decline: can cognitive training be used as a selective prevention technique? pp. 537–48. Copyright © International Psychogeriatric Association 2010. This drew on several sources (61–63) to synthesize definitions.

Cognitive Training in Major Depressive Disorder

In light of the aforementioned evidence, over the past few years, CT has attracted attention as a viable treatment for neuropsychological dysfunction in the context of MDD. Like most of the CT literature, there is significant heterogeneity in the evidence to date. Of the available evidence, there are certainly a greater number of studies investigating CT in individuals with depressive symptoms rather than clinically defined MDD. Nonetheless, we will now summarize the evidence for CT in MDD.

As shown in Table 19.1, of the 12 available studies, the majority examined computer-based CT exclusively, two studies investigated a combined approach of computer-based CT and strategy-based techniques, and one study investigated a strategy-based intervention alone. While the overwhelming majority of studies report neuropsychological outcomes, some studies do not (64, 65). A number of studies report improvements in memory (10, 11, 51, 66–68), which is aligned with the broader CT literature to date, despite considerable heterogeneity in CT programme characteristics across these trials. Positive changes are also reported in executive functioning (10, 12, 67). Two studies described improvements in working memory (67, 69) and two studies described improvements in both attention and processing speed (10, 51). With regard to affective outcomes, a number of studies do report a reduction in depressive symptoms (12, 56, 69, 70) irrespective of improvements in cognition, which is consistent with an emerging body of research that CT might improve depressed mood in MDD (64, 65). However, other studies of CT in MDD either do not measure mood as an outcome (51) or find no effect of CT on mood (10, 11, 66, 67).

Recently, a number of studies have directly compared the efficacy of CT in MDD with traditional pharmacological antidepressant treatment (12, 70), exercise (69), and more novel treatments, including tDCS (56), although these are predominantly preliminary trials with small samples. Overall, when CT is directly compared to other treatments for MDD, it seems to provide additional benefits (for example, shorter time to treatment response (12, 70), neuropsychological improvements (67, 70), or a synergistic effect) such that CT enhances the antidepressant effect of other treatments (56).

Potential mechanisms of neuropsychological benefit following CT have been examined in both animal and human trials. CT is proposed to promote neuroplastic processes that maintain neuropsychological performance and potentially mask or prevent clinical manifestation of neurocognitive disease via cellular processes, including synaptogenesis, hippocampal neurogenesis, glial activity, and upregulation of neurotrophic factors (reviewed in [71, 72]). Although the findings are promising, it is important to note that studies examining neurobiological changes associated with CT tend to include small samples, diverse methodologies, and varied imaging sequences and CT techniques.

As noted above, in line with the broader CT literature, clinical trials of CT in MDD are heterogeneous with respect to sample variability (e.g. older versus younger adults, inpatients versus outpatients, etc.), clinical factors (e.g. current versus lifetime depressive episode/s, depressive symptoms versus a major depressive episode, etc.), study design (passive versus active control, randomized versus non-randomized studies, etc.), method and format of CT delivery (strategy-based versus computer-based, individual versus group-based, supervised or not, etc.), the dose of CT (e.g. frequency, intensity, and duration), and which outcomes (e.g. neuropsychological versus psychological) are assessed. Despite this, evidence

Table 19.1 Characteristics of studies

Study	Study demographics		Intervention design				Group size	CT delivery
	Cohort	N	Mean age (years)	Design	CT target	CT duration		
Alvarez et al. 2008 (70)	MDD	T = 31 CT/noAD = 11 CT/AD = 10 AD = 11	T = 22.7 CT/noAD = 21.0, CT/ AD = 23.3, AD = 23.8	Active control	Cognition Mood Behaviour	Sessions: 2 per week Mins/session: 30 Weeks: Unspecified	Unspecified	Computer-based
Bowie et al. 2013 (51)	MDD, treatment resistant	T = 33 I = 17 C = 16	I = 49.2 C = 42.2	RCT with waitlist control	Cognition Mood Social skills	Sessions: unspecified Mins/session: 90 Weeks: 10	3	Computer- and strategy-based
Dalgleish et al. 2013 (68)	MDD, either in episode or in remission	T = 38 I = 18 C = 20	I = 43.73 C = 47.80	RCT with active control	Cognition	Sessions: 1 per week Mins/session: 60 Weeks: 2	Unspecified	Strategy-based
Elgamal et al. 2007 (10)	MDD	T = 46 I = 12 C = 12 HC = 22	I = 50.3 C = 47.4 HC = 49.1	Passive controls	Cognition	Sessions: 2 per week Mins/session: 45–60 Weeks: 10	Individual	Computer-based
Morimoto et al. 2014 (12)	MDD, treatment resistant	T = 44 I = 11 C = 33	I = 73.5 C = 73.1	Active control	Cognition Mood Disability	Sessions: Unspecified Mins/session: 30 h Weeks: 4	Individual	Computer-based
Naismith et al. 2010 (66)	History of MDD	T = 16 I = 8 C = 8	T = 33.5 I = 33.6 C = 33.	Waitlist control	Cognition (memory)	Sessions: 2 per week Mins/session: 60 Weeks: 10	Group, unspecified	Computer-based

Study	Population	N	Age	Design	Outcome	Session details	Group	Delivery
Naismith et al. 2011 (11)	History of MDD	T = 44, I = 22, C = 19	T = 64.8	Waitlist control	Cognition (memory)	Sessions: 1 per week, Mins/session: 120, Weeks: 10	Group (n<10)	Computer- and strategy-based
Oertel-Knochel et al. 2014 (69)	MDD	T = 31, CT = 9, CT + exercise = 8, CT + relaxation = 6, C=8	T = Unspecified, CT = Unspecified, CT + exercise = 36.63, CT + relaxation = 41.37, C = 42.21	RCT with active and waitlist controls	Cognition	Sessions: 3 per week, Mins/session: 75, Weeks: 4	Unspecified	Computer-based
Papageorgiou et al. 2000 (64)	MDD	T = 4	T = 25.25	Case series	Mood	Sessions: 1 per week, Mins/session: 15--45, Weeks: 5-8	Individual	Computer-based
Segrave et al. 2014 (56)	MDD	T = 29, CT + tDCS = 9 shamCT + tDCS = 9 CT + shamDCS = 9	T = 40.47, CT + tDCS = 42.6, shamCT + tDCS = 33.8, CT + shamDCS = 45.0	R(sham)CT with active controls	Mood	Sessions: 5 per week, Mins/session: 55, Weeks: 1	Unspecified	Computer-based
Siegle et al. 2007 (65)	MDD	T = 25, I = 15, C = 10	T = 18--55	Waitlist control	Mood	Unspecified	Unspecified	Computer-based
Trapp et al. 2015 (67)	MDD inpatients	T = 46, I = 23, C = 23	T = 35.57, I = 34.26, C = 36.87	RCT with one active control and one treatment as usual control	Cognition	Sessions: 3 per week, Mins/session: 60, Weeks: 4	3	Computer-based

AD, Antidepressant; C, control group of interest; CT, cognitive training; HC, healthy controls; I, intervention group of interest; MDD, major depressive episode; N, number; RCT, randomized controlled trial; tDCS, transcranial direct current stimulation; T, total.

from trials in MDD as well as in other patient cohorts have revealed particular trends that may guide our practice in applying CT as a treatment option for neuropsychological dysfunction in MDD (73, 74). However, in the context of MDD, there may be other moderating factors that need to be considered. For example, the severity of the depressive illness may dictate the approach taken.

Finally, it is important to consider the utility of CT with regard to generalization or transfer of benefit to non-trained neuropsychological functions and to instrumental activities of daily living. Multidomain CT is readily associated with transfer of benefits to distal neuropsychological domains, including memory, executive functions, information processing and attention, and global cognition (74), and there is evidence that multidomain CT generalizes to non-cognitive instrumental activities of daily living (59) as well as to psychiatric and psychological health (63).

Future directions

The preliminary evidence for CT in MDD, although encouraging, is heterogeneous. Nonetheless, this is consistent with the broader CT literature, which is affected by similar limitations. Clinical application, however, is quite widely accepted. To expand the acceptability and use of CT as a treatment option for neuropsychological dysfunction in those with MDD, the following issues will need clarification. First, CT programme characteristics should be investigated. Second, it remains to be determined whether CT is best used as a standalone or adjunctive treatment. Third, the neurobiological mechanisms underpinning CT in MDD need to be further elucidated. Fourth, the generalizability of effects to functional outcomes and the sustainability of effects over time needs further exploration, particularly in relation to recurrent major depressive episodes.

Conclusion

In conclusion, the achievement of 'cognitive or neuropsychological remission' in existing pharmacological or psychological interventions for MDD remains a distinctive unmet need. This is unacceptable given that ongoing neuropsychological impairment may mitigate the efficacy of treatment; gives rise to psychosocial, functional, and occupational impairment; persists despite depressive symptom resolution; increases an individual's risk for a relapse; and represents an independent risk factor for dementia.

Despite a relatively small and heterogeneous evidence base in MDD, the use of CT to target neuropsychological dysfunction in patients with MDD represents a promising and novel therapeutic option, which may yield neuropsychological as well as affective, functional, and behavioural benefits.

References

1. World Health Organization. *Depression and Other Common Mental Disorders: Global Health Estimates*. Geneva: World Health Organization; 2017.

2. Kessler RC, Bromet EJ. The epidemiology of depression across cultures. Annu Rev Public Health 2013;34:119–38.

3. Petersen T, Papakostas GI, Mahal Y, et al. Psychosocial functioning in patients with treatment resistant depression. Eur Psychiatry 2004;19(4):196–201.

4. Cuijpers P, Smit F. Excess mortality in depression: a meta-analysis of community studies. J Affect Disord 2002;72(3):227–36.

5. Roose SP, Schatzberg AF. The efficacy of antidepressants in the treatment of late-life depression. J Clin Psychopharmacol 2005;25(4 Suppl 1):S1–7.

6. Whyte EM, Dew MA, Gildengers A, et al. Time course of response to antidepressants in late-life major depression: therapeutic implications. Drugs Aging 2004;21(8):531–54.

7. Maj M, Veltro F, Pirozzi R, Lobrace S, Magliano L. Pattern of recurrence of illness after recovery from an episode of major depression: a prospective study. Am J Psychiatry 1992;149(6):795–800.

8. Lee RS, Hermens DF, Porter MA, Redoblado-Hodge MA. A meta-analysis of cognitive deficits in first-episode major depressive disorder. J Affect Disord 2012;140(2):113–24.

9. Rock PL, Roiser JP, Riedel WJ, Blackwell AD. Cognitive impairment in depression: a systematic review and meta-analysis. Psychol Med 2014;44(10):2029–40.

10. Elgamal S, McKinnon MC, Ramakrishnan K, Joffe RT, MacQueen G. Successful computer-assisted cognitive remediation therapy in patients with unipolar depression: a proof of principle study. *Psychol Med* 2007;37(9):1229–38.

11. Naismith SL, Diamond K, Carter PE, et al. Enhancing memory in late-life depression: the effects of a combined psychoeducation and cognitive training program. J Geriatr Psychiatry 2011;19(3):240–8.

12. Morimoto SS, Wexler BE, Liu J, Hu W, Seirup J, Alexopoulos GS. Neuroplasticity-based computerized cognitive remediation for treatment-resistant geriatric depression. Nature Comm 2014;5:4579.

13. Withall A, Harris LM, Cumming SR. The relationship between cognitive function and clinical and functional outcomes in major depressive disorder. Psychol Med 2009;39(3):393–402.

14. Jaeger J, Berns S, Uzelac S, Davis-Conway S. Neurocognitive deficits and disability in major depressive disorder. Psychiatry Res 2006;145(1):39–48.

15. Porter RJ, Gallagher P, Thompson JM, Young AH. Neurocognitive impairment in drug-free patients with major depressive disorder. Br J Psychiatry 2003;182:214–20.

16. American Psychiatric Association. *Diagnostic and Statistical Manual of Mental Disorders, 5th Edition: DSM-5.* Arlington, VA: American Psychiatric Publishing; 2013.

17. Naismith SL, Hickie IB, Turner K, et al. Neuropsychological performance in patients with depression is associated with clinical, etiological and genetic risk factors. J Clin Exp Neuropsychol 2003;25(6):866–77.

18. Ravnkilde B, Videbech P, Clemmensen K, Egander A, Rasmussen NA, Rosenberg R. Cognitive deficits in major depression. Scand J Psychol 2002;43(3):239–51.

19. Lampe IK, Sitskoorn MM, Heeren TJ. Effects of recurrent major depressive disorder on behavior and cognitive function in female depressed patients. Psychiatry Res 2004;125(2):73–9.

20. Butters MA, Whyte EM, Nebes RD, et al. The nature and determinants of neuropsychological functioning in late-life depression. Arch Gen Psychiatry 2004;61(6):587–95.

21. Hasselbalch BJ, Knorr U, Hasselbalch SG, Gade A, Kessing LV. Cognitive deficits in the remitted state of unipolar depressive disorder. Neuropsychology 2012;26(5):642–51.

22. Hasselbalch BJ, Knorr U, Kessing LV. Cognitive impairment in the remitted state of unipolar depressive disorder: a systematic review. J Affect Disord 2011;134(1–3):20–31.

23. Okada G, Okamoto Y, Morinobu S, Yamawaki S, Yokota N. Attenuated left prefrontal activation during a verbal fluency task in patients with depression. Neuropsychobiology 2003;47(1):21–6.

24. Fitzgerald PB, Srithiran A, Benitez J, et al. An fMRI study of prefrontal brain activation during multiple tasks in patients with major depressive disorder. Human Brain Mapping 2008;29(4):490–501.

25. Bremner JD, Vermetten E, Afzal N, Vythilingam M. Deficits in verbal declarative memory function in women with childhood sexual abuse-related posttraumatic stress disorder. J Nervous Mental Dis 2004;192(10):643–9.

26. Werner NS, Meindl T, Materne J, et al. Functional MRI study of memory-related brain regions in patients with depressive disorder. J Affect Disord 2009;119(1–3):124–31.

27. Bhagwagar Z, Hinz R, Taylor M, Fancy S, Cowen P, Grasby P. Increased 5-HT(2A) receptor binding in euthymic, medication-free patients recovered from depression: a positron emission study with [(11)C]MDL 100,907. Am J Psychiatry 2006;163(9):1580–7.

28. Hermens DF, Chitty KM, Lee RS, et al. Hippocampal glutamate is increased and associated with risky drinking in young adults with major depression. J Affect Disord 2015;186:95–8.

29. Duffy SL, Lagopoulos J, Cockayne N, Hermens DF, Hickie IB, Naismith SL. Oxidative stress and depressive symptoms in older adults: a magnetic resonance spectroscopy study. J Affect Disord 2015;180:29–35.

30. Jayaweera HK, Lagopoulos J, Duffy SL, et al. Spectroscopic markers of memory impairment, symptom severity and age of onset in older people with lifetime depression: discrete roles of N-acetyl aspartate and glutamate. J Affect Disord 2015;183:31–8.

31. Hickie I, Naismith S, Ward PB, et al. Reduced hippocampal volumes and memory loss in patients with early- and late-onset depression. Br J Psychiatry 2005;186:197–202.

32. Elcombe EL, Lagopoulos J, Duffy SL, et al. Hippocampal volume in older adults at risk of cognitive decline: the role of sleep, vascular risk, and depression. J Alzheimer's Dis 2015;44(4):1279–90.

33. Barch DM, Sheline YI, Csernansky JG, Snyder AZ. Working memory and prefrontal cortex dysfunction: specificity to schizophrenia compared with major depression. Biol Psychiatry 2003;53(5):376–84.

34. Arnone D, McIntosh AM, Ebmeier KP, Munafo MR, Anderson IM. Magnetic resonance imaging studies in unipolar depression: systematic review and meta-regression analyses. Eur Neuropsychopharmacol 2012;22(1):1–16.

35. Moylan S, Maes M, Wray NR, Berk M. The neuroprogressive nature of major depressive disorder: pathways to disease evolution and resistance, and therapeutic implications. Mol Psychiatry 2013;18(5):595–606.

36. Masi G, Brovedani P. The hippocampus, neurotrophic factors and depression: possible implications for the pharmacotherapy of depression. CNS Drugs 2011;25(11):913–31.

37. Naismith SL, Norrie LM, Mowszowski L, Hickie IB. The neurobiology of depression in later-life: clinical, neuropsychological, neuroimaging and pathophysiological features. Prog Neurobiol 2012;98(1):99–143.

38. Thomas AJ, O'Brien JT, Davis S, et al. Ischemic basis for deep white matter hyperintensities in major depression: a neuropathological study. Arch Gen Psychiatry 2002;59(9):785–92.

39. Alexopoulos GS, Meyers BS, Young RC, Kakuma T, Silbersweig D, Charlson M. Clinically defined vascular depression. Am J Psychiatry 1997;154(4):562–5.

40. Krishnan KR, McDonald WM, Escalona PR, et al. Magnetic resonance imaging of the caudate nuclei in depression. Preliminary observations. Arch Gen Psychiatry 1992;49(7):553–7.

41. Sheline YI, Pieper CF, Barch DM, et al. Support for the vascular depression hypothesis in late-life depression: results of a 2-site, prospective, antidepressant treatment trial. Arch Gen Psychiatry 2010;67(3):277–85.

42. Naismith SL, Rogers NL, Hickie IB, Mackenzie J, Norrie LM, Lewis SJ. Sleep well, think well: sleep–wake disturbance in mild cognitive impairment. J Geriatr Psychiatry Neurol 2010;23(2):123–30.

43. Norton S, Matthews FE, Barnes DE, Yaffe K, Brayne C. Potential for primary prevention of Alzheimer's disease: an analysis of population-based data. Lancet Neurol 2014;13(8):788–94.

44. Minzenberg MJ, Carter CS. Modafinil: a review of neurochemical actions and effects on cognition. Neuropsychopharmacology 2008;33(7):1477–502.

45. Raskin J, Wiltse CG, Siegal A, et al. Efficacy of duloxetine on cognition, depression, and pain in elderly patients with major depressive disorder: an 8-week, double-blind, placebo-controlled trial. Am J Psychiatry 2007;164(6):900–9.

46. Schrijvers D, Maas YJ, Pier MP, Madani Y, Hulstijn W, Sabbe BG. Psychomotor changes in major depressive disorder during sertraline treatment. Neuropsychobiology 2009;59(1):34–42.

47. Constant EL, Adam S, Gillain B, Seron X, Bruyer R, Seghers A. Effects of sertraline on depressive symptoms and attentional and executive functions in major depression. Depress Anxiety 2005;21(2):78–89.

48. Saczynski JS, Rosen AB, McCammon RJ, et al. Antidepressant use and cognitive decline: The Health and Retirement Study. Am J Med 2015;128(7):739–46.

49. Wykes T, Reeder C, Landau S, Matthiasson P, Haworth E, Hutchinson C. Does age matter? Effects of cognitive rehabilitation across the age span. Schizophrenia Res 2009;113(2–3):252–8.

50. Deckersbach T, Nierenberg AA, Kessler R, et al. RESEARCH: cognitive rehabilitation for bipolar disorder: an open trial for employed patients with residual depressive symptoms. CNS Neurosci Ther 2010;16(5):298–307.

51. Bowie CR, Gupta M, Holshausen K, Jokic R, Best M, Milev R. Cognitive remediation for treatment-resistant depression: effects on cognition and functioning and the role of online homework. J Nerv Ment Dis 2013;201(8):680–5.

52. Amoyal NF. Physical exercise and cognitive training clinical interventions used in slow degeneration associated with mild cognitive impairment: a review of the recent literature. Top Geriatr Rehabil 2012;28(3):208–16.

53. Sun M, Lanctot K, Herrmann N, Gallagher D. Exercise for cognitive symptoms in depression: a systematic review of interventional studies. Can J Psychiatry 2018;63(2):115–28.

54. Bouckaert F, Sienaert P, Obbels J, et al. ECT: its brain enabling effects: a review of electroconvulsive therapy-induced structural brain plasticity. J ECT. 2014;30(2):143–51.

55. Serafini G, Pompili M, Belvederi MM, et al. The effects of repetitive transcranial magnetic stimulation on cognitive performance in treatment-resistant depression. A systematic review. Neuropsychobiology 2015;71(3):125–39.

56. Segrave RA, Arnold S, Hoy K, Fitzgerald PB. Concurrent cognitive control training augments the antidepressant efficacy of tDCS: a pilot study. Brain Stim 2014;7(2):325–31.

57. Mowszowski L, Batchelor J, Naismith SL. Early intervention for cognitive decline: can cognitive training be used as a selective prevention technique? Int Psychoger 2010;22(4):537–48.

58. Gates NJ, Sachdev PS, Fiatarone Singh MA, Valenzuela M. Cognitive and memory training in adults at risk of dementia: a systematic review. BMC Ger 2011;11:55.

59. Kueider AM, Parisi JM, Gross AL, Rebok GW. Computerized cognitive training with older adults: a systematic review. PloS One 2012;7(7):e40588.

60. Liberati G, Raffone A, Olivetti Belardinelli M. Cognitive reserve and its implications for rehabilitation and Alzheimer's disease. Cogn Process 2012;13(1):1–12.

61. Medalia A, Richardson R. What predicts a good response to cognitive remediation interventions? Schizophrenia Bull 2005;31(4):942–53.

62. Sitzer DI, Twamley EW, Jeste DV. Cognitive training in Alzheimer's disease: a meta-analysis of the literature. Acta Psychiatrica Scand 2006;114(2):75–90.

63. Belleville S. Cognitive training for persons with mild cognitive impairment. Int Psychoger 2008;20(1):57–66.

64. Papageorgiou CaW. Treatment of recurrent major depression with attention training. Cogn Behav Practice 2000;7:407–13.

65. Siegle GJ, Ghinassi F, Thase ME. Neurobehavioral therapies in the 21st century: summary of an emerging field and an extended example of cognitive control training for depression. Cogn Ther Res 2007;31:235–62.

66. Naismith SL, Redoblado-Hodge MA, Lewis SJ, Scott EM, Hickie IB. Cognitive training in affective disorders improves memory: a preliminary study using the NEAR approach. J Affect Disord 2010;121(3):258–62.

67. Trapp W, Engel S, Hajak G, Lautenbacher S, Gallhofer B. Cognitive remediation for depressed inpatients: results of a pilot randomized controlled trial. Aust NZ J Psychiatry 2016;50(1):46–55.

68. Dalgleish TN, Bird E, Hill E, Dunn BD, Golden AM. Method-of-loci as a mnemonic device to facilitate access to self-affirming personal memories for individuals with depression. Clin Psychol Sci 2013;1(2):156–62.

69. Oertel-Knochel V, Mehler P, Thiel C, et al. Effects of aerobic exercise on cognitive performance and individual psychopathology in depressive and schizophrenia patients. Eur Arch Psychiatry Clin Neurosci 2014;264(7):589–604.

70. Alvarez LM, Cortés Sotres JF, León SO, Estrella J, Sosa JJS. Computer program in the treatment for major depression and cognitive impairment in university students. Computers Hum Behav 2008;24(3):816–26.

71. Mowszowski L, Hermens DF, Diamond K, et al. Cognitive training enhances pre-attentive neurophysiological responses in older adults 'at risk' of dementia. J Alzheimers Dis 2014;41(4):1095–108.

72. Grady C. The cognitive neuroscience of ageing. Nature Rev Neurosci 2012; 13(7):491–505.

73. Lampit A, Hallock H, Valenzuela M. Computerized cognitive training in cognitively healthy older adults: a systematic review and meta-analysis of effect modifiers. PLoS Med 2014;11(11):e1001756.

74. Lampit A, Hallock H, Moss R, et al. The timecourse of global cognitive gains from supervised computer-assisted cognitive training: A randomised, active-controlled trial in elderly with multiple dementia risk factors. J Prev Alzheimers Dis 2014;1:33–9.

20

Can Non-Pharmacological Antidepressant Treatments Influence the Processing of Affective Information?

Alexander Kaltenboeck and Catherine Harmer

Introduction

When the healthy human brain processes information with affective content, it typically does so in a positively biased way; that is, it exhibits a tendency to process positive (as opposed to negative) affective information preferentially (1). Such positive biases can be objectively measured with neuropsychological tasks and are observable in different cognitive domains (e.g. perception, memory, and attention) (1). In the depressed brain, in contrast, the processing of affective information is typically disturbed—positive biases are either less pronounced or are completely replaced by a tendency to prioritize negative input (1–4).

In contrast, recent research on the neuropsychological effects of antidepressant drugs has shown that they share the ability to push affective information processing more towards a preference for positive information (2–4). This has stimulated the development of a cognitive neuropsychological model of antidepressant treatment action (CNMATA) (2–4). According to this model, negatively biased affective information processing is not a mere epiphenomenon of depressed mood—rather, it plays a crucial causal role in its development (1–4). The model further suggests that the clinical effects of antidepressant interventions can be explained, at least in part, through their ability to push affective information processing back to a more normal state, thus allowing the depressed brain to harvest (i.e. notice, perceive, and remember) an increased amount of positively valenced information again, which eventually causes mood to go up (1–4).

The CNMATA is well validated for psychopharmacological treatments. Rapid changes in affective information processing have been documented for various antidepressant drugs, in multiple cognitive domains, both in patients with depression and in healthy volunteers (3). In some cases, the induction of more positively biased processing could be shown after a single dose of an antidepressant (i.e. long before effects on mood would become present) and preliminary evidence suggests that the changes in affective information processing appearing early in treatment are predictive of later clinical improvement (3).

However, drugs are not the only available option for the treatment of depressive disorders. Indeed, the past decades have seen an increasing number of non-pharmacological therapies being developed, and some of these therapies have shown promising effects in clinical trials (5). In this chapter, we will therefore extend our focus to some important non-pharmacological treatment modalities and ask whether they too can influence affective cognition in patients with depression, and, if so, what their effects look like.

We will cover cognitive behavioural therapy (CBT), electroconvulsive therapy (ECT), transcranial direct current stimulation (tDCS), bright light therapy (BLT), and negative ion treatment (NIT). For each of these treatments, we will discuss currently available studies that have assessed how they influence affective information processing in patients with depression (and, if appropriate, other mood and anxiety disorders). We will show that, for all of these treatments, preliminary evidence suggests that they can indeed impact on affective cognition, and, at least in some cases, the observed effects are directly in line with the predictions of the CNMATA. However, it will also become clear that the evidence base at the moment is still weak and in many regards incomplete, and that any conclusions drawn must therefore be considered preliminary and open to future revision.

Cognitive Behavioural Therapy

CBT is a psychological intervention that aims to correct dysfunctional ways by which patients with depression interpret, think about, and react to events in their environment. Its clinical efficacy for depression is well established and, in line with its theoretical assumptions, there is evidence that CBT does indeed change the abstract high-level mental constructs (e.g. automatic thoughts, dysfunctional attitudes) it targets (6). However, such effects are typically measured by questionnaires or interviews. Whether CBT can also induce changes in more objective measures of affective information processing, e.g. performance in neuropsychological tests or neural activity patterns, has been investigated by only a few studies to date.

Docteur et al. (7) studied free recall memory for affective words in patients with remitted bipolar disorder. The patients were allocated to either 6 months of group CBT or a waitlist. Prior to treatment, the authors did not find any differences in memory performance between the groups. However, at follow-up and compared to controls, CBT-treated patients exhibited improved recall for positive and neutral words, while showing worsened recall performance for negative words—a clear indicator that retrieval of affective information had become more biased towards positive information.

The idea that CBT can induce behaviourally measurable changes in affective information processing is also supported by Reinecke et al. (8), although they focused on patients with panic disorder. The authors randomized patients to either a single session of exposure-based CBT or a waiting list. One day after the intervention, an affective faces dot probe task was administered to measure vigilance for affective information. The authors found that participants on the waiting list exhibited significant vigilance for fearful facial expressions. However, patients who had received a single session of CBT did not show this feature, thus suggesting a rapidly induced attenuation of an attentional bias for negative affective information.

While the studies above provide direct support for the idea that CBT can influence behavioural measures of affective cognition in line with the CNMATA, they do contrast with a more recent study investigating the effects of CBT on facial expression recognition in patients with major depression (9). In this study, the authors studied the effects of 16 weeks of CBT (or schema therapy) on a broad range of neuropsychological variables. While both psychotherapies had a clear positive impact on depressive symptomatology, neither was associated with any convincing changes in facial expression recognition—or, as a matter of fact, any other neuropsychological variables. This finding is clearly at odds with the hypothesis that CBT can positively bias (or at least influence) affective cognition. However, in this study, facial expression recognition did not differ significantly between patients and healthy controls at baseline, which contrasts with findings from other studies and which might explain the lack of an observed effect (1–4, 10).

In addition to the abovementioned studies, which relied on behavioural tasks to assess affective cognition, some authors have also explored the effects of CBT on neural correlates of affective information processing.

In a functional magnetic resonance imaging (fMRI) study by Fu et al. (11), patients with acute depression were scanned before and after 16 sessions of CBT, while they were engaged in the implicit processing of sad facial expressions. The authors found that, prior to treatment and compared to healthy control subjects, patients exhibited increased activity in the right amygdala and decreased activity in the anterior cingulate cortex in response to sad facial expressions. However, at follow-up, brain activation patterns of patients did not differ from those observed in healthy controls—thus indicating that CBT was able to remediate abnormal neural activation during the processing of negative affective information.

In a similar study, Ritchey et al. (12) presented depressed patients with positive, negative, and neutral affective pictorial stimuli. At baseline and compared to healthy control subjects, patients showed a general decrease in ventromedial prefrontal cortex activity. Furthermore, they exhibited increased responses to negative (as compared to positive) stimuli in the left anterior temporal lobe, ventrolateral prefrontal cortex, and right dorsolateral prefrontal cortex (DLPFC), and showed reduced discrimination between affective and neutral stimuli in the amygdala, caudate, and hippocampus. However, after patients had undergone a naturalistic course of individual CBT, ventromedial prefrontal cortex activity was increased, amygdala and caudate activity better discriminated between emotional and neutral pictures, and the left anterior temporal lobe showed greater activity in response to positive compared to neutral stimuli—thus, again, providing support for the idea that CBT can remediate neural activity abnormalities during affective information processing.

Yoshimura et al. (13) investigated how CBT can affect brain activity associated with self-referential information processing. Patients with acute depression were scanned prior to and following 12 weekly sessions of group CBT. The authors found that, prior to CBT and compared to healthy control subjects, patients exhibited significantly decreased activation of the ventral anterior cingulate cortex, superior temporal cortex, and medial prefrontal cortex while processing positive self-referential words, and increased neural activity in the medial prefrontal cortex and ventral anterior cingulate cortex while processing negative self-referential words. At follow-up, these activation patterns had become reversed: patients exhibited increased activation of the ventral anterior cingulate cortex, superior temporal cortex, and medial prefrontal cortex during processing of positive self-referential words, but decreased activation of ventral anterior cingulate cortex, superior temporal cortex, and medial prefrontal cortex during processing of negative stimuli, thus adding further support to the idea that CBT can change abnormal affective information processing in depression.

In summary, the studies demonstrate that—in line with its core principles—CBT can change the way in which affective information is processed by patients suffering from depression and these effects have been observed both on a behavioural as well as on a neural level. Future studies would benefit from using randomized designs and appropriate control conditions and should further corroborate the mechanistic relevance of changes in affective information processing for the development of later occurring clinical effects.

Electroconvulsive Therapy

ECT is an antidepressant intervention whereby electrical currents are passed through the brain under general anaesthesia to induce a brief seizure. It is considered one of the most effective antidepressant treatments, but its working mechanisms are not well understood (14). Although it is clinically well known that ECT can have adverse effects on non-affective cognitive functions (especially memory) (14), only a handful of studies have assessed whether and how ECT impacts on affective cognition.

In a recent study, Bai et al. (15) investigated memory for affective pictorial stimuli in patients with depression prior to and 3 days after they had received individual ECT. The researchers found that, prior to ECT and compared to healthy control subjects, patients with depression exhibited a selective impairment in recognition memory for positively valenced pictures (but not neutral or negative ones), consistent with a (relative) negative bias in retrieving affective information. After treatment, patients exhibited impaired recall and recognition performance across all picture valences, which is not surprising given the well-known adverse effects of ECT on memory. However, recognition memory for negative pictures was impaired to a stronger degree than for positive and neutral pictures. Thus, it seems, ECT had pushed recognition memory towards a relative preference for positive affective information.

Miskowiak et al. (16, 17) also evaluated the effects of ECT on behavioural measures of affective information processing in patients with depression but focused on a single session of treatment and also included a sham-placebo condition. Together, these two studies considered a range of different cognitive domains (facial expression recognition, emotional face vigilance, affective word categorization, and affective word recall and recognition). However, they did not observe any clear behaviourally measurable effects of a single session of ECT[1].

Using fMRI, both studies also evaluated potential influences of a single session of ECT on neural correlates of affective information processing. Miskowiak et al. (16) studied brain activity during facial expression processing but did not find any clear effects. Miskowiak et al. (17) assessed brain activity during an incidental recognition memory task. They found that patients who had received ECT exhibited selectively reduced activity in the left frontopolar cortex during retrieval of positive words compared to those who had received sham-placebo. However, brain activity during retrieval of negative words did not differ between groups. Based on these findings, the authors suggest that ECT has acute impact on brain activity during affective information processing and this effect—potentially reflecting a decreased need for prefrontal resources and thus a relative ease of retrieving positive information—is consistent with a shift toward more positively biased memory retrieval. However, since a single session of ECT was not associated with behaviourally measurable changes in affective memory, these conclusions must be corroborated by future research.

Although Miskowiak et al. (16) could not find any acute effects of ECT on brain activity during facial expression processing, Redlich et al. (18) reported such an effect following a longer course of treatment. Using a non-randomized, naturalistic, prospective design, they studied the effects of repeated ECT on amygdala activity in response to subliminally presented happy, sad, or neutral facial expressions. Prior to treatment and compared to healthy control subjects, patients

---

[1]It is worth mentioning that both studies relied on relatively small sample sizes and studied a population of severely ill patients. Therefore, the study likely lacked sufficient statistical power to detect small to moderate effects.

with depression showed increased amygdala reactivity to sad faces, which might constitute the functional neural correlate of a negative processing bias (3). After ECT treatment, the amygdala response to sad faces had changed in patients to such an extent that it did not differ from that of healthy controls any more. In other words, excessive amygdala reactivity to negative information seemed to have become normalized. Supporting the idea that this normalization played a causal role in the development of clinical effects, the authors also report a significant correlation between changes in amygdala reactivity to sad faces and clinical improvement following ECT. Interestingly, similar observations were made in a clinical control group solely treated with antidepressant pharmacotherapy—an indicator that the two treatments might share common effects on affective information processing.

In summary, currently available evidence suggests that ECT can influence affective information processing in patients with depression. Furthermore, as predicted by the CNMATA, ECT seems to be able to remediate some of the negative processing biases inherent to depression. Future studies should use randomized designs with appropriate control conditions and larger sample sizes to interrogate the effects of ECT on affective cognition more fully.

Transcranial Direct Current Stimulation

tDCS is a non-invasive intervention whereby specific brain regions are electrically stimulated through the application of low direct currents delivered via electrodes attached to the scalp. Several studies have shown that tDCS can have clinically relevant antidepressant effects (19). Since tDCS is commonly used in neuroscientific research to perturbate neural activity for experimental purposes, a range of healthy volunteer studies is available. These have repeatedly shown that tDCS can influence affective information processing in different cognitive domains (e.g. affective valence perception, facial expression recognition, and attention to affective stimuli), and some of the reported effects of tDCS resemble those of antidepressant drugs (20–23). To our knowledge, however, only few studies to date have assessed how tDCS influences affective information processing in patients with depression.

Boggio et al. (24) studied the effect of a single session of tDCS on the performance in a go–no-go task with positive and negative affective pictures. The study compared three different conditions in patients with depression: anodal (i.e. excitability increasing) stimulation over the left DLPFC, the occipital cortex, and sham placebo stimulation. The authors found that DLPFC stimulation was associated with improved task performance after treatment, and that this effect was specific for positive affective stimuli—thus suggesting that tDCS had led to a relative prioritization of positive affective information.

Brennan et al. (25) investigated how facial expression identification was affected by tDCS over the left DLPFC in patients with depression and healthy control subjects. They reported that, under tDCS (as compared to sham-placebo treatment), healthy controls exhibited a higher overall emotion recognition accuracy. In the patient group, tDCS treatment was associated with better performance in anger recognition and happiness recognition (at the weakest presented intensity). Note, however, that these findings contrast with a more recent study that investigated the effects of anodal left DLPFC stimulation in healthy volunteers and did not find an emotion-specific effect, but rather a general slowing of emotion identification (26).

In a different study by Brunoni et al. (27), the authors assessed how patients with depression performed in an affective stroop task after they had been treated either with a single session of tDCS over both DLPFCs (left anodal and right cathodal) or sham-placebo. They observed that prior to treatment both groups exhibited higher reaction times for negative than for positive cues, consistent with an attentional bias for negative information. However, following treatment, the tDCS group showed higher reaction times for neutral and positive stimuli than for negative stimuli, thus suggesting that tDCS acutely abolished an attentional preference for negative affective information and pushed attention more towards a preference for positive information.

Moreno et al. (28) studied the effects of a single session of tDCS on working memory performance. They used a two-back task to assess non-affective working memory and a facial expression internal switch task to assess affective working memory. Patients with depression and healthy volunteers were treated with tDCS over the DLPFCs (left anodal and right cathodal) or a sham-placebo. Following verum stimulation, the authors found that two-back task performance was improved in both groups. Furthermore, patients also improved in the affective internal switch task, thus suggesting that tDCS might also be able to enhance affective working memory in depression.

In summary, the studies described above suggest that a single session of tDCS can influence emotion-related cognition in depression. Further research should elucidate the effects of (clinically more relevant) repeated treatment, shed light on the impact that tDCS has on neural correlates of affective information processing, and study whether early changes in the processing of emotional information can predict changes in depressed mood later in treatment.

Environmental therapeutics

Two further non-pharmacological treatments for which antidepressant efficacy has been suggested are bright light treatment (BLT) (29, 30) and (although less consistently) negative ion treatment (NIT) (31, 32). On a neurobiological level, different working mechanisms have been proposed for these treatments but, to date, only few studies have explored their effects on affective information processing.

To our knowledge, there are currently no studies available that have assessed the impact of BLT on affective information processing in patients with depression. However, research in healthy volunteers suggests that BLT can influence affective cognition.

Fisher et al. (33) studied the impact of repeated BLT with varying individual dosages on neural correlates of threat processing. Using fMRI, they measured neural activity in the corticolimbic circuit, before and after the intervention, while participants were viewing fearful, angry, and neutral faces. The study found that higher bright light dosages were associated with decreased neural activity in response to angry and fearful faces in the amygdala and medial prefrontal cortex and increased left amygdala–prefrontal and intra–prefrontal functional coupling. The authors conclude that BLT might dampen amygdala reactivity to negative affective stimuli (an effect that has also been observed for antidepressant drug treatments [34]) and enhance top-down regulation of the prefrontal cortex on threat-induced amygdala reactivity. However, regardless of the specific interpretation, these findings certainly suggest that BLT can have direct and dose-dependent effects on neural correlates of affective information processing.

This idea is further corroborated by Vandewalle et al. (35), who also explored how light can impact on affective information processing in healthy volunteers, although they focused on the effects of different wavelengths rather than full-spectrum white light as used for clinical purposes. In their study, they measured neural responses to angry and neutral vocal stimuli while participants were exposed to pulses of green or blue light. The authors found that exposure to blue light (as compared to green light) was associated with increased activity of the voice area (temporal cortex) and hippocampus in response to angry vocal stimuli. Furthermore, they observed increased functional connectivity between the voice area, the amygdala, and the hypothalamus during processing of these affective stimuli, thus indicating that different light spectra can directly influence neural measures of affective information processing.

In the case of NIT, only two studies to date have explored effects on affective cognition.

Harmer et al. (36) studied the influence of a single session of high-density NIT on affective information processing in patients with seasonal affective disorder (SAD) as well as healthy controls. They used a range of tasks tapping into different cognitive domains. The authors report that participants treated with NIT (both healthy controls and patients with SAD) showed increased recognition of positive and decreased recognition of negative facial expressions as well as enhanced vigilance for positive affective stimuli compared to those treated with sham-placebo.

Furthermore, participants with SAD who received NIT also showed enhanced recognition memory performance for positive affective stimuli compared to patients treated with sham-placebo. These differences were observed in the absence of any differences in mood or subjective state, thus indicating that NIT acutely pushed affective information processing toward a preferential processing of positive information. Similar effects were observed by Malcolm et al. (37), who used the same task battery as Harmer et al. (36) but focused on a sample of healthy volunteers only. They found that participants treated with negative ions, as compared to those treated with a sham-placebo, exhibited enhanced memory for positive affective information but worse memory for negative affective information. Different to Harmer et al. (36), they did not observe any effects on facial expression recognition or attention to affective cues.

Taken together, the abovementioned studies suggest that BLT and NIT might constitute further non-pharmacological means to change affective information processing in patients with depression. Future studies have to corroborate these preliminary findings by studying the effects of these treatments in healthy individuals as well as in patients, by establishing effects on a behavioural as well as on a neural level, and by exploring whether changes induced by these treatments early in treatment are predictive of later occurring clinical effects.

Conclusion

In this chapter, we have explored the current scientific literature describing how different non-pharmacological treatments can influence the processing of affective information in patients with depressive disorders. We have shown that, for each of the treatments discussed, there is at least some evidence suggesting an effect on behavioural or neural measures of affective cognitive processes. In some cases, the reported effects were directly in line with the predictions of the CNMATA; that is, the respective treatment enhanced the processing of positive affective information and/or decreased the processing of negative information—thus suggesting that, on a cognitive level, different non-drug treatments could have similar effects to antidepressant drugs.

However, as should become clear from the number of studies described, the current evidence base is very limited and incomplete in many regards. Without exclusion, for each treatment covered here, further studies are necessary to draw more definite conclusions. Therefore, while we can say with some confidence that non-pharmacological treatments can impact on the processing of affective information, future research will need to reveal what the exact nature of these induced changes is, whether they are identical to those seen with antidepressant drugs, and whether they might be useful to improve precision treatment approaches for individuals with depression.

References

1. Roiser J, Sahakian BJ. Information processing in mood disorders. In: DeRubeis RJ, Strunk DR (eds). *The Oxford Handbook of Mood Disorders.* Oxford: Oxford University Press; 2016, Chapter 16.

2. Harmer CJ, Goodwin GM, Cowen PJ. Why do antidepressants take so long to work? A cognitive neuropsychological model of antidepressant drug action. Br J Psychiatry 2009;195(2):102–8.

3. Warren MB, Pringle A, Harmer CJ. A neurocognitive model for understanding treatment action in depression. Philos Trans R Soc Lond B Biol Sci 2015;370(1677): 20140213.

4. Roiser JP, Elliott R, Sahakian BJ. Cognitive mechanisms of treatment in depression. Neuropsychopharmacology 2012;37(1):117–36.

5. Farah WH, Alsawas M, Mainou M, et al. Non-pharmacological treatment of depression: a systematic review and evidence map. Evid Based Med 2016;21(6):214–21.

6. Strunk DR, Adler AD, Hollon SD. Cognitive therapy of depression. In: DeRubeis RJ, Strunk DR (eds). *The Oxford Handbook of Mood Disorders.* Oxford: Oxford University Press; 2016, Chapter 35.

7. Docteur A, Mirabel-Sarron C, Guelfi J-D, Rouillon F, Gorwood P. The role of CBT in explicit memory bias in bipolar I patients. J Behav Ther Exp Psychiatry 2013;44(3):307–11.

8. Reinecke A, Waldenmaier L, Cooper MJ, Harmer CJ. Changes in automatic threat processing precede and predict clinical changes with exposure-based cognitive-behavior therapy for panic disorder. Biol Psychiatry 2013;73(11):1064–70.

9. Porter RJ, Bourke C, Carter JD, et al. No change in neuropsychological dysfunction or emotional processing during treatment of major depression with cognitive-behaviour therapy or schema therapy. Psychol Med 2016;46(2):393–404.

10. Elliott R, Zahn R, Deakin JF, Anderson IM. Affective cognition and its disruption in mood disorders. Neuropsychopharmacology 2011;36(1):153–82.

11. Fu CH, Williams SC, Cleare AJ, et al. Neural responses to sad facial expressions in major depression following cognitive behavioral therapy. Biol Psychiatry 2008;64(6):505–12.

12. Ritchey M, Dolcos F, Eddington KM, Strauman TJ, Cabeza R. Neural correlates of emotional processing in depression: changes with cognitive behavioral therapy and predictors of treatment response. J Psychiatr Res 2011;45(5):577–87.

13. Yoshimura S, Okamoto Y, Onoda K, et al. Cognitive behavioral therapy for depression changes medial prefrontal and ventral anterior cingulate cortex activity associated with self-referential processing. Soc Cogn Affect Neurosci 2014;9(4):487–93.

14. George MS, Short EB, Kerns SE. Brain stimulation treatments for depression. In: DeRubeis RJ, Strunk DR (eds). *The Oxford Handbook of Mood Disorders.* Oxford: Oxford University Press; 2016, Chapter 34.

15. Bai T, Xie W, Wei Q, et al. Electroconvulsive therapy regulates emotional memory bias of depressed patients. Psychiatry Res 2017;257:296–302.

16. Miskowiak KW, Kessing LV, Ott CV, et al. Does a single session of electroconvulsive therapy alter the neural response to emotional faces in depression? A randomised sham-controlled functional magnetic resonance imaging study. J Psychopharmacol 2017;31(9):1215–24.

17. Miskowiak KW, Macoveanu J, Jørgensen MB, et al. Neural response after a single ECT session during retrieval of emotional self-referent words in depression: a randomized, sham-controlled fMRI study. Int J Neuropsychopharmacol 2018;21(3):226–35.

18. Redlich R, Burger C, Dohm K, et al. Effects of electroconvulsive therapy on amygdala function in major depression—a longitudinal functional magnetic resonance imaging study. Psychol Med 2017;47(12):2166–76.

19. Meron D, Hedger N, Garner M, Baldwin DS. Transcranial direct current stimulation (tDCS) in the treatment of depression: systematic review and meta-analysis of efficacy and tolerability. Neurosci Biobehav Rev 2015;57:46–62.

20. Mondino M, Thiffault F, Fecteau S. Does non-invasive brain stimulation applied over the dorsolateral prefrontal cortex non-specifically influence mood and emotional processing in healthy individuals? Front Cell Neurosci 2015;9:399.

21. Balzarotti S, Colombo B. Effects of unilateral transcranial direct current stimulation of left prefrontal cortex on processing and memory of emotional visual stimuli. PLoS One 2016;11(7):e0159555.

22. Chen NTM, Basanovic J, Notebaert L, MacLeod C, Clarke PJF. Attentional bias mediates the effect of neurostimulation on emotional vulnerability. J Psychiatr Res 2017;93:12–19.

23. Peña-Gomez C, Vidal-Pineiro D, Clemente IC, Pascual-Leone A, Bartres-Faz D. Down-regulation of negative emotional processing by transcranial direct current stimulation: effects of personality characteristics. PLoS One 2011;6(7):e22812.

24. Boggio PS, Bermpohl F, Vergara AO, et al. Go-no-go task performance improvement after anodal transcranial DC stimulation of the left dorsolateral prefrontal cortex in major depression. J Affect Disord 2007;101(1–3):91–8.

25. Brennan S, McLoughlin DM, O'Connell R, et al. Anodal transcranial direct current stimulation of the left dorsolateral prefrontal cortex enhances emotion recognition in depressed patients and controls. J Clin Exp Neuropsychol 2017;39(4):384–95.

26. Nord CL, Forster S, Halahakoon DC, Penton-Voak IS, Munafo MR, Roiser JP. Prefrontal cortex stimulation does not affect emotional bias, but may slow emotion identification. Soc Cogn Affect Neurosci 2017;12(5):839–47.

27. Brunoni AR, Zanao TA, Vanderhasselt MA, et al. Enhancement of affective processing induced by bifrontal transcranial direct current stimulation in patients with major depression. Neuromodulation 2014;17(2):138–42.

28. Moreno ML, Vanderhasselt MA, Carvalho AF, et al. Effects of acute transcranial direct current stimulation in hot and cold working memory tasks in healthy and depressed subjects. Neurosci Lett 2015;591:126–31.

29. Golden RN, Gaynes BN, Ekstrom RD, et al. The efficacy of light therapy in the treatment of mood disorders: a review and meta-analysis of the evidence. Am J Psychiatry 2005;162(4):656–62.

30. Lam RW, Levitt AJ, Levitan RD, et al. Efficacy of bright light treatment, fluoxetine, and the combination in patients with nonseasonal major depressive disorder: a randomized clinical trial. JAMA Psychiatry 2016;73(1):56–63.

31. Goel N, Terman M, Terman JS, Macchi MM, Stewart JW. Controlled trial of bright light and negative air ions for chronic depression. Psychol Med 2005;35(7):945–55.

32. Perez V, Alexander DD, Bailey WH. Air ions and mood outcomes: a review and meta-analysis. BMC Psychiatry 2013;13:29.

33. Fisher PM, Madsen MK, McMahon B, et al. Three-week bright-light intervention has dose-related effects on threat-related corticolimbic reactivity and functional coupling. Biol Psychiatry 2014;76(4):332–9.

34. Murphy SE, Norbury R, O'Sullivan U, Cowen PJ, Harmer CJ. Effect of a single dose of citalopram on amygdala response to emotional faces. Br J Psychiatry 2009;194(6):535–40.

35. Vandewalle G, Schwartz S, Grandjean D, et al. Spectral quality of light modulates emotional brain responses in humans. Proc Natl Acad Sci U S A 2010;107(45):19549–54.

36. Harmer CJ, Charles M, McTavish S, Favaron E, Cowen PJ. Negative ion treatment increases positive emotional processing in seasonal affective disorder. Psychol Med 2012;42(8):1605–12.

37. Malcolm CP, Cowen PJ, Harmer CJ. High-density negative ion treatment increases positive affective memory. Psychol Med 2009;39(11):1930–2.

21

Social Cognitive Deficits: Impact on Psychosocial Function and Novel Treatment Opportunities in Major Depressive Disorder

Michael Weightman and Bernhard T. Baune

Introduction

The adaptive importance of social behaviours has long been the subject of academic interest. Darwin (1) first explored the biological underpinnings of emotional behaviour in detail, while Ekman and Friesen (2) later proposed six universal facial expressions that transcended cultural bounds. Contemporary research focuses on what is now termed 'social cognition'. This is broadly defined as the way in which humans identify, perceive, and interpret socially salient information (3). Social cognition therefore encompasses a broad range of verbal and non-verbal information, including facial expressions, prosody, body language, and theory of mind.

The impact of major depressive disorder (MDD) on social cognition is more nuanced than the profound performance deficits seen in other neuropsychiatric disorders, classically schizophrenia (4) and autism (5). Despite some equivocal results in the literature, it is now mostly accepted that MDD is associated with a characteristic mood-congruent interpretative bias (3). This manifests as depressed individuals being more likely to interpret neutral stimuli negatively or display greater accuracy at identifying negatively valenced emotions, while also struggling to recognize positive stimuli. This is consistent with cognitive theories of depression (6), which postulate that depressed individuals interpret social information through negative maladaptive schemata, thus distorting the perception of everyday interactions. This chapter explores the emerging body of literature suggesting that not only do such social cognitive deficits impact the psychosocial functioning of those with MDD, but that current treatments may potentially ameliorate these deficits.

Impact on Psychosocial Function

Social cognition is closely related to the concept of psychosocial functioning. The former is the mechanism by which socially relevant information is processed and used, while the latter describes more broadly the interaction between an individual and his or her environment (including social interactions and interpersonal relationships). Some authors have attempted to quantify the impact of social cognitive impairments on the psychosocial functioning of those with an MDD. These findings are summarized in the following sections within the broad domains of social performance, emotional/empathic performance, cognitive functioning, and quality of life.

Social Performance

Social performance and the quality of social interactions appear to be interrelated with social cognitive functioning. For example, Szanto et al. (7) demonstrated that elderly depressed individuals with poor facial affect recognition exhibited greater hostility and poorer interfamily communication, while also maintaining smaller social networks and fewer close friends relative to those with stronger facial affect recognition. Likewise, Derntl et al. (8) found that subjects with depression had a greater sensitivity to detect fearful emotions and that this was associated with increased withdrawal from emotionally laden stimuli. While these results indicate a negative contribution of social cognition on social performance, neither study statistically evaluated the association between these features, underscoring the need for more research in this domain.

Depression also appears to exert a negative effect on social problem-solving ability. Depressed patients are less likely than controls to generate strategies for navigating theory of mind tasks in a socially sensitive and practically effective manner (9). Interestingly, depressed patients were still able to identify such a strategy when presented with a list of different options, suggesting that problem-solving ability is not fully impeded and the deficit is one of initiation rather than recognition. Radke et al. (10) evaluated social problem-solving ability using an electronic ultimatum game where affective facial expressions were paired to in-game offers. Depressed patients rejected a significantly higher percentage of offers than controls, suggesting that facial emotion was an important mediating factor in social decisions relating to fairness. Difficulties navigating social situations are hypothesized to contribute to low mood and diminished self-esteem. This explanation is consistent with behavioural theories of depression (11), where poor social outcomes reinforce maladaptive behaviours such as withdrawal or isolation and further perpetuate the depressive state.

It is worth noting, however, that the relationship between facial affect recognition and functional outcomes is not universal in the literature, with another study failing to demonstrate any association between social cognition and social adaptation (12). Moreover, the link between social cognition and many aspects of social performance remains uninvestigated or unreplicated, suggesting that this remains a speculative area.

Emotional and Empathic Performance

While there is very limited empirical research on the relationship between social cognition and emotional processing, the response of depressed patients to social stimuli in general has received considerable attention. Individuals experiencing low mood find it more difficult than controls to ignore the emotional dimension of facial expressions (13), suggesting increased sensitivity to emotional social cues. People with depression are also more likely than controls to rate facial expressions as untrustworthy (14) and to act fearfully (such as through freezing) in response to affective facial stimuli (15). These reactions likely lead to reduced desire for social interaction or, at least, a reduction in its quality.

In addition, depressed patients report feeling less comfortable with their own reactions to such stimuli and harbour a desire to change them (15). This may indicate a level of insight into these difficulties, but may also be a function of distorted cognitive schemata. Some individuals with depression consciously suppress their own expression of emotion, although use of this coping mechanism does not explain the reduced accuracy when identifying the expressed facial emotion of others (16).

There is evidence to suggest that depressed patients may exhibit a reduced level of empathy compared to non-depressed individuals (17–19). In fact, the degree of empathy retained during the depressed phase may be a protective factor for functioning; Thoma et al. (9) found that greater empathy in depressed patients was associated with improved psychosocial functioning, particularly in social problem-solving. Empathy has also been studied in the subgroup of depressed mothers, who demonstrate increased difficulty in correctly identifying infant facial emotion (20, 21) and respond to the infant with fewer comforting behaviours or greater avoidance (22).

General Cognitive Functioning

Social cognitive performance in depressed populations also appears connected to general cognitive functioning. Impairments in theory of mind ability (23, 24) and prosody interpretation (25) are associated with impaired performance in the cognitive domains of executive functioning and working memory. In particular, these studies identified that deficits in both verbal fluency and inhibition are related to theory of mind ability. Levens and Gotlib (26) found depressed participants to be faster than controls at integrating sad content into a working memory task, but slower at linking more complex emotional stimuli into working memory. This is consistent with the negative interpretative bias often observed within depressed populations interpreting social stimuli.

Again, some conflicting results have detected no correlation between depressed patients' performances on social cognitive tasks and their neurocognitive functioning (27, 28). This remains an area requiring additional targeted research.

General Quality of Life

Impairments to social cognition also impact on quality of life measures in MDD. For example, reduced theory of mind performance in depressed patients was associated with a lower Global Assessment of Functioning score (29), while emotion-labelling ability was a strong predictor of quality of life in older depressed people (30). Moreover, increased recognition accuracy for happy facial expressions was linked with higher self-reporting of personal wellbeing, social functioning, and symptom burden (31). Impaired ability to mentalize is linked to self-reported difficulties with social adjustment in the work, leisure, and family relationship domains of psychosocial functioning (32).

Treatment Options

Numerous studies have examined the impact of different treatment modalities (pharmacological, psychotherapeutic, and procedural interventions) on the social cognitive functioning of depressed patients. This section will present the major findings according to specific domain of social cognition.

Facial Affect Recognition

By far the greatest wealth of information regarding treatments of social cognition can be found in the domain of facial affect recognition. Indeed, there is some evidence that the accuracy of interpreting facial expressions improves after effective treatment of depression. Successful trials have been conducted using citalopram (31, 33), reboxetine (31), non-specific antidepressant pharmacotherapy (34, 35), repetitive transcranial magnetic stimulation (rTMS; 36) and transcranial direct current stimulation (tDCS; 37). In the only comparative study conducted, Tranter et al. (31) found citalopram to be superior to reboxetine at 2 weeks for improving accuracy of facial expression interpretation, but there was no difference in outcome by 6 weeks of treatment.

Other treatments have been effective for improving accuracy for a specific emotional valence: a single dose of oral reboxetine improved positive face recognition (38), while an intravenous infusion of citalopram improved fearful face recognition (39). Recognition of angry faces improved following both a course of 10 rTMS treatments (40) and 6 weeks of inpatient psychiatric management (41).

There are other treatments that have not yet shown benefit for facial affect recognition performance. For example, pharmacotherapy with sertraline (42) or 4 weeks of inpatient psychotropic management (43) were not effective. A study using duloxetine found no facial affect processing differences between depressed and control participants at either baseline assessment or following treatment (44).

Treatment may also have a role in correcting the underlying negative interpretative bias observed in the processing of affective faces in MDD. Escitalopram therapy (45) was found to be effective at reducing a pretreatment bias toward negative faces. Surguladze et al. (46) suggest that this relationship could be dose-dependent, as use of high-dose antidepressants was associated with a reduction in the bias toward labelling expressions as sad. Interestingly, more frequent negative interpretations of neutral facial expressions in a treated depressed population were significantly associated with missed antidepressant doses (47), indicating that strict adherence to treatment may be a relevant factor.

Evidence is more equivocal for psychological approaches. There was no impact on overall facial affect recognition performance for depressed patients receiving cognitive behavioural therapy (48), schema therapy (48), cognitive behavioural analysis system of psychotherapy (49), or inpatient psychoanalytic-interactional group therapy (50, 51). However, psychological approaches may be more suited to addressing the negative interpretative bias. Both mindfulness-based cognitive therapy (52) and inpatient psychoanalytic-interactional group therapy (53) reduced the pretreatment bias toward negative faces. There may even be opportunity to develop psychological approaches to specifically counter this interpretative bias, with one study finding that training dysphoric students to perceive happiness over sadness in ambiguous facial expressions led to improvements in mood (54).

Notably, very few of these studies employed a randomized, clinically controlled design with a longitudinal no-treatment control group. Accordingly, the effect of treatment strategies on depression cannot be clearly disentangled from the natural course of illness. At present, evidence for a treatment effect should therefore be considered preliminary, with a need for additional controlled studies in this domain.

Affective Scenes

Another popular target of social cognitive testing is interpretation of affective pictures, such as the International Affective Picture System (55). This includes stimuli ranging from everyday objects or scenes to more intensely emotive scenes, including extremes such as erotica or mutilated bodies.

There is some emerging evidence to support the use of antidepressant medication for improving behavioural performance on affective picture tasks. Wells et al. (56) used a naturalistic sample of depressed patients taking antidepressants and observed a reduced negative interpretative bias compared to a group of unmedicated depressed patients. Similarly, Rizvi et al. (57) found that treatment non-responders rated affective pictures as more aversive compared to those who responded to therapy. Furthermore, the patients taking medication performed similarly to non-depressed controls when interpreting affective scenes. However, Wang et al. (58) found no improvement of accuracy at interpreting positively valenced pictures for depressed patients compared to controls after 8 weeks of fluoxetine.

There is limited support for the use of procedural therapies (e.g. neurostimulation). Boggio et al. (59) showed that depressed patients receiving a single session of rTMS had improved performance on an affective go-no-go task compared to sham therapy. A separate study looking at a 4-week course of electroconvulsive therapy (ECT) found no improvement for depressed subjects compared to controls in interpreting affective stimuli, although bilateral parietal hypoactivation on magnetoencephalography normalized following treatment (60).

There are also few data available on psychological therapies in this area. Ritchey et al. (61) found no overall improvement in depressed patients' ability to interpret affective pictures compared to controls following a course of cognitive behavioural therapy. However, following therapy, depressed patients exhibited increased activation of multiple brain regions involved in the processing of emotionally salient information, including the prefrontal cortex, amgydala, caudate, and hippocampus.

Theory of Mind

Another potential target of treatment is theory of mind ability, which is the capacity to infer the thoughts, intentions, and feelings of others. Treatments targeted at addressing theory of mind deficits have predominantly been psychological or procedural.

Inpatient psychoanalytic-interactional group therapy over an average period of 7 weeks improved the performance of depressed patients on a task relating to mentalization from both the self and other perspectives (62). Despite this improvement following treatment, the depressed group still did not reach the performance level of non-depressed controls. Another study (63) considered behavioural activation strategies in a subthreshold depression population, finding improved reaction times on positively valenced stimuli when performing a similar task relating to self and other mentalization.

Regarding procedural therapies, Merkl et al. (64) gave treatment-resistant depressed subjects 6 months of deep brain stimulation in the subgenual anterior cingulate cortex and found that these patients experienced a significant reduction of negative bias in their empathic responses compared to controls. Ridout et al. (65) had previously demonstrated that treatment-resistant depressed patients with pre-existing anterior cingulotomy and anterior capsulotomy had significantly impaired theory of mind performance to both depressed patients without psychosurgery and non-depressed controls. Thus, this region may prove an important target for treatment.

Auditory/Prosodic Stimuli

Very limited evidence is available to assess the role of interventions in addressing social cognitive deficits in the interpretation of prosody in MDD, although one study has investigated the impact of ECT. Christ et al. (66) found that depressed patients had significantly improved performance on interpreting affective prosody following a course of ECT. This remains an area in need of additional research to both confirm the generalizability of this finding and explore whether other treatment modalities may also play a role in correcting dysfunction in prosody interpretation in depressed populations.

Conclusions

Many existing treatments for MDD are likely also to improve social cognitive deficits. Certain medications, psychotherapy modalities, and procedural interventions appear to increase the accuracy in interpretation of social information and reduce underlying negative interpretative bias.

Interestingly, current data suggest a trend towards different applications of psychotropic and psychological therapies. Simplistically, this could be conceptualized as biological treatments for biological deficits and psychological treatments for psychological deficits.

Antidepressants, in particular citalopram and reboxetine, appear to improve overall performance on facial affect recognition tasks and, to a lesser extent, for tasks involving interpretation of affective pictures. The potential mechanisms by which antidepressants alter social cognitive processing has not been explored in this chapter, although it is worth noting that growing evidence from the functional brain imaging literature is rapidly increasing understanding in this field.

In contrast, a psychotherapeutic approach was generally better suited for treating theory of mind deficits and negative interpretative bias, with only limited benefit in improving overall accuracy rates for facial affect recognition. Intensive inpatient therapy and behavioural activation in particular were efficacious, although there is a theoretical basis for the use of cognitive and mentalization-based approaches as well.

Much scarcer data are available for other treatments. ECT may have a role in the interpretation of prosody in MDD, while rTMS and tDCS have shown promise for improving facial affect recognition in single studies. This area of investigation is very much in its infancy and needs replication in larger trials in which treatment of social cognitive deficits are considered a primary treatment outcome.

In summary, many current treatments for depression appear to have a role in the treatment of social cognitive deficits. This is of importance given the functional association between social cognitive deficits and social performance, emotional/empathic performance, general cognitive functioning, and quality of life. The impact and treatment of social cognitive deficits in MDD therefore remains an exciting emerging field for ongoing research.

References

1. Darwin C. *The Expression of the Emotions in Man and Animals*. London, UK: John Murray Publishers; 1872.

2. Ekman P, Friesen WV. Constants across cultures in the face and emotion. J Pers Soc Psychol 1971;17(2):124–9.

3. Weightman MJ, Air TM, Baune BT. A review of the role of social cognition in major depressive disorder. Front Psychiatry 2014;5(179):1–13.

4. Kandalaft MR, Didehbani N, Cullum CM, et al. The Wechsler ACS Social Perception Subtest: a preliminary comparison with other measures of social cognition. J Psychoeduc Assess 2012;30:455–65.

5. Holdnack J, Goldstein G, Drozdick L. Social perception and WAIS-IV performance in adolescents and adults diagnosed with Asperger's syndrome and autism. Assess 2011;18(2):192–200.

6. Beck AT. Thinking and depression: I. idiosyncratic content and cognitive distortions. Arch Gen Psychiatry 1963;9(4):324–33.

7. Szanto K, Dombrovski AY, Sahakian BJ, et al. Social emotion recognition, social functioning, and attempted suicide in late-life depression. Am J Geriatr Psychiatry 2012;20(3):257–65.

8. Derntl B, Seidel EM, Eickhoff SB, et al. Neural correlates of social approach and with-drawal in patients with major depression. Soc Neurosci 2011;6(5–6):482–501.

9. Thoma P, Schmidt T, Juckel G, Norra C, Suchan B. Nice or effective? Social problem solving strategies in patients with major depressive disorder. Psychiatry Res 2015;228(3):835–42.

10. Radke S, Schäfer IC, Müller BW, de Bruijn ER. Do different fairness contexts and fa-cial emotions motivate 'irrational' social decision-making in major depression? An exploratory patient study. Psychiatry Res 2013;210(2):438–43.

11. Lewinsohn PM. A behavioral approach to depression. In: Coyne JC (ed.). *Essential Papers on Depression*. New York, USA: New York University Press; 1974, pp. 150–72.

12. Loi F, Vaidya JG, Paradiso S. Recognition of emotion from body language among pa-tients with unipolar depression. Psychiatry Res 2013;209(1):40–9.

13. Gilboa-Schechtman E, Ben-Artzi E, Jeczemien P, Marom S, Hermesh H. Depression impairs the ability to ignore the emotional aspects of facial expressions: evidence from the Garner task. Cogn Emot 2004;18(2):209–31.

14. Bayliss AP, Tipper SP, Wakeley J, Cowen PJ, Rogers RD. Vulnerability to depres-sion is associated with a failure to acquire implicit social appraisals. Cogn Emot 2017;31(4):825–33.

15. Persad SM, Polivy J. Differences between depressed and nondepressed individ-uals in the recognition of and response to facial emotional cues. J Abnorm Psychol 1993;102(3):358.

16. Aldinger M, Stopsack M, Barnow S, et al. The association between depressive symp-toms and emotion recognition is moderated by emotion regulation. Psychiatry Res 2013;205(1):59–66.

17. Cusi AM, MacQueen GM, Spreng RN, McKinnon MC. Altered empathic responding in major depressive disorder: relation to symptom severity, illness burden, and psy-chosocial outcome. Psychiatry Res 2011;188(2):231–6.

18. Domes G, Spenthof I, Radtke M, Isaksson A, Normann C, Heinrichs M. Autistic traits and empathy in chronic vs. episodic depression. J Affect Disord 2016;195:144–7.

19. Schneider D, Regenbogen C, Kellermann T, et al. Empathic behavioral and physiological responses to dynamic stimuli in depression. Psychiatry Res 2012;200(2):294–305.

20. Arteche A, Joormann J, Harvey A, et al. The effects of postnatal maternal depression and anxiety on the processing of infant faces. J Affect Disord 2011;133(1):197–203.

21. Stein A, Arteche A, Lehtonen A, et al. Interpretation of infant facial expression in the context of maternal postnatal depression. Infant Behav Dev 2010;33(3):273–8.

22. Macrae J, Pearson R, Lee R, et al. The impact of depression on maternal responses to infant faces in pregnancy. Infant Ment Health J 2015;36(6):588–98.

23. Uekermann J, Channon S, Lehmkamper C, Abdel-Hamid M, Vollmoeller W, Daum I. Executive function, mentalizing and humor in major depression. J Int Neuropsychol Soc 2008;14(1):55–62.

24. Zobel I, Werden D, Linster H, et al. Theory of mind deficits in chronically depressed patients. Depress Anxiety 2010;27(9):821–8.

25. Uekermann J, Abdel-Hamid M, Lehmkaemper C, Vollmoeller W, Daum I. Perception of affective prosody in major depression: a link to executive functions? J Int Neuropsychol Soc 2008;14(4):552–61.

26. Levens SM, Gotlib IH. Updating positive and negative stimuli in working memory in depression. J Exp Psychol Gen 2010;139(4):654–64.

27. Deveney CM, Deldin PJ. Memory of faces: a slow wave ERP study of major depression. Emotion 2004;4(3):295–304.

28. Doose-Grünefeld S, Eickhoff SB, Müller VI. Audiovisual emotional processing and neurocognitive functioning in patients with depression. Front Integr Neurosci 2015;9(3):1–13.

29. Cusi AM, Nazarov A, MacQueen GM, McKinnon MC. Theory of mind deficits in patients with mild symptoms of major depressive disorder. Psychiatry Res 2013;210(2):672–4.

30. Phillips LH, Scott C, Henry JD, Mowat D, Bell JS. Emotion perception in Alzheimer's disease and mood disorder in old age. Psychol Aging 2010;25(1):38–47.

31. Tranter R, Bell D, Gutting P, Harmer C, Healy D, Anderson IM. The effect of serotonergic and noradrenergic antidepressants on face emotion processing in depressed patients. J Affect Disord 2009;118(1):87–93.

32. Segal HG, Westen D, Lohr NE, Silk KR. Clinical assessment of object relations and social cognition using stories told to the picture arrangement subtest of the WAIS-R. J Pers Assess 1993;61(1):58–80.

33. Shiroma PR, Thuras P, Johns B, Lim KO. Emotion recognition processing as early predictor of response to 8-week citalopram treatment in late-life depression. Int J Geriatr Psychiatry 2014;29(11):1132–9.

34. Anderson IM, Shippen C, Juhasz G, et al. State-dependent alteration in face emotion recognition in depression. Br J Psychiatry 2011;198(4):302–8.

35. Naudin M, Carl T, Surguladze S, et al. Perceptive biases in major depressive episode. PLoS One 2014;9(2):e86832.

36. Berlim MT, McGirr A, Beaulieu M-M, Turecki G. Theory of mind in subjects with major depressive disorder: is it influenced by repetitive transcranial magnetic stimulation? World J Biol Psychiatry 2012;13(6):474–9.

37. Brennan S, McLoughlin DM, O'Connell R, et al. Anodal transcranial direct current stimulation of the left dorsolateral prefrontal cortex enhances emotion recognition in depressed patients and controls. J Clin Exp Neuropsychol 2017;39(4):384–95.

38. Harmer C, O'Sullivan U, Favaron E, et al. Effect of acute antidepressant administration on negative affective bias in depressed patients. Am J Psychiatry 2009;166(10):1178–84.

39. Bhagwagar Z, Cowen PJ, Goodwin GM, Harmer CJ. Normalization of enhanced fear recognition by acute SSRI treatment in subjects with a previous history of depression. Am J Psychiatry 2004;161(1):166–8.

40. Schutter DJ, van Honk J, Laman M, Vergouwen AC, Koerselman F. Increased sensitivity for angry faces in depressive disorder following 2 weeks of 2-Hz repetitive transcranial magnetic stimulation to the right parietal cortex. Int J Neuropsychopharmacol 2010;13(9):1155–61.

41. Douglas KM, Porter RJ, Knight RG, Maruff P. Neuropsychological changes and treatment response in severe depression. Br J Psychiatry 2011;198(2):115–22.

42. Victor TA, Furey ML, Fromm SJ, Öhman A, Drevets WC. Changes in the neural correlates of implicit emotional face processing during antidepressant treatment in major depressive disorder. Int J Neuropsychopharmacol 2013;16(10):2195–208.

43. Gaebel W, Wölwer W. Facial expression and emotional face recognition in schizophrenia and depression. Eur Arch Psychiatry Clin Neurosci 1992;242(1):46–52.

44. Fu CH, Costafreda SG, Sankar A, et al. Multimodal functional and structural neuroimaging investigation of major depressive disorder following treatment with duloxetine. BMC Psychiatry 2015;15:82.

45. Zhou Z, Cao S, Li H, Li Y. Treatment with escitalopram improves the attentional bias toward negative facial expressions in patients with major depressive disorders. J Clin Neurosci 2015;22(10):1609–13.

46. Surguladze SA, Young AW, Senior C, Brebion G, Travis MJ, Phillips ML. Recognition accuracy and response bias to happy and sad facial expressions in patients with major depression. Neuropsychol 2004;18(2):212–18.

47. Keeley RD, Davidson AJ, Crane LA, Matthews B, Pace W. An association between negatively biased response to neutral stimuli and antidepressant nonadherence. J Psychosom Res 2007;62(5):535–44.

48. Porter R, Bourke C, Carter J, et al. No change in neuropsychological dysfunction or emotional processing during treatment of major depression with cognitive-behaviour therapy or schema therapy. Psychol Med 2016;46(02):393–404.

49. Klein JP, Becker B, Hurlemann R, Scheibe C, Colla M, Heuser I. Effect of specific psychotherapy for chronic depression on neural responses to emotional faces. J Affect Disord 2014;166:93–7.

50. Karparova SP, Kersting A, Suslow T. Disengagement of attention from facial emotion in unipolar depression. Psychiatry Clin Neurosci 2005;59(6):723–9.

51. Suslow T, Dannlowski U, Lalee-Mentzel J, Donges U-S, Arolt V, Kersting A. Spatial processing of facial emotion in patients with unipolar depression: a longitudinal study. J Affect Disord 2004;83(1):59–63.

52. de Raedt R, Baert S, Demeyer I, et al. Changes in attentional processing of emotional information following mindfulness-based cognitive therapy in people with a history of depression: towards an open attention for all emotional experiences. Cogn Ther Res 2012;36(6):612–20.

53. Dannlowski U, Kersting A, Donges US, Lalee-Mentzel J, Arolt V, Suslow T. Masked facial affect priming is associated with therapy response in clinical depression. Eur Arch Psychiatry Clin Neurosci 2006;256(4):215–21.

54. Penton-Voak IS, Bate H, Lewis G, Munafò MR. Effects of emotion perception training on mood in undergraduate students: randomised controlled trial. Br J Psychiatry 2012;201(1):71–2.

55. Lang PJ, Bradley MM, Cuthbert BN. *International Affective Picture System (IAPS): Technical Manual and Affective Ratings.* Florida, USA: NIMH Center for the Study of Emotion and Attention; 1997.

56. Wells TT, Clerkin EM, Ellis AJ, Beevers CG. Effect of antidepressant medication use on emotional information processing in major depression. Am J Psychiatry 2014;171(2):195–200.

57. Rizvi SJ, Salomons TV, Konarski JZ, et al. Neural response to emotional stimuli associated with successful antidepressant treatment and behavioral activation. J Affect Disord 2013;151(2):573–81.

58. Wang Y, Xu C, Cao X, et al. Effects of an antidepressant on neural correlates of emotional processing in patients with major depression. Neurosci Lett 2012;527(1):55–9.

59. Boggio PS, Bermpohl F, Vergara AO, et al. Go-no-go task performance improvement after anodal transcranial DC stimulation of the left dorsolateral prefrontal cortex in major depression. J Affect Disord 2007;101(1):91–8.

60. Zwanzger P, Klahn AL, Arolt V, et al. Impact of electroconvulsive therapy on magnetoencephalographic correlates of dysfunctional emotional processing in major depression. Eur Neuropsychopharmacol 2016;26(4):684–92.

61. Ritchey M, Dolcos F, Eddington KM, Strauman TJ, Cabeza R. Neural correlates of emotional processing in depression: changes with cognitive behavioral therapy and predictors of treatment response. J Psychiatr Res 2011;45(5):577–87.

62. Donges U-S, Kersting A, Dannlowski U, Lalee-Mentzel J, Arolt V, Suslow T. Reduced awareness of others' emotions in unipolar depressed patients. J Nerv Ment Dis 2005;193(5):331–7.

63. Shiota S, Okamoto Y, Okada G, et al. Effects of behavioural activation on the neural basis of other perspective self-referential processing in subthreshold depression: a functional magnetic resonance imaging study. Psychol Med 2017;47(5):877–88.

64. Merkl A, Neumann W-J, Huebl J, et al. Modulation of beta-band activity in the subgenual anterior cingulate cortex during emotional empathy in treatment-resistant depression. Cereb Cortex 2016;26:2626–38.

65. Ridout N, O'Carroll RE, Dritschel B, Christmas D, Eljamel M, Matthews K. Emotion recognition from dynamic emotional displays following anterior cingulotomy and anterior capsulotomy for chronic depression. Neuropsychologia 2007;45(8):1735–43.

66. Christ M, Michael N, Hihn H, et al. Auditory processing of sine tones before, during and after ECT in depressed patients by fMRI. J Neural Transm 2008;115(8):1199–211.

Index

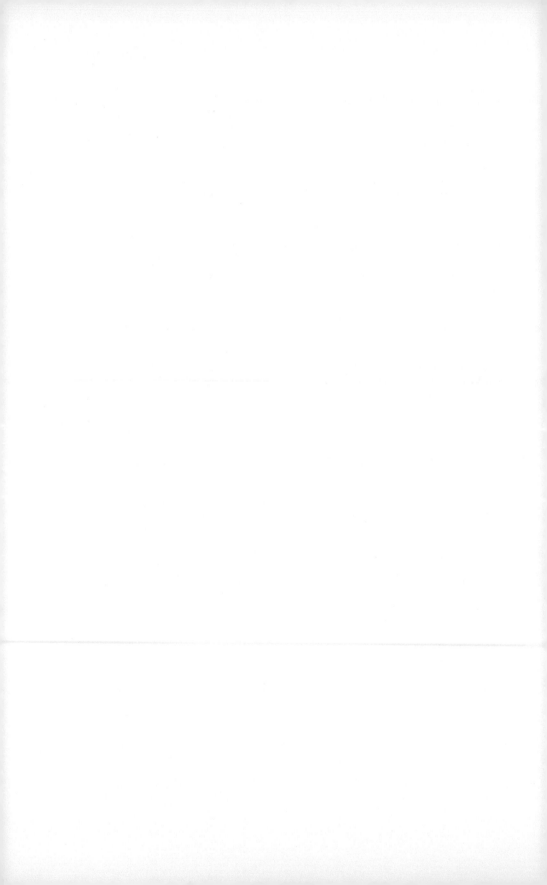

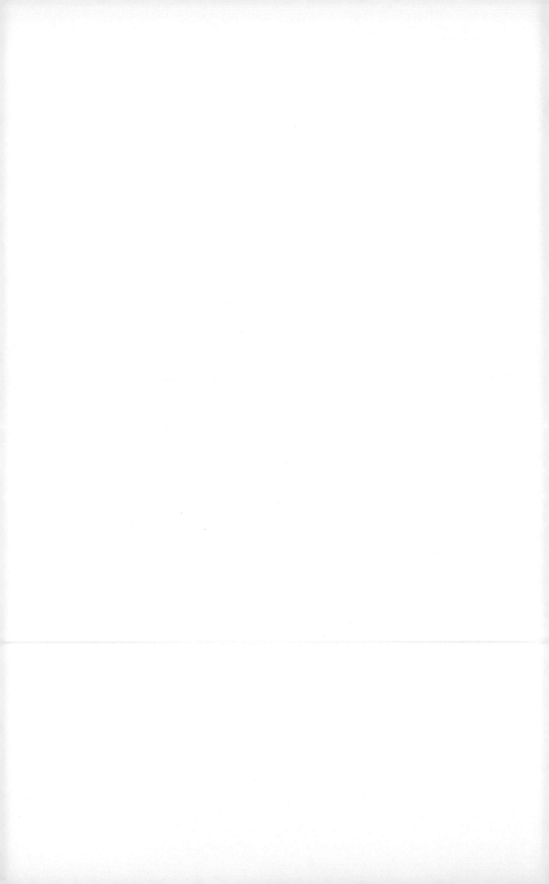

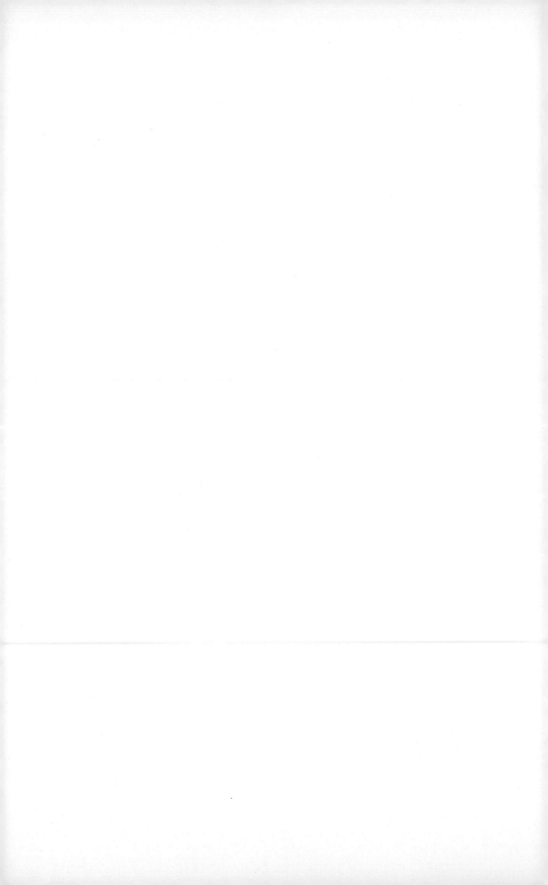